D1189950

Changes | An Insider's View

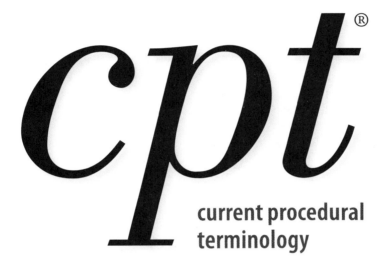

cpt®

current procedural
terminology

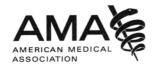

AMA
AMERICAN MEDICAL
ASSOCIATION

Contents

Foreword

The American Medical Association (AMA) is pleased to offer *CPT® Changes 2019: An Insider's View (CPT Changes)*. Since this book was first published in 2000, it has served as the definitive text on additions, revisions, and deletions to the CPT code set.

In developing this book, it was our intention to provide CPT users with a glimpse of the logic, rationale, and proposed function of the changes in the CPT code set that resulted from the decisions of the CPT Editorial Panel and the yearly update process. The AMA staff members have the unique perspective of being both participants in the CPT editorial process and users of the CPT code set.

CPT Changes is intended to bridge understanding between clinical decisions made by the CPT Editorial Panel regarding appropriate service or procedure descriptions with functional interpretations of coding guidelines, code intent, and code combinations, which are necessary for users of the CPT code set. A new edition of this book, like the codebook, is published annually.

To assist CPT users in applying the new and revised CPT codes, this book includes clinical examples that describe the typical patient who might undergo the procedure and detailed descriptions of the procedure. Both of these are required as a part of the CPT code change proposal process, which are used by the CPT Editorial Panel in crafting language, guidelines, and parenthetical notes associated with the new or revised codes. In addition, many of the clinical examples and descriptions of the procedures are used in the AMA/Specialty Society Relative Value Scale (RVS) Update (RUC) process to conduct surveys on physician work and to develop work relative value recommendations to the Centers for Medicare and Medicaid Services (CMS) as part of the Medicare Physician Fee Schedule (MPFS).

We are confident that the information provided in *CPT Changes* will prove to be a valuable resource to CPT users, not only as they apply changes for the year of publication, but also as a resource for frequent reference as they continue their education in CPT coding. The AMA makes every effort to be a voice of clarity and consistency in an otherwise confusing system of health care claims and payment, and *CPT Changes 2019: An Insider's View* demonstrates our continued commitment to assist users of the CPT code set.

Using This Book

This book is designed to serve as a reference guide to understanding the changes contained in the Current Procedural Terminology (CPT®) 2019 code set and is not intended to replace the CPT codebook. Every effort is made to ensure accuracy, however, if differences exist, you should always defer to the information in the *CPT 2019* codebook.

The Symbols

This book uses the same coding conventions as those used in the CPT nomenclature.

●   Indicates a new procedure number was added to the CPT nomenclature

▲   Indicates a code revision has resulted in a substantially altered procedure descriptor

✚   Indicates a CPT add-on code

⊘   Indicates a code that is exempt from the use of modifier 51 but is not designated as a CPT add-on procedure or service

►◄ Indicates revised guidelines, cross-references, and/or explanatory text

⇗   Indicates a code for a vaccine that is pending FDA approval

\#   Indicates a resequenced code. Note that rather than deleting and renumbering, resequencing allows existing codes to be relocated to an appropriate location for the code concept, regardless of the numeric sequence. Numerically placed references (ie, Code is out of numerical sequence. See...) are used as navigational alerts in the CPT codebook to direct the user to the location of an out-of-sequence code. Therefore, remember to refer to the CPT codebook for these references.

★   Indicates a telemedicine code

⭓   Indicates a duplicate PLA test

Whenever possible, complete segments of text from the CPT codebook are provided; however, in some instances, only pertinent text is included.

The Rationale

After listing each change or series of changes from the CPT codebook, a rationale is provided. The rationale is intended to provide a brief clarification and explanation of the changes. Nevertheless, it is important to note that they may not address every question that may arise as a result of the changes.

Reading the Clinical Examples

The clinical examples and their procedural descriptions, which reflect typical clinical situations found in the health-care setting, are included in this text with many of the codes to provide practical situations for which the new and/or revised codes in the CPT 2019 code set would be appropriately reported. It is important to note that these examples do not suggest limiting the use of a code; instead, they are meant to represent the typical patient and service or procedure, as previously stated. In addition, they do not describe the universe of patients for whom the service or procedure would be appropriate. It is important to also note that third-party payer reporting policies may differ.

Summary of Additions, Deletions, and Revisions and Indexes

A **summary of additions, deletions, and revisions** for the section is presented in a tabular format at the beginning of each section. This table provides readers with the ability to quickly search and have an overview of all of the new, revised, and deleted codes for 2019. In addition to the tabular review of changes, the coding index individually lists all of the new, revised, and deleted codes with each code's status (new, revised, deleted) in parentheses. For more information about these indexes, please read the **Instructions for the Use of the Changes Indexes** on page 243.

CPT Codebook Conventions and Styles

Similar to the CPT codebook, the guidelines and revised and new CPT code descriptors and parenthetical notes in *CPT Changes 2019* are set in green type. Any revised text, guidelines, and/or headings are indicated with the ▶ ◀ symbols. To match the style used in the codebook, the revised or new text symbol is placed at the beginning and end of a paragraph or section that contains revisions, and the use of green text visually indicates new and/or revised content. Similarly, each section's and subsections' (Surgery) complete code range are listed in the tabs, regardless if these codes are discussed in this book. In addition, all of the different level of headings in the codebook are also picked up, as appropiate, and set in the same style and color. Besides matching the convention and style used in the CPT codebook, the Rationales are placed within a shaded box to distinguish them from the rest of the content for quick and easy reference.

Evaluation and Management

There have been a number of changes made to the Evaluation and Management (E/M) section. The Critical Care Services, Inpatient Neonatal Intensive Care Services and Pediatric and Neonatal Critical Care Services, and Transitional Care Management Services subsections' guidelines have been revised because of the deletion of code 99090 in the Medicine section and codes 0188T and 0189T in the Category III section.

The most substantial changes to the E/M section include revisions and additions of codes and subsections to the Non-Face-to-Face Services subsection:

- The "Interprofessional Telephone/Internet Consultation" subsection title has been revised to "Interprofessional Telephone/Internet Consultation/Electronic Health Record." Additional changes to this subsection include revisions to numerous guidelines and codes 99446, 99447, 99448, and 99449, and the addition of two new codes (99451, 99452).

- The Digitally Stored Data Services/Remote Physiologic Monitoring subsection has been added along with introductory guidelines and two new codes (99453, 99454) to describe remote physiologic monitoring services. In addition, code 99091 has been revised, resequenced, and moved from the Medicine section to this subsection.

- The "Remote Physiologic Monitoring Treatment Management Services" subsection has been added along with new introductory guidelines, parenthetical notes, and a new code (99457).

For the Chronic Care Management Services subsection, the introductory guidelines have been revised and a new code (99491) and three new parenthetical notes have been added.

With the addition of code 99491 in the E/M section, the guidelines and parenthetical notes in the Prolonged Service Without Direct Patient Contact and Care Management Services subsections have also been revised accordingly.

The guidelines in the Inpatient Neonatal Intensive Care Services and Pediatric and Neonatal Critical Care Services subsection and a parenthetical note in the Cognitive Assessment and Care Plan Services subsection have been revised because of the deletion of Medicine and Category III codes.

The introductory guidelines to the Psychiatric Collaborative Care Management Services subsection have also been revised for clarity. The introductory guidelines in the Home Services subsection have been revised to further clarify the definition of home.

Finally, the guidelines in the Transitional Care Management Services subsection and other subsections throughout the E/M section have also been revised in accordance with the deletion of code 99090 in the Medicine section.

Summary of Additions, Deletions, and Revisions

The summary of changes shows the actual changes that have been made to the code descriptors.

New codes appear with a bullet (●) and are indicated as "Code added." Revised codes are preceded with a triangle (▲). Within revised codes, or if a code symbol has been deleted, the deleted language and code symbol appears with a s̶t̶r̶i̶k̶e̶t̶h̶r̶o̶u̶g̶h̶ (⊖), while new text appears underlined.

The ⚡ symbol is used to identify codes for vaccines that are pending FDA approval. The # symbol is used to identify codes that have been resequenced. CPT add-on codes are annotated by the ✚ symbol. The ⊘ symbol is used to identify codes that are exempt from the use of modifier 51. The ★ symbol is used to identify codes that may be used for reporting telemedicine services. The ✕ is used to identify proprietary laboratory analyses (PLA) test that has an identical descriptor as another PLA test.

Code	Description
▲99446	Interprofessional telephone/Internet/electronic health record assessment and management service provided by a consultative physician, including a verbal and written report to the patient's treating/requesting physician or other qualified health care professional; 5-10 minutes of medical consultative discussion and review
▲99447	11-20 minutes of medical consultative discussion and review
▲99448	21-30 minutes of medical consultative discussion and review
▲99449	31 minutes or more of medical consultative discussion and review
#●99451	Code added
#●99452	Code added
#●99453	Code added
#●99454	Code added
#▲99091	Collection and interpretation of physiologic data (eg, ECG, blood pressure, glucose monitoring) digitally stored and/or transmitted by the patient and/or caregiver to the physician or other qualified health care professional, qualified by education, training, licensure/regulation (when applicable) requiring a minimum of 30 minutes of time, each 30 days
#●99457	Code added
#●99491	Code added

Evaluation and Management

Critical Care Services

Critical care is the direct delivery by a physician(s) or other qualified health care professional of medical care for a critically ill or critically injured patient. A critical illness or injury acutely impairs one or more vital organ systems such that there is a high probability of imminent or life threatening deterioration in the patient's condition. Critical care involves high complexity decision making to assess, manipulate, and support vital system function(s) to treat single or multiple vital organ system failure and/or to prevent further life threatening deterioration of the patient's condition. Examples of vital organ system failure include, but are not limited to: central nervous system failure, circulatory failure, shock, renal, hepatic, metabolic, and/or respiratory failure. Although critical care typically requires interpretation of multiple physiologic parameters and/or application of advanced technology(s), critical care may be provided in life threatening situations when these elements are not present. Critical care may be provided on multiple days, even if no changes are made in the treatment rendered to the patient, provided that the patient's condition continues to require the level of attention described above.

Providing medical care to a critically ill, injured, or post-operative patient qualifies as a critical care service only if both the illness or injury and the treatment being provided meet the above requirements. Critical care is usually, but not always, given in a critical care area, such as the coronary care unit, intensive care unit, pediatric intensive care unit, respiratory care unit, or the emergency care facility.

Inpatient critical care services provided to infants 29 days through 71 months of age are reported with pediatric critical care codes 99471-99476. The pediatric critical care codes are reported as long as the infant/young child qualifies for critical care services during the hospital stay through 71 months of age. Inpatient critical care services provided to neonates (28 days of age or younger) are reported with the neonatal critical care codes 99468 and 99469. The neonatal critical care codes are reported as long as the neonate qualifies for critical care services during the hospital stay through the 28th postnatal day. The reporting of the pediatric and neonatal critical care services is not based on time or the type of unit (eg, pediatric or neonatal critical care unit) and it is not dependent upon the type of physician or other qualified health care professional delivering the care. To report critical care services provided in the outpatient setting (eg, emergency department or office),

for neonates and pediatric patients up through 71 months of age, see the critical care codes 99291, 99292. If the same individual provides critical care services for a neonatal or pediatric patient in both the outpatient and inpatient settings on the same day, report only the appropriate neonatal or pediatric critical care code 99468-99472 for all critical care services provided on that day. Also report 99291-99292 for neonatal or pediatric critical care services provided by the individual providing critical care at one facility but transferring the patient to another facility. Critical care services provided by a second individual of a different specialty not reporting a per day neonatal or pediatric critical care code can be reported with codes 99291, 99292. For additional instructions on reporting these services, see the Neonatal and Pediatric Critical Care section and codes 99468-99476.

Services for a patient who is not critically ill but happens to be in a critical care unit are reported using other appropriate E/M codes.

Critical care and other E/M services may be provided to the same patient on the same date by the same individual.

►For reporting by professionals, the following services are included in critical care when performed during the critical period by the physician(s) providing critical care: the interpretation of cardiac output measurements (93561, 93562), chest X rays (71045, 71046), pulse oximetry (94760, 94761, 94762), blood gases, and collection and interpretation of physiologic data (eg, ECGs, blood pressures, hematologic data); gastric intubation (43752, 43753); temporary transcutaneous pacing (92953); ventilatory management (94002-94004, 94660, 94662); and vascular access procedures (36000, 36410, 36415, 36591, 36600). Any services performed that are not included in this listing should be reported separately. Facilities may report the above services separately.◄

Rationale

In accordance with the deletion of code 99090, the critical care services guidelines have been revised by removing code 99090 and removing "information data stored in computers" and updating them with "collection and interpretation of physiologic data."

Refer to the codebook and the Rationale for Digitally Stored Data Services/Remote Physiologic Monitoring subsection in the Evaluation and Management section and Medicine Miscellaneous subsection for a full discussion of these changes.

Codes 99291, 99292 should be reported for the attendance during the transport of critically ill or critically injured patients older than 24 months of age to or from a facility or hospital. For transport services of critically ill or critically injured pediatric patients 24 months of age or younger, see 99466, 99467.

Codes 99291, 99292 are used to report the total duration of time spent in provision of critical care services to a critically ill or critically injured patient, even if the time spent providing care on that date is not continuous. For any given period of time spent providing critical care services, the individual must devote his or her full attention to the patient and, therefore, cannot provide services to any other patient during the same period of time.

Time spent with the individual patient should be recorded in the patient's record. The time that can be reported as critical care is the time spent engaged in work directly related to the individual patient's care whether that time was spent at the immediate bedside or elsewhere on the floor or unit. For example, time spent on the unit or at the nursing station on the floor reviewing test results or imaging studies, discussing the critically ill patient's care with other medical staff or documenting critical care services in the medical record would be reported as critical care, even though it does not occur at the bedside. Also, when the patient is unable or lacks capacity to participate in discussions, time spent on the floor or unit with family members or surrogate decision makers obtaining a medical history, reviewing the patient's condition or prognosis, or discussing treatment or limitation(s) of treatment may be reported as critical care, provided that the conversation bears directly on the management of the patient.

▶Time spent in activities that occur outside of the unit or off the floor (eg, telephone calls whether taken at home, in the office, or elsewhere in the hospital) may not be reported as critical care since the individual is not immediately available to the patient. Time spent in activities that do not directly contribute to the treatment of the patient may not be reported as critical care, even if they are performed in the critical care unit (eg, participation in administrative meetings or telephone calls to discuss other patients). Time spent performing separately reportable procedures or services should not be included in the time reported as critical care time.◀

Code 99291 is used to report the first 30-74 minutes of critical care on a given date. It should be used only once per date even if the time spent by the individual is not continuous on that date. Critical care of less than 30 minutes total duration on a given date should be reported with the appropriate E/M code.

Code 99292 is used to report additional block(s) of time, of up to 30 minutes each beyond the first 74 minutes. (See the following table.)

Total Duration of Critical Care Codes

less than 30 minutes	appropriate E/M codes
30-74 minutes (30 minutes - 1 hr. 14 min.)	99291 X 1
75-104 minutes (1 hr. 15 min. - 1 hr. 44 min.)	99291 X 1 AND 99292 X 1
105-134 minutes (1 hr. 45 min. - 2 hr. 14 min.)	99291 X 1 AND 99292 X 2
135-164 minutes (2 hr. 15 min. - 2 hr. 44 min.)	99291 X 1 AND 99292 X 3
165-194 minutes (2 hr. 45 min. - 3 hr. 14 min.)	99291 X 1 AND 99292 X 4
195 minutes or longer (3 hr. 15 min. - etc.)	99291 and 99292 as appropriate (see illustrated reporting examples above)

99291 **Critical care, evaluation and management** of the critically ill or critically injured patient; first 30-74 minutes

✚ **99292** each additional 30 minutes (List separately in addition to code for primary service)

(Use 99292 in conjunction with 99291)

Rationale

In accordance with the deletion of Category III codes 0188T and 0189T, the critical care services guidelines that are affected by this deletion have been revised accordingly.

Refer to the codebook and the Rationale for codes 0188T and 0189T for a full discussion of these changes.

Home Services

▶The following codes are used to report evaluation and management services provided in a home. Home may be defined as a private residence, temporary lodging, or short term accommodation (eg, hotel, campground, hostel, or cruise ship).◀

For definitions of key components and commonly used terms, please see **Evaluation and Management Services Guidelines.**

★ = Telemedicine ✚ = Add-on code ✔ = FDA approval pending # = Resequenced code ⊘ = Modifier 51 exempt

(For care plan oversight services provided to a patient in the home under the care of a home health agency, see 99374, 99375, and for hospice agency, see 99377, 99378. For care plan oversight provided to a patient under hospice or home health agency care, see 99339, 99340)

New Patient

99341 **Home visit** for the evaluation and management of a new patient, which requires these 3 key components:

- **A problem focused history;**

- **A problem focused examination; and**

- **Straightforward medical decision making.**

Counseling and/or coordination of care with other physicians, other qualified health care professionals, or agencies are provided consistent with the nature of the problem(s) and the patient's and/or family's needs.

Usually, the presenting problem(s) are of low severity. Typically, 20 minutes are spent face-to-face with the patient and/or family.

Rationale

The guidelines in the Home Services subsection have been revised to expand the definition of home. In addition to a private residence, home may also include temporary lodging or short-term accommodations. Short-term accommodations may include hotels, campgrounds, hostels, or cruise ships.

Prolonged Services

Prolonged Service Without Direct Patient Contact

99358 **Prolonged evaluation and management service** before and/or after direct patient care; first hour

+ 99359 each additional 30 minutes (List separately in addition to code for prolonged service)

(Use 99359 in conjunction with 99358)

▶(Do not report 99358, 99359 during the same month with 99484, 99487-99489, 99490, 99491, 99492, 99493, 99494)◀

(Do not report 99358, 99359 when performed during the service time of codes 99495 or 99496)

Rationale

In accordance with the addition of code 99491, the parenthetical note following code 99359 has been revised to include code 99491.

Refer to the codebook and the Rationale for code 99491 for a full discussion of these changes.

Non-Face-to-Face Services

▶Interprofessional Telephone/ Internet/Electronic Health Record Consultations◀

▶The consultant should use codes 99446, 99447, 99448, 99449, 99451 to report interprofessional telephone/ Internet/electronic health record consultations. An interprofessional telephone/Internet/electronic health record consultation is an assessment and management service in which a patient's treating (eg, attending or primary) physician or other qualified health care professional requests the opinion and/or treatment advice of a physician with specific specialty expertise (the consultant) to assist the treating physician or other qualified health care professional in the diagnosis and/or management of the patient's problem without patient face-to-face contact with the consultant.

The patient for whom the interprofessional telephone/ Internet/electronic health record consultation is requested may be either a new patient to the consultant or an established patient with a new problem or an exacerbation of an existing problem. However, the consultant should not have seen the patient in a face-to-face encounter within the last 14 days. When the telephone/Internet/electronic health record consultation leads to a transfer of care or other face-to-face service (eg, a surgery, a hospital visit, or a scheduled office evaluation of the patient) within the next 14 days or next available appointment date of the consultant, these codes are not reported.

Review of pertinent medical records, laboratory studies, imaging studies, medication profile, pathology specimens, etc is included in the telephone/Internet/ electronic health record consultation service and should not be reported separately when reporting 99446, 99447, 99448, 99449, 99451. The majority of the service time reported (greater than 50%) must be devoted to the medical consultative verbal or Internet discussion. If greater than 50% of the time for the service is devoted to data review and/or analysis, 99446, 99447, 99448, 99449 should not be reported. However, the service time for 99451 is based on total review and interprofessional-communication time.

If more than one telephone/Internet/electronic health record contact(s) is required to complete the consultation request (eg, discussion of test results), the entirety of the service and the cumulative discussion and information review time should be reported with a single code. Codes 99446, 99447, 99448, 99449, 99451 should not be reported more than once within a seven-day interval.

The written or verbal request for telephone/Internet/electronic health record advice by the treating/requesting physician or other qualified health care professional should be documented in the patient's medical record, including the reason for the request. Codes 99446, 99447, 99448, 99449 conclude with a verbal opinion report and written report from the consultant to the treating/requesting physician or other qualified health care professional. Code 99451 concludes with only a written report.

Telephone/Internet/electronic health record consultations of less than five minutes should not be reported. Consultant communications with the patient and/or family may be reported using 98966, 98967, 98968, 98969, 99441, 99442, 99443, 99444, and the time related to these services is not used in reporting 99446, 99447, 99448, 99449. Do not report 99358, 99359 for any time within the service period, if reporting 99446, 99447, 99448, 99449, 99451.

When the sole purpose of the telephone/Internet/electronic health record communication is to arrange a transfer of care or other face-to-face service, these codes are not reported.

The treating/requesting physician or other qualified health care professional may report 99452 if spending 16-30 minutes in a service day preparing for the referral and/or communicating with the consultant. Do not report 99452 more than once in a 14-day period. The treating/requesting physician or other qualified health care professional may report the prolonged service codes 99354, 99355, 99356, 99357 for the time spent on the interprofessional telephone/Internet/electronic health record discussion with the consultant (eg, specialist) if the time **exceeds 30 minutes** beyond the typical time of the appropriate E/M service performed and the patient is present (on-site) and accessible to the treating/requesting physician or other qualified health care professional. If the interprofessional telephone/Internet/electronic health record assessment and management service occurs when the patient is not present and the time spent in a day **exceeds 30 minutes,** then the non-face-to-face prolonged service codes 99358, 99359 may be reported by the treating/requesting physician or other qualified health care professional.◄

(For telephone services provided by a physician to a patient, see 99441, 99442, 99443)

(For telephone services provided by a qualified health care professional to a patient, see 98966, 98967, 98968)

(For an on-line medical evaluation provided by a physician to a patient, use 99444)

(For an on-line assessment and management service provided by a qualified health care professional to a patient, use 98969)

▲ **99446** Interprofessional telephone/Internet/electronic health record assessment and management service provided by a consultative physician, including a verbal and written report to the patient's treating/requesting physician or other qualified health care professional; 5-10 minutes of medical consultative discussion and review

▲ **99447** 11-20 minutes of medical consultative discussion and review

▲ **99448** 21-30 minutes of medical consultative discussion and review

▲ **99449** 31 minutes or more of medical consultative discussion and review

#● **99451** Interprofessional telephone/Internet/electronic health record assessment and management service provided by a consultative physician, including a written report to the patient's treating/requesting physician or other qualified health care professional, 5 minutes or more of medical consultative time

#● **99452** Interprofessional telephone/Internet/electronic health record referral service(s) provided by a treating/requesting physician or other qualified health care professional, 30 minutes

Rationale

A revision has been made to the heading for Interprofessional Telephone/Internet Consultation and the guidelines have also been revised. The current codes 99446-99449 have been revised to include electronic health record and two new codes have been added to this subsection. Code 99451 has been established to report interprofessional consultation services provided by a consultative physician and code 99452 to report interprofessional referral services provided by a treating/requesting physician or other qualified health care professional (QHP).

Prior to 2019, codes 99446-99449 were available to report an assessment and management consultation service in which a patient's treating (eg, attending or primary) physician/QHP requests the opinion and/or treatment advice of a physician with specific specialty expertise (ie, the consultant) to assist the treating physician/QHP in the diagnosis and/or management of the patient's problem, with a verbal and written component as the vehicle for the consultant to convey the assessment. There were no codes for the consultant to report the service of sending the results of a consultation, without the additional verbal component. Therefore, code 99451 was established to allow reporting of telephone/Internet/electronic health record consultation services without a verbal component. The service described by code 99451 concludes with only a written report. Code 99452 should be reported for interprofessional telephone/Internet/electronic health record referral services provided either by a treating/requesting physician or QHP. Report 16-30 mins of a service day for time spent preparing for the referral and/or communicating with the consultant using code 99452. If the time spent exceeds 30 minutes, the treating/requesting physician/QHP may report the prolonged services codes.

The revisions to the guidelines in this subsection now align with modern medicine practice and specify what is included when reporting these new and revised codes. This form of consultation can assist in serving patients in areas in need of services, who may otherwise not be able to receive them (eg, due to lack of specialists in the geographic area).

Clinical Example (99451)

A 54-year-old female with dyspnea on exertion has been evaluated by her primary physician with normal chest X ray and pulmonary function tests (flow, volumes and diffusing capacity of the lungs for carbon monoxide [DLCO]) and an echocardiogram with increased pulmonary pressures. The referring clinician asks a colleague pulmonologist (via shared electronic record) for advice on management of the patient.

Description of Procedure (99451)

The intraservice period includes clarifying nature of patient's problem; obtaining and reviewing data or relevant information; presenting an analysis of patient's problem, including likely diagnosis and suggested management; responding to questions to clarify diagnostic and treatment approach; relaying relevant scientific background on the diagnosis; outlining suggestions for long-term handling of patient's problem; and completing literature review in response to issues raised during communication.

Clinical Example (99452)

A 10-year-old boy with attention deficit disorder has become increasingly aggressive at home and in school.

Description of Procedure (99452)

The intraservice period includes physician work reviewing records, assembling pertinent materials, developing clinical questions/concerns, and transmitting this information to the appropriate consultant. As needed, the treating/requesting physician directly communicates with the consultant.

▶Digitally Stored Data Services/ Remote Physiologic Monitoring◀

▶Codes 99453 and 99454 are used to report remote physiologic monitoring services (eg, weight, blood pressure, pulse oximetry) during a 30-day period. To report 99453, 99454, the device used must be a medical device as defined by the FDA, and the service must be ordered by a physician or other qualified health care professional. Code 99453 may be used to report the set-up and patient education on use of the device(s). Code 99454 may be used to report supply of the device for daily recording or programmed alert transmissions. Codes 99453, 99454 are not reported if monitoring is less than 16 days. Do not report 99453, 99454 when these services are included in other codes for the duration of time of the physiologic monitoring service (eg, 95250 for continuous glucose monitoring requires a minimum of 72 hours of monitoring).

Code 99091 should be reported no more than once in a 30-day period to include the physician or other qualified health care professional time involved with data accession, review and interpretation, modification of care plan as necessary (including communication to patient and/or caregiver), and associated documentation.

If the services described by 99091 are provided on the same day the patient presents for an Evaluation and Management (E/M) service, these services should be considered part of the E/M service and not reported separately.

Do not report 99091 in the same calendar month as care plan oversight services (99374, 99375, 99377, 99378, 99379, 99380), home, domiciliary, or rest home care plan oversight services (99339, 99340), and remote physiologic monitoring services (99457). Do not report 99091 if other more specific codes exist (eg, 93227, 93272 for cardiographic services; 95250 for continuous glucose monitoring). Do not report 99091 for transfer and interpretation of data from hospital or clinical laboratory computers.

Code 99453 is reported for each episode of care. For coding remote monitoring of physiologic parameters, an episode of care is defined as beginning when the remote monitoring physiologic service is initiated, and ends with attainment of targeted treatment goals.◀

#● 99453 Remote monitoring of physiologic parameter(s) (eg, weight, blood pressure, pulse oximetry, respiratory flow rate), initial; set-up and patient education on use of equipment

▶(Do not report 99453 more than once per episode of care)◀

▶(Do not report 99453 for monitoring of less than 16 days)◀

#● 99454 device(s) supply with daily recording(s) or programmed alert(s) transmission, each 30 days

▶(For physiologic monitoring treatment management services, use 99457)◀

▶(Do not report 99454 for monitoring of less than 16 days)◀

▶(Do not report 99453, 99454 in conjunction with codes for more specific physiologic parameters [eg, 93296, 94760])◀

#▲ 99091 Collection and interpretation of physiologic data (eg, ECG, blood pressure, glucose monitoring) digitally stored and/or transmitted by the patient and/or caregiver to the physician or other qualified health care professional, qualified by education, training, licensure/regulation (when applicable) requiring a minimum of 30 minutes of time, each 30 days

▶(Do not report 99091 in conjunction with 99457)◀

▶(Do not report 99091 if it occurs within 30 days of 99339, 99340, 99374, 99375, 99377, 99378, 99379, 99380, 99457)◀

Rationale

A new subsection (Digitally Stored Data Services/Remote Physiologic Monitoring) and guidelines have been added to the Evaluation and Management Services section. With the addition of this new subsection, two new codes have been added, one code deleted, and one code resequenced.

Prior to 2019, the CPT code set had very general codes related to collection and analysis of electronic data. These new codes are specific to physiologic monitoring services (eg, weight, blood pressure, and pulse oximetry). The guidelines specify that the device used must be a medical device as defined by the Food and Drug Administration and ordered by the physician/QHP.

Code 99453 has been added to report the remote monitoring of physiologic parameter(s) initial set-up and patient education, specifically on the use of the device. This code should be reported once for each episode of care, as defined in the new guidelines. Code 99454 has been established to report the device supply for daily

recordings or programmed alert transmissions for 30-day periods.

To allow a more robust reporting of remote services, the current code 99091 (collection and interpretation of physiologic data) has been resequenced to this new subsection from the Medicine Miscellaneous subsection. If the services described by code 99091 are performed on the same day a patient presents for an E/M service, code 99091 is not reported separately.

Finally, code 99090, *Analysis of clinical data stored in computers (eg, ECGs, blood pressures, hematologic data)*, has been deleted due to low utilization.

Clinical Example (99453)

A 75-year-old female with a chronic condition presents to her primary care practice with increased distress. Following the visit, she is enrolled in a remote physiologic patient monitoring program to enable data collection and monitoring to facilitate treatment management.

Description of Procedure (99453)

N/A

Clinical Example (99454)

A 75-year-old female with a chronic condition presents to her primary care practice with increased distress. Following the visit, she is enrolled in a remote physiologic patient monitoring program to enable data collection and monitoring to facilitate treatment management.

Description of Procedure (99454)

N/A

▶Remote Physiologic Monitoring Treatment Management Services◀

▶Remote physiologic monitoring treatment management services are provided when clinical staff/physician/other qualified health care professional use the results of remote physiological monitoring to manage a patient under a specific treatment plan. To report remote physiological monitoring, the device used must be a medical device as defined by the FDA, and the service must be ordered by a physician or other qualified health care professional. Use 99457 for time spent managing care when patients or the practice do not meet the requirements to report more specific services. Code 99457 may be reported during the same service period as chronic care management services (99487, 99489,

99490), transitional care management services (99495, 99496), and behavioral health integration services (99484, 99492, 99493, 99494). However, time spent performing these services should remain separate and no time should be counted toward the required time for both services in a single month. Code 99457 requires a live, interactive communication with the patient/caregiver and 20 minutes or more of clinical staff/physician/other qualified health care professional time in a calendar month. Report 99491 one time regardless of the number of physiologic monitoring modalities performed in a given calendar month.

Do not count any time on a day when the physician or other qualified health care professional reports an E/M service (office or other outpatient services 99201, 99202, 99203, 99204, 99205, 99211, 99212, 99213, 99214, 99215, domiciliary, rest home services 99324, 99325, 99326, 99327, 99328, 99334, 99335, 99336, 99337, home services 99341, 99342, 99343, 99344, 99345, 99347, 99348, 99349, 99350). Do not count any time related to other reported services (eg, 93290).◄

#● 99457   Remote physiologic monitoring treatment management services, 20 minutes or more of clinical staff/physician/other qualified health care professional time in a calendar month requiring interactive communication with the patient/caregiver during the month

      ►(Report 99457 once each 30 days, regardless of the number of parameters monitored)◄

      ►(Do not report 99457 in conjunction with 99091)◄

Rationale

A new subsection (Remote Physiologic Monitoring Treatment Management Services) and guidelines have been added to the Evaluation and Management Services section. In addition, a new code (99457) has been established to report remote physiologic monitoring treatment management services for 20 minutes or more in a calendar month. Code 99457 requires interactive communication with the patient/caregiver during the month. As indicated in the guidelines, it is important to note that the device used to provide these services must be a medical device defined by the FDA, and it must be ordered by a physician/QHP.

Clinical Example (99457)

An 82-year-old female with systolic dysfunction heart failure is enrolled in a heart failure management program that uses remote physiologic monitoring services.

Description of Procedure (99457)

Based on interpreted data, the physician or other qualified health care professional uses medical decision making to assess the patient's clinical stability, communicates the results to the patient, and oversees the management and/or coordination of services as needed, for all medical conditions.

Special Evaluation and Management Services

Basic Life and/or Disability Evaluation Services

99451   Code is out of numerical sequence. See 99448-99455

99452   Code is out of numerical sequence. See 99448-99455

99453   Code is out of numerical sequence. See 99448-99455

99454   Code is out of numerical sequence. See 99448-99455

Work Related or Medical Disability Evaluation Services

99457   Code is out of numerical sequence. See 99448-99455

Inpatient Neonatal Intensive Care Services and Pediatric and Neonatal Critical Care Services

Pediatric Critical Care Patient Transport

Codes 99466, 99467 are used to report the physical attendance and direct face-to-face care by a physician during the interfacility transport of a critically ill or critically injured pediatric patient 24 months of age or younger. Codes 99485, 99486 are used to report the control physician's non-face-to-face supervision of interfacility transport of a critically ill or critically injured pediatric patient 24 months of age or younger. These codes are not reported together for the same patient by the same physician. For the purpose of reporting 99466 and 99467, face-to-face care begins when the physician assumes primary responsibility of the pediatric patient at the referring facility, and ends when the receiving facility accepts responsibility for the pediatric patient's care. Only the time the physician spends in direct face-to-face contact with the patient during the transport should be reported. Pediatric patient transport services involving less than 30 minutes of face-to-face physician care should not be reported using 99466, 99467. Procedure(s) or service(s) performed by other members of the transporting team may not be reported by the supervising physician.

Codes 99485, 99486 may be used to report control physician's non-face-to-face supervision of interfacility pediatric critical care transport, which includes all two-way communication between the control physician and the specialized transport team prior to transport, at the referring facility and during transport of the patient back to the receiving facility. The "control" physician is the physician directing transport services. These codes do not include pretransport communication between the control physician and the referring facility before or following patient transport. These codes may only be reported for patients 24 months of age or younger who are critically ill or critically injured. The control physician provides treatment advice to a specialized transport team who are present and delivering the hands-on patient care. The control physician does not report any services provided by the specialized transport team. The control physician's non-face-to-face time begins with the first contact by the control physician with the specialized transport team and ends when the patient's care is handed over to the receiving facility team. Refer to 99466 and 99467 for face-to-face transport care of the critically ill/injured patient. Time spent with the individual patient's transport team and reviewing data submissions should be recorded. Code 99485 is used to report the first 16-45 minutes of direction on a given date and should only be used once even if time spent by the physician is discontinuous. Do not report services of 15 minutes or less or any time when another physician is reporting 99466, 99467. Do not report 99485 or 99486 in conjunction with 99466, 99467 when performed by the same physician.

For the definition of the critically injured pediatric patient, see the **Neonatal and Pediatric Critical Care Services** section.

The non-face-to-face direction of emergency care to a patient's transporting staff by a physician located in a hospital or other facility by two-way communication is not considered direct face-to-face care and should not be reported with 99466, 99467. Physician-directed non-face-to-face emergency care through outside voice communication to transporting staff personnel is reported with 99288 or 99485, 99486 based upon the age and clinical condition of the patient.

Emergency department services (99281-99285), initial hospital care (99221-99223), critical care (99291, 99292), initial date neonatal intensive (99477) or critical care (99468) may only be reported after the patient has been admitted to the emergency department, the inpatient floor, or the critical care unit of the receiving facility. If inpatient critical care services are reported in the referring facility prior to transfer to the receiving hospital, use the critical care codes (99291, 99292).

▶The following services are included when performed during the pediatric patient transport by the physician providing critical care and may not be reported separately: routine monitoring evaluations (eg, heart rate, respiratory rate, blood pressure, and pulse oximetry), the interpretation of cardiac output measurements (93562), chest X rays (71045, 71046), pulse oximetry (94760, 94761, 94762), blood gases and information data stored in computers (eg, ECGs, blood pressures, hematologic data), gastric intubation (43752, 43753), temporary transcutaneous pacing (92953), ventilatory management (94002, 94003, 94660, 94662), and vascular access procedures (36000, 36400, 36405, 36406, 36415, 36591, 36600). Any services performed which are not listed above should be reported separately.◀

Services provided by the specialized transport team during non-face-to-face transport supervision are not reported by the control physician.

Rationale

In accordance with the deletion of code 99090, the guidelines for care management services have been revised by removing this code.

Refer to the codebook and the Rationale for code 99090 for a full discussion of these changes.

Inpatient Neonatal and Pediatric Critical Care

The same definitions for critical care services apply for the adult, child, and neonate.

Codes 99468, 99469 may be used to report the services of directing the inpatient care of a critically ill neonate or infant 28 days of age or younger. They represent care starting with the date of admission (99468) for critical care services and all subsequent day(s) (99469) that the neonate remains in critical care. These codes may be reported only by a single individual and only once per calendar day, per patient. Initial inpatient neonatal critical care (99468) may only be reported once per hospital admission. If readmitted for neonatal critical care services during the same hospital stay, then report the subsequent inpatient neonatal critical care code (99469) for the first day of readmission to critical care, and 99469 for each day of critical care following readmission.

The initial inpatient neonatal critical care code (99468) can be used in addition to 99464 or 99465 as appropriate, when the physician or other qualified health care professional is present for the delivery (99464) or resuscitation (99465) is required. Other procedures performed as a necessary part of the resuscitation (eg, endotracheal intubation [31500]) may also be reported separately, when performed as part of the pre-admission delivery room care. In order to report these procedures separately, they must be performed as a necessary component of the resuscitation and not simply as a convenience before admission to the neonatal intensive care unit.

Codes 99471-99476 may be used to report the services of directing the inpatient care of a critically ill infant or young child from 29 days of postnatal age through 5 years of age. They represent care starting with the date of admission (99471, 99475) for pediatric critical care services and all subsequent day(s) (99472, 99476) that the infant or child remains in critical condition. These codes may only be reported by a single individual and only once per calendar day, per patient. Services for the critically ill or critically injured child 6 years of age or older would be reported with the time-based critical care codes (99291, 99292). Initial inpatient critical care (99471, 99475) may only be reported once per hospital admission. If readmitted to the pediatric critical care unit during the same hospital stay, then report the subsequent inpatient pediatric critical care code 99472 or 99476 for the first day of readmission to critical care and 99472 or 99476 for each day of critical care following readmission.

The pediatric and neonatal critical care codes include those procedures listed for the critical care codes (99291, 99292). In addition, the following procedures are also included (and are not separately reported by professionals, but may be reported by facilities) in the pediatric and neonatal critical care service codes (99468-99472, 99475, 99476) and the intensive care services codes (99477-99480).

Any services performed that are not included in these listings may be reported separately. For initiation of selective head or total body hypothermia in the critically ill neonate, report 99184. Facilities may report the included services separately.

Invasive or non-invasive electronic monitoring of vital signs

Vascular access procedures

  Peripheral vessel catheterization (36000)

  Other arterial catheters (36140, 36620)

  Umbilical venous catheters (36510)

  Central vessel catheterization (36555)

  Vascular access procedures (36400, 36405, 36406)

  Vascular punctures (36420, 36600)

  Umbilical arterial catheters (36660)

Airway and ventilation management

  Endotracheal intubation (31500)

  Ventilatory management (94002-94004)

  Bedside pulmonary function testing (94375)

  Surfactant administration (94610)

  Continuous positive airway pressure (CPAP) (94660)

Monitoring or interpretation of blood gases or oxygen saturation (94760-94762)

Car Seat Evaluation (94780-94781)

Transfusion of blood components (36430, 36440)

Oral or nasogastric tube placement (43752)

Suprapubic bladder aspiration (51100)

Bladder catheterization (51701, 51702)

Lumbar puncture (62270)

Any services performed which are not listed above may be reported separately.

When a neonate or infant is not critically ill but requires intensive observation, frequent interventions, and other intensive care services, the Continuing Intensive Care Services codes (99477-99480) should be used to report these services.

To report critical care services provided in the outpatient setting (eg, emergency department or office) for neonates and pediatric patients of any age, see the Critical Care codes 99291, 99292. If the same individual provides critical care services for a neonatal or pediatric patient less than 6 years of age in both the outpatient and inpatient settings on the same day, report only the appropriate Neonatal or Pediatric Critical Care codes 99468-99476 for all critical care services provided on that day. Critical care services provided by a second individual of a different specialty not reporting a per-day neonatal or pediatric critical care code can be reported with 99291, 99292.

When critical care services are provided to neonates or pediatric patients less than 6 years of age at two separate institutions by an individual from a different group on the same date of service, the individual from the referring institution should report their critical care services with the time-based critical care codes (99291, 99292) and the receiving institution should report the appropriate initial day of care code 99468, 99471, 99475 for the same date of service.

Critical care services to a pediatric patient 6 years of age or older are reported with the time based critical care codes 99291, 99292.

When the critically ill neonate or pediatric patient improves and is transferred to a lower level of care to another individual in another group within the same facility, the transferring individual does not report a per day critical care service. Subsequent hospital care (99231-99233) or time-based critical care services (99291-99292) is reported, as appropriate based upon the condition of the neonate or child. The receiving individual reports subsequent intensive care (99478-99480) or subsequent hospital care (99231-99233) services, as appropriate based upon the condition of the neonate or child.

When the neonate or infant becomes critically ill on a day when initial or subsequent intensive care services (99477-99480), hospital services (99221-99233), or normal newborn services (99460, 99461, 99462) have been performed by one individual and is transferred to a critical care level of care provided by a different individual in a different group, the transferring individual reports either the time-based critical care services performed (99291, 99292) for the time spent providing critical care to the patient, the intensive care service (99477-99480), hospital care services (99221-99233), or normal newborn service (99460, 99461, 99462) performed, but only one service. The receiving individual reports initial or subsequent inpatient neonatal or pediatric critical care (99468-99476), as appropriate based upon the patient's age and whether this is the first or subsequent admission to the critical care unit for the hospital stay.

When a newborn becomes critically ill on the same day they have already received normal newborn care (99460, 99461, 99462), and the same individual or group assumes critical care, report initial critical care service (99468) with modifier 25 in addition to the normal newborn code.

When a neonate, infant, or child requires initial critical care services on the same day the patient already has received hospital care or intensive care services by the same individual or group, only the initial critical care service code (99468, 99471, 99475) is reported.

Time-based critical care services (99291, 99292) are not reportable by the same individual or different individual of the same specialty and same group, when neonatal or pediatric critical care services (99468-99476) may be reported for the same patient on the same day. Time-based critical care services (99291, 99292) may be reported by an individual of a different specialty from either the same or different group on the same day that neonatal or pediatric critical care services are reported. Critical care interfacility transport face-to-face (99466, 99467) or supervisory (99485, 99486) services may be

reported by the same or different individual of the same specialty and same group, when neonatal or pediatric critical care services (99468-99476) are reported for the same patient on the same day.

Rationale

In accordance with the deletion of Category III codes 0188T and 0189T, the paragraph in the guidelines for inpatient neonatal and pediatric critical care that included these codes has been deleted.

Refer to the codebook and the Rationale for codes 0188T and 0189T for a full discussion of these changes.

Cognitive Assessment and Care Plan Services

99483 Assessment of and care planning for a patient with cognitive impairment, requiring an independent historian, in the office or other outpatient, home or domiciliary or rest home, with all of the following required elements:

- Cognition-focused evaluation including a pertinent history and examination;

- Medical decision making of moderate or high complexity;

- Functional assessment (eg, basic and instrumental activities of daily living), including decision-making capacity;

- Use of standardized instruments for staging of dementia (eg, functional assessment staging test [FAST], clinical dementia rating [CDR]);

- Medication reconciliation and review for high-risk medications;

- Evaluation for neuropsychiatric and behavioral symptoms, including depression, including use of standardized screening instrument(s);

- Evaluation of safety (eg, home), including motor vehicle operation;

- Identification of caregiver(s), caregiver knowledge, caregiver needs, social supports, and the willingness of caregiver to take on caregiving tasks;

- Development, updating or revision, or review of an Advance Care Plan;

★ = Telemedicine   ✦ = Add-on code   ✗ = FDA approval pending   # = Resequenced code   ⊘ = Modifier 51 exempt

- Creation of a written care plan, including initial plans to address any neuropsychiatric symptoms, neuro-cognitive symptoms, functional limitations, and referral to community resources as needed (eg, rehabilitation services, adult day programs, support groups) shared with the patient and/or caregiver with initial education and support.

Typically, 50 minutes are spent face-to-face with the patient and/or family or caregiver.

►(Do not report 99483 in conjunction with E/M services [99201, 99202, 99203, 99204, 99205, 99211, 99212, 99213, 99214, 99215, 99241, 99242, 99243, 99244, 99245, 99324, 99325, 99326, 99327, 99328, 99334, 99335, 99336, 99337, 99341, 99342, 99343, 99344, 99345, 99347, 99348, 99349, 99350, 99366, 99367, 99368, 99497, 99498]; psychiatric diagnostic procedures [90785, 90791, 90792]; brief emotional/behavioral assessment [96127]; health risk assessment administration [96160, 96161]; medication therapy management services [99605, 99606, 99607])◄

Rationale

In accordance with the deletion of codes 96103 and 96120, the parenthetical note following code 99483 has been revised to remove this code from its listing. Refer to the codebook and the Rationale for code 96101 for a full discussion of these changes.

Care Management Services

►Care management services are management and support services provided by clinical staff, under the direction of a physician or other qualified health care professional, or may be provided personally by a physician or other qualified health care professional to a patient residing at home or in a domiciliary, rest home, or assisted living facility. Services include establishing, implementing, revising, or monitoring the care plan, coordinating the care of other professionals and agencies, and educating the patient or caregiver about the patient's condition, care plan, and prognosis. The physician or other qualified health care professional provides or oversees the management and/or coordination of services, as needed, for all medical conditions, psychosocial needs, and activities of daily living.◄

A plan of care must be documented and shared with the patient and/or caregiver. A care plan is based on a physical, mental, cognitive, social, functional, and environmental assessment. It is a comprehensive plan of care for all health problems. It typically includes, but is

not limited to, the following elements: problem list, expected outcome and prognosis, measurable treatment goals, symptom management, planned interventions, medication management, community/social services ordered, how the services of agencies and specialists unconnected to the practice will be directed/coordinated, identification of the individuals responsible for each intervention, requirements for periodic review, and, when applicable, revision of the care plan.

►Codes 99487, 99489, 99490, 99491 are reported only once per calendar month and may only be reported by the single physician or other qualified health care professional who assumes the care management role with a particular patient for the calendar month.

For 99487, 99489, 99490 the face-to-face and non-face-to-face time spent by the clinical staff in communicating with the patient and/or family, caregivers, other professionals, and agencies; creating, revising, documenting, and implementing the care plan; or teaching self-management is used in determining the care management clinical staff time for the month. Only the time of the clinical staff of the reporting professional is counted. Only count the time of one clinical staff member when two or more clinical staff members are meeting about the patient. For 99491, only count the time personally spent by the physician or other qualified health care professional. Do not count any of the clinical staff time spent on the day of an initiating visit (the creation of the care plan, initial explanation to the patient and/or caregiver, and obtaining consent).

Care management activities performed by clinical staff, or personally by the physician or other qualified health care professional, typically include:◄

- communication and engagement with patient, family members, guardian or caretaker, surrogate decision makers, and/or other professionals regarding aspects of care;

- communication with home health agencies and other community services utilized by the patient;

- collection of health outcomes data and registry documentation;

- patient and/or family/caregiver education to support self-management, independent living, and activities of daily living;

- assessment and support for treatment regimen adherence and medication management;

- identification of available community and health resources;

- facilitating access to care and services needed by the patient and/or family;

- management of care transitions not reported as part of transitional care management (99495, 99496);

- ongoing review of patient status, including review of laboratory and other studies not reported as part of an E/M service, noted above;

- development, communication, and maintenance of a comprehensive care plan.

The care management office/practice must have the following capabilities:

- provide 24/7 access to physicians or other qualified health care professionals or clinical staff including providing patients/caregivers with a means to make contact with health care professionals in the practice to address urgent needs regardless of the time of day or day of week;

- provide continuity of care with a designated member of the care team with whom the patient is able to schedule successive routine appointments;

- provide timely access and management for follow-up after an emergency department visit or facility discharge;

- utilize an electronic health record system so that care providers have timely access to clinical information;

- use a standardized methodology to identify patients who require care management services;

- have an internal care management process/function whereby a patient identified as meeting the requirements for these services starts receiving them in a timely manner;

- use a form and format in the medical record that is standardized within the practice;

- be able to engage and educate patients and caregivers as well as coordinate care among all service professionals, as appropriate for each patient.

▶E/M services may be reported separately by the same physician or other qualified health care professional during the same calendar month. A physician or other qualified health care professional who reports codes 99487, 99489, 99490, may not report care plan oversight services (99339, 99340, 99374-99380), prolonged services without direct patient contact (99358, 99359), home and outpatient INR monitoring (93792, 93793), medical team conferences (99366, 99367, 99368), education and training (98960, 98961, 98962, 99071, 99078), telephone services (99366, 99367, 99368, 99441, 99442, 99443), on-line medical evaluation (98969, 99444), preparation of special reports (99080), analysis of data (99091), transitional care management services (99495, 99496), medication therapy management services (99605, 99606, 99607) and, if performed, these services may not be reported separately during the month for which 99487, 99489, 99490 are reported. All other services may be reported. Do not report 99487, 99489, 99490, 99491 if reporting ESRD

services (90951-90970) during the same month. If the care management services are performed within the postoperative period of a reported surgery, the same individual may not report 99487, 99489, 99490, 99491.

Care management may be reported in any calendar month during which the clinical staff time or physician or other qualified health care professional personal time requirements are met. If care management resumes after a discharge during a new month, start a new period or report transitional care management services (99495, 99496) as appropriate. If discharge occurs in the same month, continue the reporting period or report Transitional Care Management Services. Do not report 99487, 99489, 99490 for any post-discharge care management services for any days within 30 days of discharge, if reporting 99495, 99496.

When behavioral or psychiatric collaborative care management services are also provided, 99484, 99492, 99493, 99494 may be reported in addition.◀

Chronic Care Management Services

▶Chronic care management services are provided when medical and/or psychosocial needs of the patient require establishing, implementing, revising, or monitoring the care plan. Patients who receive chronic care management services have two or more chronic continuous or episodic health conditions that are expected to last at least 12 months, or until the death of the patient, and that place the patient at significant risk of death, acute exacerbation/decompensation, or functional decline. Code 99490 is reported when, during the calendar month, at least 20 minutes of clinical staff time is spent in care management activities. Code 99491 is reported when 30 minutes of physician or other qualified health care professional personal time is spent in care management activities. Do not report 99490 in the same month as 99491.◀

 # 99490 Chronic care management services, at least 20 minutes of clinical staff time directed by a physician or other qualified health care professional, per calendar month, with the following required elements:

- multiple (two or more) chronic conditions expected to last at least 12 months, or until the death of the patient;

- chronic conditions place the patient at significant risk of death, acute exacerbation/decompensation, or functional decline;

- comprehensive care plan established, implemented, revised, or monitored.

(Chronic care management services of less than 20 minutes duration, in a calendar month, are not reported separately)

▶(Do not report 99490 in the same calendar month as 99487, 99489, 99491)◀

#● **99491**   Chronic care management services, provided personally by a physician or other qualified health care professional, at least 30 minutes of physician or other qualified health care professional time, per calendar month, with the following required elements:

- multiple (two or more) chronic conditions expected to last at least 12 months, or until the death of the patient;

- chronic conditions place the patient at significant risk of death, acute exacerbation/decompensation, or functional decline;

- comprehensive care plan established, implemented, revised, or monitored.

▶(Do not report 99491 in the same calendar month as 99487, 99489, 99490)◀

▶(Do not report 99491 in conjunction with 99339, 99340)◀

Rationale

Code 99491 has been established to report chronic care management provided by a physician/QHP of at least 30 minutes per calendar month, with establishment/ implementation/revision/monitoring of comprehensive care plan.

Currently, there is no specific CPT code to report chronic care management provided by a physician/QHP of at least 30 minutes per calendar month. This service may only be reported by one physician/QHP at a given time within the calendar month. This service is different from the prolonged services codes because this is for a calendar month and it requires documentation of services throughout the calendar month as described in the code descriptor.

In a continuing effort to update the chronic care management services guidelines to reflect current clinical practice, these guidelines have been revised to include code 99491 and indicate that it should only be reported when 30 minutes of a physician's/QHP's personal time is spent in care management activities and may not be reported with code 99490.

Clinical Example (99491)

Adult Patient: An 83-year-old female with congestive heart failure and early cognitive dysfunction, who has been hospitalized twice in the prior 12 months, is becoming increasingly confused and refuses an office visit. She has a certified nursing assistant supervised by a home care agency, participates in a remote weight and

vital signs monitoring program, and sees a cardiologist and neurologist.

Child Patient: A 6-year-old child with spastic quadriplegia, gastrostomy, gastroesophageal reflux with recurrent bouts of aspiration pneumonia and reactive airway disease, chronic seizure disorder, failure to thrive, and severe neurodevelopment delay. He receives home occupational, physical, and speech therapy services.

Description of Procedure (99491)

A physician or other qualified health care professional personally provides these chronic care management (CCM) services, which are management and support services, to a patient residing at home or in a domiciliary, rest home, or assisted living facility. These services typically include establishing, implementing, revising, or monitoring the care plan; coordinating the care of other professionals and agencies; and educating the patient or caregiver about the patient's condition, care plan, and prognosis. The physician or other qualified health care professional provides and/or oversees the coordination of services as needed for all medical conditions, psychosocial needs, and activities of daily living. Document and share a plan of care with the patient and/or caregiver. A care plan is based on a physical, mental, cognitive, social, functional, and environmental assessment. It is a comprehensive plan of care for all health problems. It typically includes, but is not limited to, the following elements:

- Problem list;

- Expected outcome and prognosis;

- Measurable treatment goals;

- Symptom management;

- Planned interventions;

- Medication management;

- Community and social services ordered;

- How the services of agencies and specialists not associated with the practice will be directed and coordinated;

- Identification of the individuals responsible for each intervention;

- Requirements for periodic review; and

- When applicable, revision of the care plan.

In addition, the care management office/practice must have the following capabilities:

- Provide 24/7 access to physicians or other qualified health care professionals or clinical staff, including providing patients and caregivers with a means to make contact with health care professionals in the

Evaluation / Management 99201-99499

practice to address urgent needs, regardless of the time of day or day of week;

- Provide continuity of care with a designated member of the care team with whom the patient is able to schedule successive routine appointments;

- Provide timely access and management for follow-up after an emergency department visit or facility discharge;

- Use an electronic health record system so that care providers have timely access to clinical information;

- Use a standardized methodology to identify patients who require care management services;

- Have an internal care management process/function whereby a patient identified as meeting the requirements for these services starts receiving them in a timely manner;

- Use a form and format in the medical record that is standardized within the practice; and

- Engage and educate patients and caregivers as well as coordinate care among all service professionals, as appropriate for each patient.

Complex Chronic Care Management Services

99487   Complex chronic care management services, with the following required elements:

- multiple (two or more) chronic conditions expected to last at least 12 months, or until the death of the patient,

- chronic conditions place the patient at significant risk of death, acute exacerbation/decompensation, or functional decline,

- establishment or substantial revision of a comprehensive care plan,

- moderate or high complexity medical decision making;

- 60 minutes of clinical staff time directed by a physician or other qualified health care professional, per calendar month.

(Complex chronic care management services of less than 60 minutes duration, in a calendar month, are not reported separately)

+ 99489   each additional 30 minutes of clinical staff time directed by a physician or other qualified health care professional, per calendar month (List separately in addition to code for primary procedure)

(Report 99489 in conjunction with 99487)

(Do not report 99489 for care management services of less than 30 minutes additional to the first 60 minutes of complex chronic care management services during a calendar month)

►(Do not report 99487, 99489, 99490 during the same month with 90951-90970, 93792, 93793, 98960-98962, 98966-98969, 99071, 99078, 99080, 99091, 99339, 99340, 99358, 99359, 99366-99368, 99374-99380, 99441-99444, 99495, 99496, 99605-99607)◄

99490   Code is out of numerical sequence. See 99480-99489

99491   Code is out of numerical sequence. See 99480-99489

Rationale

In accordance with the deletion of code 99090, the parenthetical note following code 99489 has been revised to remove this code.

Refer to the codebook and the Rationale for code 99090 for a full discussion of these changes.

Psychiatric Collaborative Care Management Services

►Psychiatric collaborative care services are provided under the direction of a treating physician or other qualified health care professional (see definitions below) during a calendar month. These services are reported by the treating physician or other qualified health care professional and include the services of the treating physician or other qualified health care professional, the behavioral health care manager (see definition below), and the psychiatric consultant (see definition below), who has contracted directly with the treating physician or other qualified health care professional, to provide consultation. Patients directed to the behavioral health care manager typically have behavioral health signs and/or symptoms or a newly diagnosed behavioral health condition, may need help in engaging in treatment, have not responded to standard care delivered in a nonpsychiatric setting, or require further assessment and engagement, prior to consideration of referral to a psychiatric care setting.

These services are provided when a patient requires a behavioral health care assessment; establishing, implementing, revising, or monitoring a care plan; and provision of brief interventions.

The following definitions apply to this section:◄

★ = Telemedicine   ✚ = Add-on code   ✔ = FDA approval pending   # = Resequenced code   ⊘ = Modifier 51 exempt

Definitions

Episode of care patients are treated for an episode of care, which is defined as beginning when the patient is directed by the treating physician or other qualified health care professional to the behavioral health care manager and ending with:

- the attainment of targeted treatment goals, which typically results in the discontinuation of care management services and continuation of usual follow-up with the treating physician or other qualified healthcare professional; or

- ▶failure to attain targeted treatment goals culminating in referral to a psychiatric care provider for ongoing treatment of the behavioral health condition; or◀

- lack of continued engagement with no psychiatric collaborative care management services provided over a consecutive six month calendar period (break in episode).

Rationale

The introductory guidelines for psychiatric collaborative care management services have been revised to clarify that psychiatric collaborative care management services are provided to patients who typically have behavioral health signs and/or symptoms or a newly diagnosed behavioral health condition. This revision aligns the psychiatric collaborative care management services codes with Centers for Medicare & Medicaid Services (CMS) guidance.

Transitional Care Management Services

Codes 99495 and 99496 are used to report transitional care management services (TCM). These services are for a new or established patient whose medical and/or psychosocial problems require moderate or high complexity medical decision making during transitions in care from an inpatient hospital setting (including acute hospital, rehabilitation hospital, long-term acute care hospital), partial hospital, observation status in a hospital, or skilled nursing facility/nursing facility to the patient's community setting (home, domiciliary, rest home, or assisted living). TCM commences upon the date of discharge and continues for the next 29 days.

TCM is comprised of one face-to-face visit within the specified timeframes, in combination with non-face-to-face services that may be performed by the physician or other qualified health care professional and/or licensed clinical staff under his/her direction.

Non-face-to-face services provided by clinical staff, under the direction of the physician or other qualified health care professional, may include:

- communication (with patient, family members, guardian or caretaker, surrogate decision makers, and/or other professionals) regarding aspects of care,

- communication with home health agencies and other community services utilized by the patient,

- patient and/or family/caretaker education to support self-management, independent living, and activities of daily living,

- assessment and support for treatment regimen adherence and medication management,

- identification of available community and health resources,

- facilitating access to care and services needed by the patient and/or family

Non-face-to-face services provided by the physician or other qualified health care provider may include:

- obtaining and reviewing the discharge information (eg, discharge summary, as available, or continuity of care documents);

- reviewing need for or follow-up on pending diagnostic tests and treatments;

- interaction with other qualified health care professionals who will assume or reassume care of the patient's system-specific problems;

- education of patient, family, guardian, and/or caregiver;

- establishment or reestablishment of referrals and arranging for needed community resources;

- assistance in scheduling any required follow-up with community providers and services.

TCM requires a face-to-face visit, initial patient contact, and medication reconciliation within specified time frames. The first face-to-face visit is part of the TCM service and not reported separately. Additional E/M services provided on subsequent dates after the first face-to-face visit may be reported separately. TCM requires an interactive contact with the patient or caregiver, as appropriate, within two business days of discharge. The contact may be direct (face-to-face), telephonic, or by electronic means. Medication reconciliation and management must occur no later than the date of the face-to-face visit.

These services address any needed coordination of care performed by multiple disciplines and community service agencies. The reporting individual provides or oversees the management and/or coordination of services, as needed, for all medical conditions, psychosocial needs and activity of daily living support by providing first contact and continuous access.

Medical decision making and the date of the first face-to-face visit are used to select and report the appropriate TCM code. For 99496, the face-to-face visit must occur within 7 calendar days of the date discharge and medical decision making must be of high complexity. For 99495, the face-to-face visit must occur within 14 calendar days of the date of discharge and medical decision making must be of at least moderate complexity.

Type of Medical Decision Making	Face-to-Face Visit Within 7 Days	Face-to-Face Visit Within 8 to 14 Days
Moderate Complexity	99495	99495
High Complexity	99496	99495

Medical decision making is defined by the E/M Services Guidelines. The medical decision making over the service period reported is used to define the medical decision making of TCM. Documentation includes the timing of the initial post discharge communication with the patient or caregivers, date of the face-to-face visit, and the complexity of medical decision making.

Only one individual may report these services and only once per patient within 30 days of discharge. Another TCM may not be reported by the same individual or group for any subsequent discharge(s) within the 30 days. The same individual may report hospital or observation discharge services and TCM. However, the discharge service may not constitute the required face-to-face visit. The same individual should not report TCM services provided in the postoperative period of a service that the individual reported.

▶A physician or other qualified health care professional who reports codes 99495, 99496 may not report care plan oversight services (99339, 99340, 99374-99380), prolonged services without direct patient contact (99358, 99359), home and outpatient INR monitoring (93792, 93793), medical team conferences (99366-99368), education and training (98960-98962, 99071, 99078), telephone services (98966-98968, 99441-99443), end stage renal disease services (90951-90970), online medical evaluation services (98969, 99444), preparation of special reports (99080), analysis of data (99091), complex chronic care coordination services (99487-99489), medication therapy management services (99605-99607), during the time period covered by the transitional care management services codes.◄

Rationale

In accordance with the deletion of code 99090, the guidelines for transitional care management services have been revised to remove this code.

Refer to the codebook and the Rationale for code 99090 for a full discussion of these changes.

99495 **Transitional Care Management Services** with the following required elements:

- Communication (direct contact, telephone, electronic) with the patient and/or caregiver within 2 business days of discharge

- Medical decision making of at least moderate complexity during the service period

- Face-to-face visit, within 14 calendar days of discharge

99496 **Transitional Care Management Services** with the following required elements:

- Communication (direct contact, telephone, electronic) with the patient and/or caregiver within 2 business days of discharge

- Medical decision making of high complexity during the service period

- Face-to-face visit, within 7 calendar days of discharge

(Do not report 99495, 99496 in conjunction with 93792, 93793)

▶(Do not report 90951-90970, 98960-98962, 98966-98969, 99071, 99078, 99080, 99091, 99339, 99340, 99358, 99359, 99366-99368, 99374-99380, 99441-99444, 99487-99489, 99605-99607, when performed during the service time of codes 99495 or 99496)◄

Rationale

In accordance with the deletion of code 99090, the parenthetical note following code 99496 has been revised to remove this code.

Refer to the codebook and the Rationale for code 99090 for a full discussion of these changes.

★ = Telemedicine   ✚ = Add-on code   ✇ = FDA approval pending   # = Resequenced code   ⊘ = Modifier 51 exempt

Anesthesia

A new subsection together with an unlisted code have been added to the Anesthesia Guidelines section.

Summary of Additions, Deletions, and Revisions

The summary of changes shows the actual changes that have been made to the code descriptors.

New codes appear with a bullet (●) and are indicated as "Code added." Revised codes are preceded with a triangle (▲). Within revised codes, or if a code symbol has been deleted, the deleted language and code symbol appears with a ~~strikethrough~~ (Ө), while new text appears <u>underlined</u>.

The ⚺ symbol is used to identify codes for vaccines that are pending FDA approval. The # symbol is used to identify codes that have been resequenced. CPT add-on codes are annotated by the ✚ symbol. The ⊘ symbol is used to identify codes that are exempt from the use of modifier 51. The ★ symbol is used to identify codes that may be used for reporting telemedicine services. The ✖ is used to identify proprietary laboratory analyses (PLA) test that has an identical descriptor as another PLA test.

Heading	New and/or Revised Guidelines
►Unlisted Service or Procedure◄	►A service or procedure may be provided that is not listed in this edition of the CPT codebook. When reporting such a service, the appropriate "Unlisted Procedure" code may be used to indicate the service, identifying it by "Special Report" as discussed in the section below. The "Unlisted Procedures" and accompanying code for **Anesthesia** is as follows:◄

Anesthesia Guidelines

►Unlisted Service or Procedure◄

►A service or procedure may be provided that is not listed in this edition of the CPT codebook. When reporting such a service, the appropriate "Unlisted Procedure" code may be used to indicate the service, identifying it by "Special Report" as discussed in the section below. The "Unlisted Procedures" and accompanying code for **Anesthesia** is as follows:◄

01999   Unlisted anesthesia procedure(s)

Rationale

For consistency, the subsection of "Unlisted Service or Procedure" and the corresponding unlisted anesthesia code have been added to the Anesthesia Guidelines section.

Surgery

In the General Surgery section, a new subsection, Fine Needle Aspiration (FNA) Biopsy, has been added along with new guidelines, parenthetical notes, and nine new codes (10004, 10005, 10006, 10007, 10008, 10009, 10010, 10011, 10012). In addition, code 10021 has been revised and code 10022 has been deleted. Multiple parenthetical notes throughout the code set have also been revised to incorporate the code revision and additions.

In the Biopsy subsection of the Integumentary System section, the Biopsy guidelines have been revised to specify distinct biopsy modalities. In addition, six new codes (11102, 11103, 11104, 11105, 11106, 11107) have been added, and two codes (11100, 11101) have been deleted. Multiple parenthetical notes and a new table to assist with appropriate biopsy code selection have been added. In the Skin Replacement Surgery subsection, the skin substitute graft definition has been editorially revised to clarify the nonreporting of nongraft wound dressings.

In the General subsection of the Musculoskeletal System section, one code (20005) has been deleted and three codes (20932, 20933, 20934) have been added. Multiple parenthetical notes have also been added and/or revised in support of these changes. In the Head and Spine (Vertebral Column) subsections, two parenthetical notes have been revised and one parenthetical note has been deleted in accordance with the deletion of other codes throughout the code set. In the Femur (Thigh Region) and Knee Joint subsection, code 27370 has been deleted and new code 27369 added. Several parenthetical notes have been added following code 27369 too. In the Foot and Toes and Application of Casts and Strapping subsections, multiple parenthetical notes have also been added and revised.

In the Respiratory System section, code 31595 has been deleted. Multiple parenthetical notes throughout the section have been revised in support of other new, revised, and/or deleted codes throughout the code set accordingly as well.

Numerous changes have been made to the Cardiovascular System section. In the Pacemaker or Implantable Defibrillator subsection, two codes (33274, 33275) have been added to report transcatheter insertion or replacement/removal of a permanent leadless ventricular pacemaker. These changes follow the deletion of their corresponding Category III codes. In response to these changes, guidelines and parenthetical notes and revision of the pacemaker and implantable defibrillator system table have similarly been made. The title of "Patient-Activated Event Recorder" subsection has been revised to "Subcutaneous Cardiac Rhythm Monitor." Two codes (33282, 33284) in this subsection have been deleted and two codes (33285, 33286) have been added to report insertion and removal of a subcutaneous cardiac rhythm monitor. Guidelines and parenthetical notes were also added throughout the code set regarding the reporting of subcutaneous cardiac rhythm monitor services. A new subsection, "Implantable Hemodynamic Monitors," has been added along with guidelines, parenthetical notes, and code 33289 to report implantation of wireless pulmonary artery pressure sensors. In the Aortic Valve subsection, one code (33440) and multiple parenthetical notes have been added. New guidelines and parenthetical notes along with code 33866 have been added to the Thoracic Aortic Aneurysm subsection to report the use of an aortic hemiarch graft as well. Parenthetical notes in the Arteries and Veins and Bypass Graft subsections have also been added and revised. A number of changes have also taken place regarding peripherally inserted central venous catheter (PICC) procedures in the Central Venous Access Procedures and Insertion of Central Venous Access Device subsections. In addition, three codes (36568, 36569, 36584) have been revised and two new codes (36572, 36573) have been added. Similarly, guidelines and parenthetical notes have been added and revised as accordingly.

In the Hemic and Lymphatic Systems section, a new code (38531) has been added. As a result, code 38531 and other pelvic and vulvar codes have also been added to the parenthetical note following code 38900. Similarly, multiple parenthetical notes have been revised throughout this section in support of other new and/or revised codes throughout the code set.

In the Digestive System section, two codes (41500, 46762) have been deleted. In the Stomach subsection, one code (43760) has been deleted and two new codes (43762, 43763) have been added along with three parenthetical notes. Multiple parenthetical notes have also been revised throughout this section in support of other new and/or revised codes throughout the code set.

In the Other Introduction (Injection/Change/Removal) Procedures subsection of the Urinary System section, one code (50395) has been replaced with two new codes (50436, 50437) to describe dilation of an existing urinary tract. Multiple parenthetical notes and guidelines have been added and revised to further support these changes. In the Urethra subsection, a new code (53854) to report water vapor thermotherapy for destruction of prostate issue has been added.

In the Male Genital System, Female Genital System, and Endocrine System sections, parenthetical notes have been added and revised in support of other new and/or revised codes throughout the code set.

In the Nervous System section, six codes (61332, 61480, 61610, 61612, 63615, 64508) have been deleted. Two codes (61641, 61642) in the Endovascular Therapy subsection have been revised. The guidelines in the Neurostimulators (Intracranial), (Spinal), and (Peripheral Nerve) subsections have been revised in conjunction with changes made to reporting services for neurostimulator services in the Medicine section. Multiple parenthetical notes have also been revised in this section.

In the Ocular section, one code (66220) has been deleted and various parenthetical notes have also been revised in this section.

Summary of Additions, Deletions, and Revisions

The summary of changes shows the actual changes that have been made to the code descriptors.

New codes appear with a bullet (●) and are indicated as "Code added." Revised codes are preceded with a triangle (▲). Within revised codes, or if a code symbol has been deleted, the deleted language and code symbol appears with a ~~strikethrough~~ (⊖), while new text appears underlined.

The ⁄ symbol is used to identify codes for vaccines that are pending FDA approval. The # symbol is used to identify codes that have been resequenced. CPT add-on codes are annotated by the ✚ symbol. The ⊘ symbol is used to identify codes that are exempt from the use of modifier 51. The ★ symbol is used to identify codes that may be used for reporting telemedicine services. The ⵋ is used to identify proprietary laboratory analyses (PLA) test that has an identical descriptor as another PLA test.

Code	Description
▲10021	Fine needle aspiration biopsy, without imaging guidance; ~~without imaging guidance~~first lesion
~~10022~~	~~with imaging guidance~~
#✚●10004	Code added
#●10005	Code added
#✚●10006	Code added

Code	Description
#●**10007**	Code added
#+●**10008**	Code added
#●**10009**	Code added
#+●**10010**	Code added
#●**10011**	Code added
#+●**10012**	Code added
~~**11100**~~	~~Biopsy of skin, subcutaneous tissue and/or mucous membrane (including simple closure), unless otherwise listed; single lesion~~
~~**11101**~~	~~each separate/additional lesion (List separately in addition to code for primary procedure)~~
●**11102**	Code added
+●**11103**	Code added
●**11104**	Code added
+●**11105**	Code added
●**11106**	Code added
+●**11107**	Code added
~~**20005**~~	~~Incision and drainage of soft tissue abscess, subfascial (ie, involves the soft tissue below the deep fascia)~~
+●**20932**	Code added
+●**20933**	Code added
+●**20934**	Code added
●**27369**	Code added
~~**27370**~~	~~Injection of contrast for knee arthrography~~
~~**31595**~~	~~Section recurrent laryngeal nerve, therapeutic (separate procedure), unilateral~~
#●**33274**	Code added
#●**33275**	Code added
~~**33282**~~	~~Implantation of patient-activated cardiac event recorder~~
~~**33284**~~	~~Removal of an implantable, patient-activated cardiac event recorder~~
●**33285**	Code added
●**33286**	Code added
●**33289**	Code added
#●**33440**	Code added
+●**33866**	Code added
▲**36568**	Insertion of peripherally inserted central venous catheter (PICC), without subcutaneous port or pump, without imaging guidance; younger than 5 years of age

Code	Description
▲36569	age 5 years or older
#●36572	Code added
#●36573	Code added
▲36584	Replacement, complete, of a peripherally inserted central venous catheter (PICC), without subcutaneous port or pump, through same venous access, including all imaging guidance, image documentation, and all associated radiological supervision and interpretation required to perform the replacement
●38531	Code added
41500	Fixation of tongue, mechanical, other than suture (eg, K-wire)
43760	Change of gastrostomy tube, percutaneous, without imaging or endoscopic guidance
●43762	Code added
●43763	Code added
46762	implantation artificial sphincter
50395	Introduction of guide into renal pelvis and/or ureter with dilation to establish nephrostomy tract, percutaneous
#●50436	Code added
#●50437	Code added
●53854	Code added
61332	Exploration of orbit (transcranial approach); with biopsy
61480	for mesencephalic tractotomy or pedunculotomy
61610	Transection or ligation, carotid artery in cavernous sinus, with repair by anastomosis or graft (List separately in addition to code for primary procedure)
61612	with repair by anastomosis or graft (List separately in addition to code for primary procedure)
+▲61641	each additional vessel in same vascular familyterritory (List separately in addition to code for primary procedure)
+▲61642	each additional vessel in different vascular familyterritory (List separately in addition to code for primary procedure)
63615	Stereotactic biopsy, aspiration, or excision of lesion, spinal cord
64508	carotid sinus (separate procedure)
64550	Application of surface (transcutaneous) neurostimulator (eg, TENS unit)
66220	Repair of scleral staphyloma; without graft

★ = Telemedicine   ✚ = Add-on code   ✗ = FDA approval pending   # = Resequenced code   ⊘ = Modifier 51 exempt

Surgery Guidelines

Imaging Guidance

▶When imaging guidance or imaging supervision and interpretation is included in a surgical procedure, guidelines for image documentation and report, included in the guidelines for Radiology (Including Nuclear Medicine and Diagnostic Ultrasound), will apply. Imaging guidance should not be reported for use of a nonimaging-guided tracking or localizing system (eg, radar signals, electromagnetic signals). Imaging guidance should only be reported when an imaging modality (eg, radiography, fluoroscopy, ultrasonography, magnetic resonance imaging, computed tomography, or nuclear medicine) is used and is appropriately documented.◀

Rationale

Guidelines in the Surgery/Imaging Guidance subsection have been revised to clarify reporting for nonimaging guidance. Imaging guidance should not be reported when a nonimaging-guided modality (eg, radar signals, electromagnetic signals) is used. Instead, it should only be reported when an imaging modality (eg, radiography, fluoroscopy, ultrasonography, magnetic resonance imaging, computed tomography, or nuclear medicine) is used and is appropriately documented.

Surgery

General

►Fine Needle Aspiration (FNA) Biopsy◄

►A **fine needle aspiration** (FNA) biopsy is performed when material is aspirated with a fine needle and the cells are examined cytologically. A **core needle biopsy** is typically performed with a larger bore needle to obtain a core sample of tissue for histopathologic evaluation. FNA biopsy procedures are performed with or without imaging guidance. Imaging guidance codes (eg, 76942, 77002, 77012, 77021) may not be reported separately with 10004, 10005, 10006, 10007, 10008, 10009, 10010, 10011, 10012, 10021. Codes 10004, 10005, 10006, 10007, 10008, 10009, 10010, 10011, 10012, 10021 are reported once per lesion sampled in a single session. When more than one FNA biopsy is performed on separate lesions at the same session, same day, same imaging modality, use the appropriate imaging modality add-on code for the second and subsequent lesion(s). When more than one FNA biopsy is performed on separate lesions, same session, same day, using different imaging modalities, report the corresponding primary code with modifier 59 for each additional imaging modality and corresponding add-on codes for subsequent lesions sampled. This instruction applies regardless of whether the lesions are ipsilateral or contralateral to each other, and/or whether they are in the same or different organs/structures. When FNA biopsy and core needle biopsy both are performed on the same lesion, same session, same day using the same type of imaging guidance, do not separately report the imaging guidance for the core needle biopsy. When FNA biopsy is performed on one lesion and core needle biopsy is performed on a separate lesion, same session, same day using the same type of imaging guidance, both the core needle biopsy and the imaging guidance for the core needle biopsy may be reported separately with modifier 59. When FNA biopsy is performed on one lesion and core needle biopsy is performed on a separate lesion, same session, same day using different types of imaging guidance, both the core needle biopsy and the imaging guidance for the core needle biopsy may be reported with modifier 59.◄

10004   Code is out of numerical sequence. See 10021-10035

10005   Code is out of numerical sequence. See 10021-10035

10006   Code is out of numerical sequence. See 10021-10035

10007   Code is out of numerical sequence. See 10021-10035

10008   Code is out of numerical sequence. See 10021-10035

10009   Code is out of numerical sequence. See 10021-10035

10010   Code is out of numerical sequence. See 10021-10035

10011   Code is out of numerical sequence. See 10021-10035

10012   Code is out of numerical sequence. See 10021-10035

▲ 10021   Fine needle aspiration biopsy, without imaging guidance; first lesion

►(10022 has been deleted. To report, see 10005, 10006, 10007, 10008, 10009, 10010, 10011, 10012)◄

\#+● 10004   each additional lesion (List separately in addition to code for primary procedure)

►(Use 10004 in conjunction with 10021)◄

►(Do not report 10004, 10021 in conjunction with 10005, 10006, 10007, 10008, 10009, 10010, 10011, 10012 for the same lesion)◄

►(For evaluation of fine needle aspirate, see 88172, 88173, 88177)◄

\#● 10005   Fine needle aspiration biopsy, including ultrasound guidance; first lesion

\#+● 10006   each additional lesion (List separately in addition to code for primary procedure)

►(Use 10006 in conjunction with 10005)◄

►(Do not report 10005, 10006 in conjunction with 76942)◄

►(For evaluation of fine needle aspirate, see 88172, 88173, 88177)◄

\#● 10007   Fine needle aspiration biopsy, including fluoroscopic guidance; first lesion

\#+● 10008   each additional lesion (List separately in addition to code for primary procedure)

►(Use 10008 in conjunction with 10007)◄

►(Do not report 10007, 10008 in conjunction with 77002)◄

►(For evaluation of fine needle aspirate, see 88172, 88173, 88177)◄

\#● 10009   Fine needle aspiration biopsy, including CT guidance; first lesion

\#+● 10010   each additional lesion (List separately in addition to code for primary procedure)

►(Use 10010 in conjunction with 10009)◄

►(Do not report 10009, 10010 in conjunction with 77012)◄

►(For evaluation of fine needle aspirate, see 88172, 88173, 88177)◄

\#● 10011   Fine needle aspiration biopsy, including MR guidance; first lesion

\#+● 10012   each additional lesion (List separately in addition to code for primary procedure)

►(Use 10012 in conjunction with 10011)◄

★ = Telemedicine   + = Add-on code   ⫽ = FDA approval pending   # = Resequenced code   ⊘ = Modifier 51 exempt

►(Do not report 10011, 10012 in conjunction with 77021)◄

►(For evaluation of fine needle aspirate, see 88172, 88173, 88177)◄

(For percutaneous needle biopsy other than fine needle aspiration, see 19081-19086 for breast, 20206 for muscle, 32400 for pleura, 32405 for lung or mediastinum, 42400 for salivary gland, 47000 for liver, 48102 for pancreas, 49180 for abdominal or retroperitoneal mass, 50200 for kidney, 54500 for testis, 54800 for epididymis, 60100 for thyroid, 62267 for nucleus pulposus, intervertebral disc, or paravertebral tissue, 62269 for spinal cord)

►(For percutaneous image-guided fluid collection drainage by catheter of soft tissue [eg, extremity, abdominal wall, neck], use 10030)◄

Rationale

Rather significant changes have been made to the codes for fine needle aspiration (FNA) biopsy procedures, which now include imaging guidance as part of the procedure: new subsection entitled Fine Needle Aspiration [FNA] Biopsy; nine new Category I codes (10004-10012); one revised code (10021); and one deleted code (10022). In addition, new guidelines have been added to the new subsection and a number of parenthetical notes have been added and/or revised throughout the CPT code set to accommodate these changes.

Codes 10021 and 10022 were reviewed because of a survey requested by the AMA/Specialty Relative Value Scale (RVS) Update Committee (RUC) Relativity Assessment Workgroup (RAW), which identified these codes as part of a family of codes that were potentially misvalued. The review revealed that codes 10021 and 10022 were actually being misused (ie, reported for each pass rather than per lesion as intended). In addition, it was also noted that code 10022 was reported with ultrasound imaging more than 75% of the time. As a result, this section has been revised to update (10021) and replace (10022) these two codes with more descriptive codes and to provide instructions that better reflect the intended use for FNA procedures. The addition of the guidelines, parenthetical notes, and replacement/revision of the codes—all serves to provide a better reporting mechanism for these services.

To provide better instruction regarding reporting, new guidelines have been added within the subsection. These guidelines provide a number of clarifications, which includes:

1. Provision of a definition of "fine needle aspiration" vs "core needle biopsy";

2. Separate direction regarding exclusion of separate reporting of imaging for these procedures;

3. Direction that these codes may only be reported once per lesion sampled, which inherently restricts: separate reporting for multiple passes into a single lesion; separate reporting for use of different types of imaging on the same lesion; and separate reporting for attempts at nonimaged biopsy that later requires some type of imaging; and

4. Instruction for reporting biopsies performed on different lesions; reporting for different types of biopsies; and/or using different types of imaging procedures. When reporting multiple biopsies and/or multiple methods for imaging, instructions have been provided to assist users in identifying when the procedure should be reported with an add-on code for services that may include certain shared tasks and when the use of separate codes appended with modifier 59 may be appropriate.

Code 10021 has been revised to specify that the procedure reported is intended as a biopsy and is used to report the first lesion biopsied. This is accomplished by adding the terms "biopsy" and "first lesion" to the descriptor. Addition of "biopsy" to the code descriptor (and as part of the language for the newly added FNA biopsy codes) helps specify that these codes are intended for reporting biopsy procedures with cytopathologic evaluation and not simple aspiration procedures. Retaining the acronym/language "FNA/fine needle aspiration" helps to differentiate these procedures from core needle biopsies that are used more for histopathological analyses, which require a different technique to obtain the sample.

Code 10022 has been deleted and new codes (10004-10012) that identify the specific imaging and biopsy procedures have been added. The addition of these new codes enables multiple lesion biopsy procedures reporting. Codes 10005, 10007, 10009, and 10011 each identify FNA biopsies performed for the first lesion using the imaging technique specified in the descriptor (fluoroscopy, ultrasound, computed tomography [CT], or magnetic resonance [MR] guidance, respectively). The inclusion of new add-on codes (10004, 10006, 10008, 10010, 10012) for each type of biopsy and imaging procedure enable reporting for any additional lesions that may be biopsied during the same session. Parenthetical notes provide instructions regarding the appropriate reporting for these add-on codes.

Parenthetical notes have been added, moved, and/or deleted according to instruction that is needed for the surrounding codes. Exclusionary parenthetical notes restrict reporting for procedures that are mutually excluded, such as the reporting of imaging for these services. This is also explained in the guidelines for this subsection. Some instructional parenthetical notes have been moved to areas for better visibility, such as for evaluation of fine needle aspirates (88172, 88173, 88177) or the instruction for percutaneous image-guided fluid collection by catheter of soft tissue. Therefore, these parenthetical notes provide instructions about reporting procedures that are not reported by codes in this new section. Conversely, other parenthetical notes, such as the parenthetical note that provides instruction regarding placement of localization devices, have been removed. Relocation of these parenthetical notes allows users the ability to focus on instruction regarding FNA for biopsies. Similarly, all parenthetical notes that used to provide instructions regarding separate reporting for imaging have been deleted.

Essentially, all of the changes made in the codes and the associated parenthetical notes are to inherently include imaging guidance with all FNA biopsy or core biopsy procedures that are usually provided with imaging. In order to accommodate the revisions made for reporting FNA procedures, additional parenthetical notes have been revised throughout the CPT code set to direct users to these codes when it is appropriate to report FNA procedures. This includes the addition of the term "biopsy" when needed for the FNA language and deletion of code 10022.

Clinical Example (10004)

A 68-year-old male presents with a palpable lesion in the submandibular region and second palpable lesion in the contralateral lower neck. After a fine needle aspiration (FNA) biopsy of the first lesion is performed (reported separately), a FNA biopsy without imaging guidance is performed on the second lesion.

Description of Procedure (10004)

Insert a needle with attached syringe into the lesion. Perform a FNA biopsy without imaging guidance of the lesion by making multiple passes with the same needle under suction with the syringe. Withdraw the needle and express the material onto slides. Smear the slides and inspect for adequacy and apply a slide fixative. Aspirate the appropriate solution into the syringe and needle and express in cell block fixative solution for purposes of cell block preparation. Repeat the previous process in the same lesion (typically repeated two additional times). Between each aspiration, apply compression at the FNA biopsy site and observe the patient for bleeding, hematoma, or other complication(s). Apply a dressing and hold compression for several minutes. Document the

procedure for the medical record. Monitor the patient for any evidence of hematoma.

Clinical Example (10005)

A 59-year-old female presents with a nonpalpable thyroid nodule previously identified with diagnostic ultrasound. The patient undergoes an ultrasound-guided FNA biopsy of the lesion.

Description of Procedure (10005)

Perform a preliminary ultrasound (US) to identify the appropriate approach for initial needle placement. Use US to confirm the correct trajectory for needle advancement to the target anatomic lesion and to avoid vascular structures and nontarget organs. Mark the site. Position and prepare the patient. Clean the biopsy site with disinfectant. Inject a local anesthetic. Using concurrent real-time US visualization, insert a needle with attached syringe into the lesion. Perform a FNA biopsy of the lesion. Intermittent US visualization may take place during the intervention, which necessitated the needle placement. Withdraw the needle and express the material onto slides, into fixative, and/or in the appropriate solution for the pathology workup. Repeat the previous process in the same lesion (typically a total of three or four samples are obtained). A pathology representative (pathologist or cytotechnologist) evaluates the sample to assess adequacy. Obtain additional FNA biopsy samples as needed. Apply compression at the FNA biopsy site. Observe patient for bleeding, hematoma, or other complication(s). Record permanent image(s).

Clinical Example (10006)

A 59-year-old male presents with nonpalpable nodules in both the left and right lobes of the thyroid previously identified by diagnostic ultrasound. After a FNA biopsy of the first lesion is performed (reported separately) using ultrasound guidance, an ultrasound-guided FNA biopsy is performed on the second lesion.

Description of Procedure (10006)

Explain the additional procedure and its purpose to the patient, including potential complications. Clarify the differences between the subsequent procedure and the first FNA biopsy procedure for the patient. Obtain informed consent. Perform a preliminary US to identify the appropriate approach for initial needle placement. Use US to confirm the correct trajectory for needle advancement to the target anatomic lesion and to avoid vascular structures and nontarget organs. Mark the site. Reposition the patient and prepare again. Cleanse the biopsy site with disinfectant. Inject a local anesthetic. Using concurrent real-time US visualization, insert a needle with attached syringe into the lesion. Perform a FNA biopsy of the lesion. Intermittent US visualization may take place during the intervention, which necessitated the needle placement. Withdraw the needle and express the material expressed onto slides, into fixative, and/or in the appropriate solution. Repeat the previous process in the same lesion (typically, a total of three or four samples are obtained). A cytopathologist evaluates the sample to assess adequacy. Obtain additional FNA biopsy samples as needed. Apply compression at the FNA biopsy site and observe the patient for bleeding, hematoma, or other complication(s). Record permanent image(s). Dictate a report of the additional procedure for the medical record (which may be included in the report for 10005). Dictate an addendum to the report when the final pathology results are received (which may be included in the report for 10005). Call the referring physician or other qualified health care professional and provide the report if the test results are significant or if final pathology disagrees with imaging results.

Clinical Example (10007)

A 62-year-old female presents with a lung lesion visible on chest radiographs. The patient undergoes a fluoroscopic-guided FNA biopsy of the lesion.

Description of Procedure (10007)

Place the patient on a fluoroscopy table and position appropriately. Perform targeted fluoroscopy, including angulation of the image intensifier, to identify the appropriate level and approach for the initial needle placement. Prepare and mark the skin entry site. Apply sterile drapes. Determine approach to the lesion. Inject local anesthetic with fluoroscopic guidance. During needle placement, use intermittent fluoroscopy and angulation of the image intensifier to confirm the correct approach and the need for needle repositioning or realignment. If the position is not correct, use additional fluoroscopy to guide repositioning until the proper position is achieved. Administer intermittent contrast material injection as needed. Using fluoroscopic guidance, insert a needle with attached syringe into the lesion. Perform a FNA biopsy of the lesion. Intermittent fluoroscopic visualization may take place during the intervention, which necessitated the needle placement. Withdraw the needle and express the material expressed onto slides, into fixative, and/or in the appropriate solution for further pathology workup. Repeat the previous process in the same lesion (typically, three or four samples are acquired). A pathology representative (pathologist or cytotechnologist) evaluates the sample to assess adequacy. Obtain additional FNA biopsy samples as needed. Apply compression at the FNA biopsy site and observe the patient for bleeding, hematoma, or other complication(s). Record permanent image(s).

Clinical Example (10008)

A 79-year-old male is found to have two lung lesions on chest radiographs. After a fluoroscopic-guided FNA biopsy of the first lesion is performed (reported separately), a fluoroscopic-guided FNA biopsy is performed on the second lesion.

Description of Procedure (10008)

Explain the additional procedure and its purpose to the patient, including potential complications. Clarify the differences between the subsequent procedure and the first FNA biopsy procedure for the patient. Obtain informed consent. Reposition the patient on the fluoroscopy table. Perform targeted fluoroscopy, including angulation of the image intensifier, to identify the appropriate level and approach for the initial needle placement. Prepare and mark the skin entry site. Apply sterile drapes. Determine approach to the lesion. Inject a local anesthetic with fluoroscopic guidance. During needle placement, use intermittent fluoroscopy and angulation of the image intensifier to confirm the correct approach and the need for needle repositioning or realignment. If the position is not correct, use additional fluoroscopy to guide repositioning until the proper position is achieved. Perform an intermittent contrast material injection as needed. Using fluoroscopic guidance, insert a needle with attached syringe into the lesion. Perform a FNA biopsy of the lesion. Intermittent fluoroscopic visualization may take place during the intervention, which necessitated the needle placement. Withdraw the needle and express the material onto slides, into fixative, and/or in the appropriate solution. Repeat the previous process in the same lesion (typically, three or four samples are obtained). A pathology representative (pathologist or cytotechnologist) evaluates the sample to assess adequacy. Obtain additional FNA biopsy samples as needed. Apply compression at the FNA biopsy site and observe the patient for bleeding, hematoma, or other complication(s). Record permanent image(s). Dictate a report of the additional procedure for the medical record (which may be included in the report for 10007). Dictate an addendum to the report when the final pathology results are received (which may be included in the report for 10007). Call the referring physician or other qualified health care professional and provide the report if the test results are significant or if final pathology disagrees with imaging results.

Clinical Example (10009)

A 58-year-old male presents with a lesion in the left lung identified on a previous computerized tomography (CT) chest scan. The patient undergoes a CT-guided FNA biopsy of the lesion.

Description of Procedure (10009)

Perform targeted CT to identify the appropriate approach for the initial needle placement. Reposition patient as necessary to facilitate the safest CT-guided access to the lesion. Prepare and mark the skin entry site. Apply sterile drapes. Determine approach to the lesion. Inject a local anesthetic with CT guidance. Use CT guidance to confirm the correct trajectory for needle advancement to the target anatomic lesion, avoiding vascular structures and nontarget organs. During needle placement, use intermittent CT to confirm the correct approach and the need for needle repositioning or realignment. If the position is not correct, use additional CT guidance to facilitate repositioning until the proper position is achieved. Perform intermittent contrast material injection as needed. Using CT guidance, insert a needle with attached syringe into the lesion. Perform a FNA biopsy of the lesion. Intermittent CT visualization may take place during the intervention, which necessitated the needle placement. Withdraw the needle and express the material expressed onto slides, into fixative, and/or in the appropriate solution. Repeat the previous process in the same lesion (typically, three or four samples are obtained). A pathology representative (pathologist or cytotechnologist) evaluates the sample to assess adequacy. Obtain additional FNA biopsy samples as needed. Apply compression at the FNA biopsy site and observe the patient for bleeding, hematoma, or other complication(s). Record permanent image(s). Obtain post-procedural CT scan and interpret to evaluate for complications. Interpret all images resulting from the study, including dedicated review of the target(s) as well as all visualized viscera, fascial planes, vasculature, soft tissues, and osseous structures. Assess for complications or other unexpected findings. Compare to all pertinent available prior studies.

Clinical Example (10010)

A 67-year-old male is found to have two lung lesions identified on a previous chest CT scan. After a CT-guided FNA biopsy of the first lesion is performed (reported separately), a CT-guided FNA biopsy is performed on the second lesion.

Description of Procedure (10010)

Explain the additional procedure and its purpose to the patient, including potential complications. Clarify the differences between the subsequent procedure and the first FNA biopsy procedure for the patient. Obtain informed consent. Reposition the patient on the CT scanner as needed. Perform targeted CT to identify the appropriate level and approach for the initial needle placement. Reposition the patient as necessary to facilitate the safest CT-guided access to the lesion. Prepare and mark the skin entry site. Apply sterile

drapes. Determine approach to the lesion. Inject a local anesthetic with CT guidance. Use CT guidance to confirm the correct trajectory for needle advancement to the target anatomic lesion, avoiding vascular structures and nontarget organs. During needle placement, use intermittent CT to confirm the correct approach and the need for needle repositioning or realignment. If the position is not correct, use additional CT guidance to facilitate repositioning until the proper position is achieved. Perform intermittent contrast material injection as needed. Using CT guidance, insert a needle with attached syringe into the lesion. Perform a FNA biopsy of the lesion. Intermittent CT visualization may take place during the intervention, which necessitated the needle placement. Withdraw the needle and express the material expressed onto slides, into fixative, and/or in the appropriate solution. Repeat the previous process in the same lesion (typically, three or four samples are obtained). A pathology representative (pathologist or cytotechnologist) evaluates the sample to assess adequacy. Obtain additional FNA biopsy samples as needed. Apply compression at the FNA biopsy site and observe the patient for bleeding, hematoma, or other complication(s). Record permanent image(s). Obtain post-procedural CT scan and interpret to evaluate for complications. Interpret all images resulting from the study, including dedicated review of the target(s) as well as all visualized viscera, fascial planes, vasculature, soft tissues, and osseous structures. Assess for complications or other unexpected findings. Compare to all pertinent available prior studies.

Dictate a report of the additional procedure for the medical record (which may be included in the report for 10009). Dictate an addendum to the report when the final pathology results are received (which may be included in the report for 10009). Call the referring physician or other qualified health care professional and provide the report if the test results are significant or if final pathology disagrees with imaging results.

Clinical Example (10011)

A 55-year-old male presents with a skull-based lesion identified on a previous magnetic resonance (MRI) image. The patient undergoes an MRI-guided FNA biopsy of the lesion.

Description of Procedure (10011)

Perform targeted MRI to identify the appropriate approach for the initial needle placement. Reposition the patient as needed for the best MRI-guided access to the lesion. Prepare and mark the skin entry site. Apply sterile drapes. Determine approach to the lesion. Inject a local anesthetic with MRI guidance. Use MRI guidance to confirm the correct trajectory for needle advancement to the target anatomic lesion, avoiding vascular structures and nontarget organs. During needle placement, use intermittent MRI to confirm the correct approach and the need for needle repositioning or realignment. If the position is not correct, use additional MRI guidance to facilitate repositioning until the proper position is achieved. Perform intermittent contrast material injection as needed.

Using MRI guidance, insert a needle with attached syringe into the lesion. Perform a FNA biopsy of the lesion. Intermittent MRI visualization may take place during the intervention, which necessitated the needle placement. Withdraw the needle and express the material onto slides, into fixative, and/or in the appropriate solution. Repeat the previous process in the same lesion (typically, a total of three or four samples are acquired). A pathology representative (pathologist or cytotechnologist) evaluates the sample to assess adequacy. Obtain additional FNA biopsy samples as needed. Apply compression at the FNA biopsy site and observe the patient for bleeding, hematoma, or other complication(s). Record permanent image(s). Obtain post-procedural MRI and interpret to evaluate for complications. Interpret all images resulting from the study, including dedicated review of the target(s) as well as all visualized viscera, fascial planes, vasculature, soft tissues, and osseous structures. Assess for complications or other unexpected findings. Compare to all pertinent available prior studies.

Clinical Example (10012)

A 59-year-old male is found to have bilateral neck lesions detected on MRI. After an MRI-guided FNA biopsy of the first lesion is performed (reported separately), an MRI-guided FNA biopsy is performed on the second lesion.

Description of Procedure (10012)

Reposition the patient on the MRI scanner. Perform targeted MRI to identify the appropriate level and approach for the initial needle placement. Reposition the patient for the best MRI-guided access to the lesion. Prepare and mark the skin entry site. Apply sterile drapes. Determine approach to the lesion. Inject a local anesthetic with MRI guidance. Use MRI guidance to confirm the correct trajectory for needle advancement to the target anatomic lesion, avoiding vascular structures and nontarget organs. During needle placement, use intermittent MRI to confirm the correct approach and the need for needle repositioning or realignment. If the position is not correct, use additional MRI guidance to facilitate repositioning until the proper position is achieved. Perform intermittent contrast material injection as needed. Using MRI guidance, insert a needle with attached syringe into the lesion. Perform a FNA biopsy of the lesion. Intermittent MRI

visualization may take place during the intervention, which necessitated the needle placement. Withdraw the needle and express the material onto slides, into fixative, and/or in the appropriate solution. Repeat the previous process in the same lesion (typically, three or four samples are acquired). A pathology representative (pathologist or cytotechnologist) evaluates the sample to assess adequacy. Obtain additional FNA biopsy samples as needed. Apply compression at the FNA biopsy site and observe the patient for bleeding, hematoma, or other complication(s). Record permanent image(s). Obtain post-procedural MRI and interpret to evaluate for complications. Interpret all images resulting from the study, including dedicated review of the target(s) as well as all visualized viscera, fascial planes, vasculature, soft tissues, and osseous structures. Assess for complications or other unexpected findings. Compare to all pertinent available prior studies.

Clinical Example (10021)

A 68-year-old male presents with a palpable lesion in the submandibular region. A FNA biopsy of the lesion is performed without imaging guidance.

Description of Procedure (10021)

Insert a needle with attached syringe into the lesion. Perform a FNA biopsy without imaging guidance of the lesion by making multiple passes with the same needle under suction with the syringe. Withdraw the needle and express the material onto slides. Smear the slides, inspect for adequacy, and apply slide fixative. Aspirate the appropriate solution into the syringe and needle and express in cell block fixative solution for purposes of cell block preparation. Repeat the previous process in the same lesion (typically repeated two additional times). Between each aspiration, apply compression at the FNA biopsy site and observe the patient for bleeding, hematoma, or other complication(s). Apply a dressing and compress for several minutes.

Integumentary System

Skin, Subcutaneous, and Accessory Structures

Biopsy

▶The use of a biopsy procedure code (eg, 11102, 11103, 11104, 11105, 11106, 11107) indicates that the procedure to obtain tissue solely for diagnostic histopathologic examination was performed independently, or was unrelated or distinct from other procedures/services provided at that time. Biopsies performed on different lesions or different sites on the same date of service may be reported separately, as they are not considered components of other procedures.

During certain surgical procedures in the integumentary system, such as excision, destruction, or shave removals, the removed tissue is often submitted for pathologic examination. The obtaining of tissue for pathology during the course of these procedures is a routine component of such procedures. This obtaining of tissue is not considered a separate biopsy procedure and is not separately reported.

Partial-thickness biopsies are those that sample a portion of the thickness of skin or mucous membrane and do not penetrate below the dermis or lamina propria. Full-thickness biopsies penetrate into tissue deep to the dermis or lamina propria, into the subcutaneous or submucosal space.

Sampling of stratum corneum only, by any modality (eg, skin scraping, tape stripping) does not constitute a skin biopsy procedure and is not separately reportable.

An appropriate biopsy technique is selected based on optimal tissue-sampling considerations for the type of neoplastic, inflammatory, or other lesion requiring a tissue diagnosis. Biopsy of the skin is reported under three distinct techniques:

***Tangential biopsy* (eg, shave, scoop, saucerize, curette)** is performed with a sharp blade, such as a flexible biopsy blade, obliquely oriented scalpel or curette to remove a sample of epidermal tissue with or without portions of underlying dermis. The intent of a tangential biopsy (11102, 11103) is to obtain a tissue sample from a lesion for the purpose of diagnostic pathologic examination. Biopsy of lesions by tangential technique (11102, 11103) is not considered an excision. Tangential biopsy technique may be represented by a superficial sample and does not involve the full thickness of the dermis, which could result in portions of the lesion remaining in the deeper layers of the dermis.

For therapeutic removal of epidermal or dermal lesion(s) using shave technique, see 11300-11313.

An indication for a shave removal (11300-11313) procedure may include a symptomatic lesion that rubs on waistband or bra, or any other reason why an elevated lesion is being completely removed with the shave technique, suggesting a therapeutic intent. It is the responsibility of the physician or qualified health care professional performing the procedure to clearly indicate the purpose of the procedure.

Punch biopsy requires a punch tool to remove a full-thickness cylindrical sample of skin. The intent of a

punch biopsy (11104, 11105) is to obtain a cylindrical tissue sample of a cutaneous lesion for the purpose of diagnostic pathologic examination. Simple closure of the defect is included in the service. Manipulation of the biopsy defect to improve wound approximation is included in simple closure.

Incisional biopsy requires the use of a sharp blade (not a punch tool) to remove a full-thickness sample of tissue via a vertical incision or wedge, penetrating deep to the dermis, into the subcutaneous space. The intent of an incisional biopsy (11106, 11107) is to obtain a full-thickness tissue sample of a skin lesion for the purpose of diagnostic pathologic examination. This type of biopsy may sample subcutaneous fat, such as those performed for the evaluation of panniculitis. Although closure is usually performed on incisional biopsies, simple closure is not separately reported.

(For complete lesion excision with margins, see 11400-11646)

When multiple biopsy techniques are performed during the same encounter, only one primary lesion biopsy code (11102, 11104, 11106) is reported. Additional biopsy codes should be selected based on the following convention:

If multiple biopsies of the same type are performed, the primary code for that biopsy should be used along with the corresponding add-on code(s).

If an incisional biopsy is performed, report 11106 in combination with a tangential (11103), punch (11105), or incisional biopsy (11107) for the additional biopsy procedures.

If a punch biopsy is performed, report 11104 in combination with a tangential (11103), or punch (11105), for the additional biopsy procedures.

If multiple tangential biopsies are performed, report tangential biopsy (11102) in combination with 11103 for the additional tangential biopsy procedures.

When two or more biopsies of the same technique (ie, tangential, punch, or incisional) are performed on separate/additional lesions, use the appropriate add-on code (11103, 11105, 11107) to specify each additional biopsy. When two or three different biopsy techniques (ie, tangential, punch, or incisional) are performed to sample separate/additional lesions, select the appropriate biopsy code (11102, 11104, 11106) plus an additional add-on code (11103, 11105, 11107) for each additional biopsy performed.

The following table provides an illustration of the appropriate use of these codes for multiple biopsies:

Procedures Performed	CPT Code(s) Reported
2 tangential biopsies	11102 X 1, 11103 X 1
3 punch biopsies	11104 X 1, 11105 X 2
2 incisional biopsies	11106 X 1, 11107 X 1
1 incisional biopsy, 1 tangential biopsy and 1 punch biopsy	11106 X 1, 11103 X 1, 11105 X 1
1 punch biopsy and 2 tangential biopsies	11104 X 1, 11103 X 2◄

▶(For biopsy of nail unit, use 11755)◄

▶(For biopsy, intranasal, use 30100)◄

▶(For biopsy of lip, use 40490)◄

▶(For biopsy of vestibule of mouth, use 40808)◄

▶(For biopsy of tongue, anterior two-thirds, use 41100)◄

▶(For biopsy of floor of mouth, use 41108)◄

▶(For biopsy of penis, use 54100)◄

▶(For biopsy of vulva or perineum, see 56605, 56606)◄

▶(For biopsy of eyelid skin including lid margin, use 67810)◄

▶(For biopsy of conjunctiva, use 68100)◄

▶(For biopsy of ear, use 69100)◄

▶(11100 has been deleted. To report, see 11102, 11104, 11106)◄

▶(11101 has been deleted. To report, see 11103, 11105, 11107)◄

● **11102** Tangential biopsy of skin (eg, shave, scoop, saucerize, curette); single lesion

+● **11103** each separate/additional lesion (List separately in addition to code for primary procedure)

▶(Report 11103 in conjunction with 11102, 11104, 11106, when different biopsy techniques are performed to sample separate/additional lesions for each type of biopsy technique used)◄

● **11104** Punch biopsy of skin (including simple closure, when performed); single lesion

+● **11105** each separate/additional lesion (List separately in addition to code for primary procedure)

▶(Report 11105 in conjunction with 11104, 11106, when different biopsy techniques are performed to sample separate/additional lesions for each type of biopsy technique used)◄

● **11106** Incisional biopsy of skin (eg, wedge) (including simple closure, when performed); single lesion

+● **11107** each separate/additional lesion (List separately in addition to code for primary procedure)

▶(Report 11107 in conjunction with 11106)◄

Rationale

Codes 11102, 11103, 11104, 11105, 11106, and 11107 have been established to describe distinct biopsy modalities, such as tangential, punch, and incisional biopsies. Guidelines and a table have been added to the Biopsy subsection to define and describe the use of these three modalities of biopsy. Codes 11100 and 11101 have been deleted as the new codes that provide more specificity to the biopsy procedures have been established. Several parenthetical notes have also been added directing users to specific anatomic biopsy codes located throughout the code set.

The previous codes (11100, 11101) did not distinguish between the biopsy techniques used for sampling tissue. Therefore, these new codes (11102, 11104, 11106) individually define three distinct biopsy modalities in order to provide optimal description of the services performed: tangential, punch, and incisional biopsies. The modalities are reported based on the biopsy technique and the thickness of the sample. Add-on code 11103 may be reported in conjunction with codes 11102, 11104, and 11106, when additional biopsies of the same or different techniques are performed to sample separate/additional lesions. Add-on code 11105 may be reported in conjunction with codes 11104 and 11106, when additional biopsies of the same or different techniques are performed to sample separate/additional lesions. Add-on code 11107 may only be reported in conjunction with code 11106 for incisional biopsy.

It is important to note that a shave removal is different from these modalities. A shave removal (11300-11313) is therapeutic removal of an epidermal or epidermal-dermal lesion with the shave technique. Histopathologic evaluation is incidental to the removal. A tangential biopsy is a sampling of a lesion for the purpose of a diagnostic pathologic evaluation.

Clinical Example (11102)

A 65-year-old patient presents with a raised, translucent, telangiectatic papule. Following examination, a nodular basal cell carcinoma is suspected. A tangential biopsy is performed.

Description of Procedure (11102)

While providing firm traction on the surrounding skin and using a tangential biopsy technique, sharply remove a sample of the lesion with a scalpel or other suitable

Surgery / Integumentary System   10021-19499

instrument. This is accomplished by advancing the cutting instrument at an oblique angle relative to the skin surface with a fine slicing motion, yielding a saucer or bowl-shaped skin specimen. Inspect removed tissue and base of biopsy for adequacy of biopsy, evidence of pigmentation, and gross presence and extent of tumor at bottom of defect. Collect specimen in labeled formalin container. Achieve hemostasis.

Clinical Example (11103)

A 65-year-old patient presents with multiple raised, translucent, telangiectatic papules. Following examination, a squamous cell carcinoma is suspected. A tangential biopsy is performed for each additional lesion. (**Note:** This is an add-on code for the additional physician work related to the biopsy of one additional lesion. The physician work for the biopsy of the first lesion would be reported separately with code 11102.)

Description of Procedure (11103)

While providing firm traction on the surrounding skin and using a tangential biopsy technique, sharply remove a sample of the lesion with a scalpel or other suitable instrument. This is accomplished by advancing the cutting instrument at an oblique angle relative to the skin surface with a fine slicing motion, yielding a saucer or bowl-shaped skin specimen. Inspect removed tissue and base of biopsy for adequacy, evidence of pigmentation, and gross presence and extent of tumor at bottom of defect. Collect specimen in labeled formalin container. Achieve hemostasis.

Clinical Example (11104)

A 68-year-old patient presents with an indurated plaque, which may represent a deeply invasive basal or squamous cell carcinoma. A punch biopsy is performed and the wound is sutured.

Description of Procedure (11104)

Using a punch technique, remove a sample of the lesion with a punch instrument suitable for the depth and width of tissue needed. This is accomplished by firmly pressing a perpendicularly oriented punch instrument into the skin and rotating the instrument in an alternating clockwise/counterclockwise twisting motion while providing firm traction on the surrounding skin. The punch instrument is advanced using this twisting motion to the desired depth. Using scissors, carefully separate the deep biopsy margin and remove tissue sample using forceps. Inspect removed tissue and base of biopsy for adequacy, evidence of pigmentation, and gross presence and extent of tumor at bottom of defect. Collect specimen in labeled formalin container. Achieve hemostasis. Undermine wound edges as needed to

facilitate repair. Suture to approximate wound edges. Determine the adequacy of closure.

Clinical Example (11105)

A 68-year-old patient presents with multiple indurated plaques, which may represent deeply invasive basal or squamous cell carcinomas. A punch biopsy is performed on each additional lesion. The biopsy wound is sutured. (**Note:** This is an add-on code for the additional physician work related to the biopsy of one additional lesion. The physician work for the biopsy of the first lesion would be reported separately with code 11104.)

Description of Procedure (11105)

Using a punch technique, remove a sample of the lesion with a punch instrument suitable for the depth and width of tissue needed. This is accomplished by firmly pressing a perpendicularly oriented punch instrument into the skin and rotating the instrument in an alternating clockwise/counterclockwise twisting motion while providing firm traction on the surrounding skin. The punch instrument is advanced using this twisting motion to the desired depth. Using scissors, carefully separate the deep biopsy margin and remove tissue sample using forceps. Inspect removed tissue and base of biopsy for adequacy, evidence of pigmentation, and gross presence and extent of tumor at bottom of defect. Collect specimen in labeled formalin container. Achieve hemostasis. Undermine wound edges as needed to facilitate repair. Suture to approximate wound edges. Determine the adequacy of closure.

Clinical Example (11106)

A 40-year-old female patient presents with multiple tender, indurated nodules consistent with a subcutaneous inflammatory process, such as panniculitis. An incisional biopsy is performed and the wound is sutured.

Description of Procedure (11106)

Using a vertical incisional technique, sharply remove an optimally deep and wide sample of the lesion with a scalpel. This is accomplished by a vertically oriented incision passing through the epidermis and dermis into the subcutis to remove a fusiform sample of skin or a sample of subcutaneous tissue. Appropriate dissection is performed to free the tissue sample from the defect. Inspect removed tissue and base of biopsy for adequacy, depth of inflammatory or neoplastic process, and gross presence and extent of inflammation, necrosis, or tumor at bottom of defect. Collect specimen in labeled formalin container. Achieve hemostasis. Undermine wound edges to facilitate repair through decreased tension on tissue margins. Suture to approximate wound edges. Determine the adequacy of closure.

Clinical Example (11107)

A 40-year-old female patient presents with multiple tender, indurated nodules consistent with a subcutaneous inflammatory process, such as panniculitis. An incisional biopsy is performed and the wound is sutured. (**Note:** This is an add-on code for the additional physician work related to the biopsy of one additional lesion. The physician work for the biopsy of the first lesion would be reported separately with code 11106.)

Description of Procedure (11107)

Using a vertical incisional technique, sharply remove an optimally deep and wide sample of the lesion with a scalpel. This is accomplished by a vertically oriented incision passing through the epidermis and dermis into the subcutis to remove a fusiform sample of skin or a sample of subcutaneous tissue. Appropriate dissection is performed to free the tissue sample from the defect. Inspect removed tissue and base of biopsy for adequacy, depth of inflammatory or neoplastic process, and gross presence and extent of inflammation, necrosis, or tumor at bottom of defect. Collect specimen in labeled formalin container. Achieve hemostasis. Undermine wound edges to facilitate repair through decreased tension on tissue margins. Suture to approximate wound edges. Determine the adequacy of closure.

Repair (Closure)

Skin Replacement Surgery

Definitions

Surgical preparation codes 15002-15005 for skin replacement surgery describe the initial services related to preparing a clean and viable wound surface for placement of an autograft, flap, skin substitute graft or for negative pressure wound therapy. In some cases, closure may be possible using adjacent tissue transfer (14000-14061) or complex repair (13100-13153). In all cases, appreciable nonviable tissue is removed to treat a burn, traumatic wound or a necrotizing infection. The clean wound bed may also be created by incisional release of a scar contracture resulting in a surface defect from separation of tissues. The intent is to heal the wound by primary intention, or by the use of negative pressure wound therapy. Patient conditions may require the closure or application of graft, flap, or skin substitute to be delayed, but in all cases the intent is to include these treatments or negative pressure wound therapy to heal the wound. Do not report 15002-15005 for removal of nonviable tissue/debris in a chronic wound (eg, venous or diabetic) when the wound is left to heal by

secondary intention. See active wound management codes (97597, 97598) and debridement codes (11042-11047) for this service. For necrotizing soft tissue infections in specific anatomic locations, see 11004-11008.

Select the appropriate code from 15002-15005 based upon location and size of the resultant defect. For multiple wounds, sum the surface area of all wounds from all anatomic sites that are grouped together into the same code descriptor. For example, sum the surface area of all wounds on the trunk and arms. Do not sum wounds from different groupings of anatomic sites (eg, face and arms). Use 15002 or 15004, as appropriate, for excisions and incisional releases resulting in wounds up to and including 100 sq cm of surface area. Use 15003 or 15005 for each additional 100 sq cm or part thereof. For example: Surgical preparation of a 20 sq cm wound on the right hand and a 15 sq cm wound on the left hand would be reported with a single code, 15004. Surgical preparation of a 75 sq cm wound on the right thigh and a 75 sq cm wound on the left thigh would be reported with 15002 for the first 100 sq cm and 15003 for the second 50 sq cm. If all four wounds required surgical preparation on the same day, use modifier 59 with 15002, and 15004.

Autografts/tissue cultured autografts include the harvest and/or application of an autologous skin graft. Repair of donor site requiring skin graft or local flaps is reported separately. Removal of current graft and/or simple cleansing of the wound is included, when performed. Do not report 97602. Debridement is considered a separate procedure only when gross contamination requires prolonged cleansing, when appreciable amounts of devitalized or contaminated tissue are removed, or when debridement is carried out separately without immediate primary closure.

Select the appropriate code from 15040-15261 based upon type of autograft and location and size of the defect. The measurements apply to the size of the recipient area. For multiple wounds, sum the surface area of all wounds from all anatomic sites that are grouped together into the same code descriptor. For example, sum the surface area of all wounds on the trunk and arms. Do not sum wounds from different groupings of anatomic sites (eg, face and arms).

▶***Skin substitute grafts*** include non-autologous human skin (dermal or epidermal, cellular and acellular) grafts (eg, homograft, allograft), non-human skin substitute grafts (ie, xenograft), and biological products that form a sheet scaffolding for skin growth. These codes are not to be reported for application of non-graft wound dressings (eg, gel, powder, ointment, foam, liquid) or injected skin substitutes. Application of non-graft wound dressings is not separately reportable. Removal of current graft and/or simple cleansing of the wound is included, when performed. Do not report 97602. Debridement is considered a separate procedure only when gross contamination requires prolonged cleansing, when appreciable amounts of devitalized or contaminated tissue are removed, or when debridement is carried out separately without immediate primary closure.

Select the appropriate code from 15271-15278 based upon location and size of the defect. For multiple wounds, sum the surface area of all wounds from all anatomic sites that are grouped together into the same code descriptor. For example, sum the surface area of all wounds on the trunk and arms. Do not sum wounds from different groupings of anatomic sites (eg, face and arms). The supply of skin substitute graft(s) should be reported separately in conjunction with 15271, 15272, 15273, 15274, 15275, 15276, 15277, 15278. For biologic implant for soft tissue reinforcement, use 15777 in conjunction with code for primary procedure.◄

Rationale

The guidelines for skin-substitute graft have been editorially revised to define non-graft wound dressings. The guidelines now indicate that application of a non-graft wound dressing is not reported separately. In addition, the guidelines now specify that the skin-substitute graft codes may not be reported for powder application. The supply of skin-substitute graft(s) should be reported separately in conjunction with codes 15271-15278. For biologic implant for soft-tissue reinforcement, use code 15777 in conjunction with the primary procedure code.

Destruction

Mohs Micrographic Surgery

Mohs micrographic surgery is a technique for the removal of complex or ill-defined skin cancer with histologic examination of 100% of the surgical margins. It requires the integration of an individual functioning in two separate and distinct capacities: surgeon and pathologist. If either of these responsibilities is delegated to another physician or other qualified health care professional who reports the services separately, these codes should not be reported. The Mohs surgeon removes the tumor tissue and maps and divides the tumor specimen into pieces, and each piece is embedded into an individual tissue block for histopathologic examination. Thus a tissue block in Mohs surgery is defined as an individual tissue piece embedded in a mounting medium for sectioning.

►If repair is performed, use separate repair, flap, or graft codes. If a biopsy of a suspected skin cancer is performed on the same day as Mohs surgery because there was no prior pathology confirmation of a diagnosis, then report a diagnostic skin biopsy (11102, 11104, 11106) and frozen section pathology (88331) with modifier 59 to distinguish from the subsequent definitive surgical procedure of Mohs surgery.◄

(If additional special pathology procedures, stains or immunostains are required, see 88311-88314, 88342)

Rationale

In support of the establishment of codes for tangential, punch, and incisional biopsies (11102, 11103, 11104, 11105, 11106, 11107), the guidelines for Mohs Micrographic Surgery have been revised to include these codes.

Refer to the codebook and the Rationale for codes 11102, 11103, 11104, 11105, 11106, and 11107 for a full discussion of these changes.

Breast

Excision

19100   Biopsy of breast; percutaneous, needle core, not using imaging guidance (separate procedure)

►(For fine needle aspiration biopsy, see 10004, 10005, 10006, 10007, 10008, 10009, 10010, 10011, 10012, 10021)◄

Rationale

A parenthetical note following code 19100 (breast biopsy) within the Excision subsection has been revised to direct users to the codes 10004-10012 and 10021 for FNA biopsy procedures.

Refer to the codebook and the Rationale for codes 10004-10012 and 10021 for a full discussion of these changes.

Musculoskeletal System

General

Incision

▶(20005 has been deleted)◀

▶(For incision and drainage of subfascial soft tissue abscess, see appropriate incision and drainage for specific anatomic sites)◀

Rationale

Code 20005, *Incision and drainage of soft tissue abscess, subfascial,* has been deleted because it was identified as potentially misvalued by the AMA/RVS RUC RAW. It was determined that other codes in the Musculoskeletal subsection are more precise and apt in their descriptions of the procedure represented by code 20005. Therefore, a parenthetical note has been added to direct users to see more appropriate incision and drainage codes for specific anatomic sites for reporting incision and drainage of subfascial soft tissue abscesses.

Excision

20206   Biopsy, muscle, percutaneous needle

(If imaging guidance is performed, see 76942, 77002, 77012, 77021)

▶(For fine needle aspiration biopsy, see 10004, 10005, 10006, 10007, 10008, 10009, 10010, 10011, 10012, 10021)◀

(For evaluation of fine needle aspirate, see 88172-88173)

(For excision of muscle tumor, deep, see specific anatomic section)

Rationale

A parenthetical note following code 20206 (muscle biopsy) within the Excision subsection has been revised to direct users to codes 10004-10012 and 10021 for FNA biopsy procedures.

Refer to the codebook and the Rationale for codes 10004-10012 and 10021 for a full discussion of these changes.

Introduction or Removal

20610   Arthrocentesis, aspiration and/or injection, major joint or bursa (eg, shoulder, hip, knee, subacromial bursa); without ultrasound guidance

20611   with ultrasound guidance, with permanent recording and reporting

▶(Do not report 20610, 20611 in conjunction with 27369, 76942)◀

(If fluoroscopic, CT, or MRI guidance is performed, see 77002, 77012, 77021)

Rationale

In accordance with the deletion of code 27370, the parenthetical note following code 20611 has been revised to remove this code from its listing.

Refer to the codebook and the Rationale for code 27370 for a full discussion of these changes.

20670   Removal of implant; superficial (eg, buried wire, pin or rod) (separate procedure)

20680   deep (eg, buried wire, pin, screw, metal band, nail, rod or plate)

▶(For removal of sinus tarsi implant, use 0510T)◀

▶(For removal and reinsertion of sinus tarsi implant, use 0511T)◀

Rationale

In support of the establishment of Category III codes 0510T and 0511T (removal of a sinus tarsi implant), parenthetical notes following codes 20670 and 20680 have been added to direct users to the appropriate codes to report removal of a sinus tarsi implant.

Refer to the codebook and the Rationale for codes 0335T, 0510T, and 0511T for a full description of these changes.

Grafts (or Implants)

+ 20931   Allograft, structural, for spine surgery only (List separately in addition to code for primary procedure)

(Use 20931 in conjunction with 22319, 22532-22533, 22548-22558, 22590-22612, 22630, 22633, 22634, 22800-22812)

+● **20932**   Allograft, includes templating, cutting, placement and internal fixation, when performed; osteoarticular, including articular surface and contiguous bone (List separately in addition to code for primary procedure)

▶(Do not report 20932 in conjunction with 20933, 20934, 23200, 24152, 27078, 27090, 27091, 27448, 27646, 27647, 27648)◀

+● **20933**   hemicortical intercalary, partial (ie, hemicylindrical) (List separately in addition to code for primary procedure)

▶(Do not report 20933 in conjunction with 20932, 20934, 23200, 24152, 27078, 27090, 27091, 27448, 27646, 27647, 27648)◀

+● **20934**   intercalary, complete (ie, cylindrical) (List separately in addition to code for primary procedure)

▶(Do not report 20934 in conjunction with 20932, 20933, 20955, 20956, 20957, 20962, 23146, 23156, 23200, 24116, 24126, 24152, 25126, 25136, 27078, 27090, 27091, 27130, 27132, 27134, 27138, 27236, 27244, 27356, 27448, 27638, 27646, 27647, 27648, 28103, 28107)◀

▶(Insertion of joint prosthesis may be separately reported)◀

▶(Use 20932, 20933, 20934 in conjunction with 23210, 23220, 24150, 25170, 27075, 27076, 27077, 27365, 27645, 27704)◀

+ **20936**   Autograft for spine surgery only (includes harvesting the graft); local (eg, ribs, spinous process, or laminar fragments) obtained from same incision (List separately in addition to code for primary procedure)

(Use 20936 in conjunction with 22319, 22532, 22533, 22548-22558, 22590-22612, 22630, 22633, 22634, 22800-22812)

Rationale

Codes 20932, 20933, and 20934 have been established to more accurately describe structural allograft procedures. These services are add-on services for fashioning and fixation of the allograft that should be reported in addition to the primary procedure.

This new family of allograft services is unique because the parent code (20932), which is also an add-on code, and the child codes (20933, 20934) should not be reported in conjunction with each other. Several parenthetical notes have been added providing instruction in the use of these codes with other procedures.

Clinical Example (20932)

During a radical resection of the humerus, a 9-year-old male with a proximal humeral osteosarcoma has an osteoarticular allograft procedure performed. The tumor is resected and a complete proximal humerus osteoarticular allograft is templated, cut, and inserted to fill the defect. (**Note:** This is an add-on code. Only consider the additional work related to fashioning and fixation of the allograft.)

Description of Procedure (20932)

Thaw the allograft in sterile fashion in antibiotic solution in the operating room (OR) and inspect. After a radical resection of the osteosarcoma (reported separately), bring the allograft up to the wound and make initial cuts to approximate the defect in the proximal humerus. Temporarily place the allograft in the defect and make additional cuts on the allograft for fit, using a burr and saw to achieve optimal bone apposition. Then rotate the allograft to accommodate the retro-version of the patient's humerus. When it is determined that the position and length of the allograft is optimal, turn attention to fixation, which is typically accomplished with two plates. Extend the wound, as necessary, to accommodate the length of the plates. Once fixation is complete and the allograft is stable, put the joint through a series of maneuvers to assess joint and allograft stability. Use imaging to confirm final allograft alignment and bone contact.

Clinical Example (20933)

During a radical resection of femur operation, a 30-year-old male with painful parosteal osteosarcoma of the posterior distal femur has a hemicortical intercalary allograft procedure performed. A resection is performed. A hemicortical intercalary allograft is templated, cut, and inserted to fill the bone defect. (**Note:** This is an add-on code. Only consider the additional work related to fashioning and fixation of the allograft.)

Description of Procedure (20933)

Thaw the allograft in sterile fashion in antibiotic solution in the OR and inspect. After a radical resection of the osteosarcoma (reported separately), bring the allograft up to the wound and make initial cuts to approximate the length of the femur and to adjust the fit into the distal femoral condyles. Temporarily place the allograft in the defect and make additional cuts on the allograft for fit, using a burr and saw to achieve optimal bone contact. When it is determined that the position and length of the allograft is optimal, turn attention to fixation, which is typically accomplished with two plates. Extend the wound, as necessary, to accommodate the length of the plates. Once fixation is complete and the allograft is stable, put the joint through a series of maneuvers to assess joint and allograft stability. Use imaging to confirm final allograft alignment and bone contact.

Clinical Example (20934)

During a radical resection of femur operation, a 21-year-old female with a diaphyseal Ewing sarcoma of the femur has a resection performed leaving a 14-cm defect. She has an intercalary allograft procedure performed. A full circumference allograft is templated, cut, and inserted to fill the bone defect. (**Note:** This is an add-on code. Only consider the additional work related to fashioning and fixation of the allograft.)

Description of Procedure (20934)

Thaw the allograft in sterile fashion in antibiotic solution in the OR and inspect. After a radical resection of the osteosarcoma (reported separately), bring up the allograft to the wound and make initial cuts to approximate the defect in the femur. Temporarily place the allograft in the defect and make additional cuts on the allograft for fit, using a burr and saw to achieve optimal bone apposition on the proximal and distal bone surfaces. Then rotate the allograft so that it is fixed relative to the proximal and distal host bone. When it is determined that the position and length of the allograft is optimal, turn attention to fixation, which is typically accomplished with intramedullary nail and unicortical plates. The intramedullary nail is typically placed at the proximal end of the femur through a separate incision. Additional incisions are also made for distal screw fixation of the intramedullary nail. Once fixation is complete, irrigate all wounds and achieve hemostasis. Close the proximal wound created for insertion of the intramedullary nail in a layered fashion (closure of the wound for the resection is included in the work of that procedure). Use imaging to confirm final allograft alignment and bone contact, as well as to check the position of the plates and intramedullary nail.

Head

Incision

▶(For incision and drainage procedures, cutaneous/subcutaneous, see 10060, 10061)◀

(For removal of embedded foreign body from dentoalveolar structure, see 41805, 41806)

21010   Arthrotomy, temporomandibular joint

(To report bilateral procedure, report 21010 with modifier 50)

Rationale

In support of the deletion of code 20005, one cross-reference parenthetical note for incision and drainage procedures that precedes code 21010 has been revised and one cross-reference parenthetical note has been deleted.

Refer to the codebook and the Rationale for code 20005 for a full discussion of these changes.

Spine (Vertebral Column)

Arthrodesis

Anterior or Anterolateral Approach Technique

22554   Arthrodesis, anterior interbody technique, including minimal discectomy to prepare interspace (other than for decompression); cervical below C2

(Do not report 22554 in conjunction with 63075, even if performed by a separate individual. To report anterior cervical discectomy and interbody fusion at the same level during the same session, use 22551)

22556   thoracic

22558   lumbar

▶(For arthrodesis using pre-sacral interbody technique, use 22586)◀

Rationale

In accordance with the deletion of Category III codes 0195T and 0196T, the parenthetical note that follows code 22558 has been updated to reflect these deletions.

Refer to the codebook and the Rationale for codes 0195T and 0196T for a full discussion of these changes.

Femur (Thigh Region) and Knee Joint

Introduction or Removal

● **27369**   Injection procedure for contrast knee arthrography or contrast enhanced CT/MRI knee arthrography

▶(Use 27369 in conjunction with 73580, 73701, 73702, 73722, 73723)◀

▶(Do not report 27369 in conjunction with 20610, 20611, 29871)◀

►(For arthrocentesis of the knee or injection of any material other than contrast for subsequent arthrography, see 20610, 20611)◄

►(When fluoroscopic guided injection is performed for enhanced CT arthrography, use 27369, 77002, and 73701 or 73702)◄

►(When fluoroscopic guided injection is performed for enhanced MR arthrography, use 27369, 77002, and 73722 or 73723)◄

►(For arthroscopic lavage and drainage of the knee, use 29871)◄

►(For radiographic arthrography, radiological supervision and interpretation, use 73580)◄

►(27370 has been deleted)◄

►(For arthrocentesis of the knee or injection of any material other than contrast for subsequent arthrography, see 20610, 20611)◄

►(For injection procedure for contrast knee arthrography or contrast enhanced CT/MRI knee arthrography, use 27369)◄

27372 Removal of foreign body, deep, thigh region or knee area

(For removal of knee prosthesis including "total knee," use 27488)

(For surgical arthroscopic knee procedures, see 29870-29887)

Rationale

Code 27370 (injection of contrast for knee arthrography) has been deleted and code 27369 has been established to report injection procedure for knee arthrography or enhanced CT/MRI knee arthrography.

The AMA RUC RAW screen identified code 27370 for high-volume growth, and a recommendation was made to revise this code to reflect current practice. It was determined that if such extensive revisions were needed, a new code should be created and to delete code 27370. Code 27370 did not include contrast enhanced CT/MRI knee arthrography. However, code 27369 can be reported for a knee injection for contrast knee arthrography or contrast enhanced CT/MRI knee arthrography.

Instructional parenthetical notes describing the appropriate reporting of fluoroscopic-guided injections have been added following code 27369. An exclusionary parenthetical note has been added to preclude the use of code 27369 in addition to codes 20610, 20611, and 29871.

Clinical Example (27369)

A 45-year-old male with a prior meniscal tear repair presents with new onset knee pain. There is clinical concern for recurrent meniscal tear. A contrast injection into the knee joint is requested for a subsequent arthrographic examination.

Description of Procedure (27369)

Position the patient on the fluoroscopy table. Perform a time-out procedure to ensure correct patient, procedure, and site. Prepare contrast mixtures for the test injection and the arthrogram injection. The affected knee is prepared and sterilely draped. Under fluoroscopic guidance (separately reported with code 73580 for plain film arthrography or with code 77002 for subsequent CT or MR arthrography), the needle is inserted into the knee joint. Perform a test injection to confirm intra-articular positioning of the needle tip and proper distribution of contrast (needle is repositioned as necessary). Inject the arthrogram contrast material into knee joint (typically 40 to 60 mL). Confirm proper distribution of contrast in the joint and adequate joint distention with intermittent imaging. Remove the needle and apply a dressing at the injection site.

Foot and Toes

Other Procedures

28890 Extracorporeal shock wave, high energy, performed by a physician or other qualified health care professional, requiring anesthesia other than local, including ultrasound guidance, involving the plantar fascia

(For extracorporeal shock wave therapy involving musculoskeletal system not otherwise specified, see 0101T, 0102T)

►(For extracorporeal shock wave therapy involving integumentary system not otherwise specified, see 0512T, 0513T)◄

►(Do not report 28890 in conjunction with 0512T, 0513T, when treating the same area)◄

28899 Unlisted procedure, foot or toes

Rationale

In support of the establishment of new codes 0512T and 0513T, two parenthetical notes have been added following code 28890. The first parenthetical note directs users to new codes 0512T and 0513T for extracorporeal shock wave therapy. The second parenthetical note precludes reporting codes 0512T and 0513T with code 28890, when treating the same area.

★ = Telemedicine   ✚ = Add-on code   ✔ = FDA approval pending   # = Resequenced code   ⊘ = Modifier 51 exempt

Refer to the codebook and the Rationale for codes 0512T and 0513T for a full discussion of these changes.

Application of Casts and Strapping

Lower Extremity

Strapping—Any Age

29520   Strapping; hip

29530   knee

29540   ankle and/or foot

   ►(Do not report 29540 in conjunction with 29580, 29581, for the same extremity)◄

29550   toes

29580   Unna boot

   ►(Do not report 29580 in conjunction with 29540, 29581, for the same extremity)◄

29581   Application of multi-layer compression system; leg (below knee), including ankle and foot

   ►(Do not report 29581 in conjunction with 29540, 29580, for the same extremity)◄

   ►(Do not report 29520, 29530, 29540, 29550, 29580, 29581 in conjunction with 36465, 36466, 36468, 36470, 36471, 36473, 36474, 36475, 36476, 36478, 36479, 36482, 36483, for the same extremity)◄

29584   upper arm, forearm, hand, and fingers

   ►(Do not report 29584 in conjunction with 36465, 36466, 36468, 36470, 36471, 36473, 36474, 36475, 36476, 36478, 36479, 36482, 36483, for the same extremity)◄

Rationale

Changes have been made throughout the CPT code set within different subsections of Surgery to clarify the intended use of "for the same extremity" in the instructions. Code 29580 (strapping; Unna boot) has been added to the exclusionary parenthetical note following code 29540 (strapping; ankle and/or foot) along with "for the same extremity" to preclude reporting these services together for the same extremity.

Similarly, code 29540 has been added to the exclusionary parenthetical note following code 29580 along with "for the same extremity" to preclude reporting these services together for the same extremity. To ensure consistency across the CPT code set that these services are not reported together when they are performed for the same extremity, codes 36468, 36470, 36471, 36475, 36476,

36478, and 36479 have been broken up from the exclusionary parenthetical note following code 29581 to identify the specific codes that are intended for exclusion as part of the exclusionary parenthetical listing. In addition, a new parenthetical note has been added to provide instruction on appropriate reporting of codes 29581 and 29584 with other services performed on the same extremity.

Endoscopy/Arthroscopy

29871   Arthroscopy, knee, surgical; for infection, lavage and drainage

   ►(Do not report 29871 in conjunction with 27369)◄

   (For implantation of osteochondral graft for treatment of articular surface defect, see 27412, 27415, 29866, 29867)

Rationale

In accordance with the deletion of code 27370 and the addition of code 27369, the parenthetical note following code 29871 has been revised to remove the deleted code from its listing.

Refer to the codebook and the Rationale for codes 27370 and 27369 for a full discussion of these changes.

Respiratory System

Nose

Excision

30100   Biopsy, intranasal

   ►(For biopsy skin of nose, see 11102, 11103, 11104, 11105, 11106, 11107)◄

Rationale

In support of the establishment of codes for tangential, punch, and incisional biopsies (11102, 11103, 11104, 11105, 11106, 11107), the parenthetical note following code 30100 has been revised.

Refer to the codebook and the Rationale for codes 11102, 11103, 11104, 11105, 11106, and 11107 for a full discussion of these changes.

Accessory Sinuses

Endoscopy

31235   Nasal/sinus endoscopy, diagnostic with sphenoid sinusoscopy (via puncture of sphenoidal face or cannulation of ostium)

(Do not report 31235 in conjunction with 31297 when performed on the same sinus)

►(To report endoscopic placement of a drug-eluting implant in the ethmoid sinus without any other nasal/sinus endoscopic surgical service, use 31299. To report endoscopic placement of a drug-eluting implant in the ethmoid sinus in conjunction with biopsy, polypectomy, or debridement, use 31237)◄

31237   Nasal/sinus endoscopy, surgical; with biopsy, polypectomy or debridement (separate procedure)

31254   Nasal/sinus endoscopy, surgical with ethmoidectomy; partial (anterior)

►(Do not report 31254 in conjunction with 31253, 31255, 31257, 31259, when performed on the ipsilateral side)◄

31255   total (anterior and posterior)

►(Do not report 31255 in conjunction with 31253, 31254, 31257, 31259, 31276, 31287, 31288, when performed on the ipsilateral side)◄

 # 31253   total (anterior and posterior), including frontal sinus exploration, with removal of tissue from frontal sinus, when performed

►(Do not report 31253 in conjunction with 31237, 31254, 31255, 31276, 31296, 31298, when performed on the ipsilateral side)◄

 # 31257   total (anterior and posterior), including sphenoidotomy

►(Do not report 31257 in conjunction with 31235, 31237, 31254, 31255, 31259, 31287, 31288, 31297, 31298, when performed on the ipsilateral side)◄

 # 31259   total (anterior and posterior), including sphenoidotomy, with removal of tissue from the sphenoid sinus

►(Do not report 31259 in conjunction with 31235, 31237, 31254, 31255, 31257, 31287, 31288, 31297, 31298, when performed on the ipsilateral side)◄

Rationale

Two identical parenthetical notes to direct users to report code 31299 for endoscopic placement of a drug-eluting implant in the ethmoid sinus without any other nasal/sinus endoscopic surgical service have been added to the subsections of Category I Surgery Endoscopy and the Category III Codes. Code 31237 should be reported for endoscopic placement of a drug-eluting implant in the ethmoid sinus in conjunction with biopsy, polypectomy, or debridement. In accordance with the deletion of codes 0406T and 0407T, several parenthetical notes have been revised with the removal of these codes.

Refer to the codebook and the Rationale for codes 0406T and 0407T for a full discussion of these changes.

Larynx

Destruction

►(31595 has been deleted)◄

Rationale

To ensure that the CPT code set reflects current clinical practice, code 31595, *Section recurrent laryngeal nerve, therapeutic (separate procedure), unilateral,* has been deleted due to low utilization.

Lungs and Pleura

Excision/Resection

32400   Biopsy, pleura, percutaneous needle

(If imaging guidance is performed, see 76942, 77002, 77012, 77021)

►(For fine needle aspiration biopsy, see 10004, 10005, 10006, 10007, 10008, 10009, 10010, 10011, 10012, 10021)◄

32405   Biopsy, lung or mediastinum, percutaneous needle

(For open biopsy of lung, see 32096, 32097. For open biopsy of mediastinum, see 39000 or 39010. For thoracoscopic [VATS] biopsy of lung, pleura, pericardium, or mediastinal space structure, see 32604, 32606, 32607, 32608, 32609)

(For radiological supervision and interpretation, see 76942, 77002, 77012, 77021)

►(For fine needle aspiration biopsy, see 10005, 10006, 10007, 10008, 10009, 10010, 10011, 10012)◄

Rationale

Parenthetical notes following codes 32400 (pleura biopsy) and 32405 (lung biopsy) within the Excision/Resection subsection have been revised to direct users to codes 10004-10012 and 10021 for FNA biopsy procedures.

Refer to the codebook and the Rationale for codes 10004-10012 and 10021 for a full discussion of these changes.

Introduction and Removal

32551   Tube thoracostomy, includes connection to drainage system (eg, water seal), when performed, open (separate procedure)

▶(Do not report 32551 in conjunction with 33020, 33025, if pleural drain/chest tube is placed on the ipsilateral side)◀

32552   Removal of indwelling tunneled pleural catheter with cuff

Rationale

An exclusionary parenthetical note following code 32551 (tube thoracostomy) has been added to prevent users from reporting code 32551 with code 33020 (pericardiotomy) or code 33025 (creation of pericardial window), if a pleural drain or chest tube is placed on the ipsilateral (same) side.

Cardiovascular System

Selective vascular catheterizations should be coded to include introduction and all lesser order selective catheterizations used in the approach (eg, the description for a selective right middle cerebral artery catheterization includes the introduction and placement catheterization of the right common and internal carotid arteries).

Additional second and/or third order arterial catheterizations within the same family of arteries supplied by a single first order artery should be expressed by 36218 or 36248. Additional first order or higher catheterizations in vascular families supplied by a first order vessel different from a previously selected and coded family should be separately coded using the conventions described above.

(For monitoring, operation of pump and other nonsurgical services, see 99190-99192, 99291, 99292, 99354-99360)

(For other medical or laboratory related services, see appropriate section)

(For radiological supervision and interpretation, see 75600-75970)

▶(For anatomic guidance of arterial and venous anatomy, see Appendix L)◀

Rationale

A parenthetical has been added to direct users to Appendix L for anatomic guidance for arterial and venous anatomy. This is intended to assist with instruction for catheterization procedures.

Refer to the codebook and the Rationale within Appendix L for a full description of these changes regarding vascular branching.

Heart and Pericardium

Pericardium

33020   Pericardiotomy for removal of clot or foreign body (primary procedure)

33025   Creation of pericardial window or partial resection for drainage

▶(Do not report 33020, 33025 in conjunction with 32551, if pleural drain/chest tube is placed on the ipsilateral side)◀

(For thoracoscopic (VATS) pericardial window, use 32659)

Rationale

A new exclusionary parenthetical note following code 33025 has been added to instruct users not to report codes 33020 and 33025 with code 32551 (tube thoracostomy), if a pleural drain or chest tube is placed on the ipsilateral (same) side.

Pacemaker or Implantable Defibrillator

A pacemaker system with lead(s) includes a pulse generator containing electronics, a battery, and one or more leads. A lead consists of one or more electrodes, as well as conductor wires, insulation, and a fixation mechanism. Pulse generators are placed in a subcutaneous "pocket" created in either a subclavicular site or just above the abdominal muscles just below the ribcage. Leads may be inserted through a vein (transvenous) or they may be placed on the surface of the heart (epicardial). The epicardial location of leads requires a thoracotomy for insertion.

A single chamber pacemaker system with lead includes a pulse generator and one electrode inserted in either the atrium or ventricle. A dual chamber pacemaker system with two leads includes a pulse generator and one lead inserted in the right atrium and one lead inserted in the right ventricle. In certain circumstances, an additional lead may be required to achieve pacing of the left ventricle (bi-ventricular pacing). In this event, transvenous (cardiac vein) placement of the lead should be separately reported using code 33224 or 33225. Epicardial placement of the lead should be separately reported using 33202, 33203.

▶A leadless cardiac pacemaker system includes a pulse generator with built-in battery and electrode for implantation in a cardiac chamber via a transcatheter approach. For implantation of a leadless pacemaker system, use 33274. Insertion, replacement, or removal of a leadless pacemaker system includes insertion of a catheter into the right ventricle.

Right heart catheterization (93451, 93453, 93456, 93457, 93460, 93461, 93530, 93531, 93532, 93533) may not be reported in conjunction with leadless pacemaker insertion and removal codes 33274, 33275 unless complete right heart catheterization is performed for an indication distinct from the leadless pacemaker procedure.◀

Like a pacemaker system, an implantable defibrillator system includes a pulse generator and electrodes. Two general categories of implantable defibrillators exist: transvenous implantable pacing cardioverter-defibrillator (ICD) and subcutaneous implantable defibrillator (S-ICD). Implantable pacing cardioverter-defibrillator devices use a combination of antitachycardia pacing, low-energy cardioversion or defibrillating shocks to treat ventricular tachycardia or ventricular fibrillation. The subcutaneous implantable defibrillator uses a single subcutaneous electrode to treat ventricular tachyarrhythmias. Subcutaneous implantable defibrillators differ from transvenous implantable pacing cardioverter-defibrillators in that subcutaneous defibrillators do not provide antitachycardia pacing or chronic pacing.

Implantable defibrillator pulse generators may be implanted in a subcutaneous infraclavicular, axillary, or abdominal pocket. Removal of an implantable defibrillator pulse generator requires opening of the existing subcutaneous pocket and disconnection of the pulse generator from its electrode(s). A thoracotomy (or laparotomy in the case of abdominally placed pulse generators) is not required to remove the pulse generator.

The electrodes (leads) of an implantable defibrillator system may be positioned within the atrial and/or ventricular chambers of the heart via the venous system (transvenously), or placed on the surface of the heart (epicardial), or positioned under the skin overlying the heart (subcutaneous). Electrode positioning on the epicardial surface of the heart requires a thoracotomy or

thoracoscopic placement of the leads. Epicardial placement of electrode(s) may be separately reported using 33202, 33203. The electrode (lead) of a subcutaneous implantable defibrillator system is tunneled under the skin to the left parasternal margin. Subcutaneous placement of electrode may be reported using 33270 or 33271. In certain circumstances, an additional electrode may be required to achieve pacing of the left ventricle (bi-ventricular pacing). In this event, transvenous (cardiac vein) placement of the electrode may be separately reported using 33224 or 33225.

▶Removal of a transvenous electrode(s) may first be attempted by transvenous extraction (33234, 33235, or 33244). However, if transvenous extraction is unsuccessful, a thoracotomy may be required to remove the electrodes (33238 or 33243). Use 33212, 33213, 33221, 33230, 33231, 33240 as appropriate, in addition to the thoracotomy or endoscopic epicardial lead placement codes (33202 or 33203) to report the insertion of the generator if done by the same physician during the same session. Removal of a subcutaneous implantable defibrillator electrode may be separately reported using 33272. For removal of a leadless pacemaker system without replacement, use 33275. For removal and replacement of a leadless pacemaker system during the same session, use 33274.◀

When the "battery" of a pacemaker system with lead(s) or implantable defibrillator is changed, it is actually the pulse generator that is changed. Removal of only the pacemaker or implantable defibrillator pulse generator is reported with 33233 or 33241. If only a pulse generator is inserted or replaced without any right atrial and/or right ventricular lead(s) inserted or replaced, report the appropriate code for only pulse generator insertion or replacement based on the number of final existing lead(s) (33227, 33228, 33229 and 33262, 33263, 33264). Do not report removal of a pulse generator (33233 or 33241) separately for this service. Insertion of a new pulse generator, when existing lead(s) are already in place and when no prior pulse generator is removed, is reported with 33212, 33213, 33221, 33230, 33231, 33240. When a pulse generator insertion involves the insertion or replacement of one or more right atrial and/or right ventricular lead(s) or subcutaneous lead(s), use system codes 33206, 33207, 33208 for pacemaker, 33249 for implantable pacing cardioverter-defibrillator, or 33270 for subcutaneous implantable defibrillator. When reporting the system insertion or replacement codes, removal of a pulse generator (33233 or 33241) may be reported separately, when performed. In addition, extraction of leads 33234, 33235 or 33244 for transvenous or 33272 for subcutaneous may be reported separately, when performed. An exception involves a pacemaker upgrade from single to dual system that

Procedure	System	
	Pacemaker	**Implantable Defibrillator**
Insert transvenous single lead only without pulse generator	33216	33216
Insert transvenous dual leads without pulse generator	33217	33217
Insert transvenous multiple leads without pulse generator	33217 + 33224	33217 + 33224
Insert subcutaneous defibrillator electrode only without pulse generator	N/A	33271
Initial pulse generator insertion only with existing single lead, includes transvenous or subcutaneous defibrillator lead	33212	33240
Initial pulse generator insertion only with existing dual leads	33213	33230
Initial pulse generator insertion only with existing multiple leads	33221	33231
Initial pulse generator insertion or replacement plus insertion of transvenous single lead	33206 (atrial) or 33207 (ventricular)	33249
Initial pulse generator insertion or replacement plus insertion of transvenous dual leads	33208	33249
Initial pulse generator insertion or replacement plus insertion of transvenous multiple leads	33208 + 33225	33249 + 33225
Initial pulse generator insertion or replacement plus insertion of subcutaneous defibrillator electrode	N/A	33270
►Insertion, replacement, or removal and replacement of permanent leadless pacemaker	33274	N/A◄
Upgrade single chamber system to dual chamber system	33214 (includes removal of existing pulse generator)	33241 + 33249
Removal pulse generator only (without replacement)	33233	33241
Removal pulse generator with replacement pulse generator only single lead system, includes transvenous or subcutaneous defibrillator lead	33227	33262
Removal pulse generator with replacement pulse generator only dual lead system (transvenous)	33228	33263
Removal pulse generator with replacement pulse generator only multiple lead system (transvenous)	33229	33264
Removal transvenous electrode only single lead system	33234	33244
Removal transvenous electrode only dual lead system	33235	33244
Removal subcutaneous defibrillator lead only	N/A	33272
Removal and replacement of pulse generator and transvenous electrodes	33233 + (33234 or 33235) + (33206, 33207, or 33208) and 33225, when appropriate	33241 + 33244 + 33249 and 33225, when appropriate
Removal and replacement of implantable defibrillator pulse generator and subcutaneous electrode	N/A	33272 + 33241 + 33270
►Removal of permanent leadless pacemaker	33275	N/A◄
Conversion of existing system to bi-ventricular system (addition of LV lead and removal of current pulse generator with insertion of new pulse generator with bi-ventricular pacing capabilities)	33225 + 33228 or 33229	33225 + 33263 or 33264

Surgery / Cardiovascular System 33010-39599

includes removal of pulse generator, replacement of new pulse generator, and insertion of new lead, reported with 33214.

Revision of a skin pocket is included in 33206-33249, 33262, 33263, 33264, 33270, 33271, 33272, 33273. When revision of a skin pocket involves incision and drainage of a hematoma or complex wound infection, see 10140, 10180, 11042, 11043, 11044, 11045, 11046, 11047, as appropriate.

Relocation of a skin pocket for a pacemaker (33222) or implantable defibrillator (33223) is necessary for various clinical situations such as infection or erosion. Relocation of an existing pulse generator may be performed as a stand-alone procedure or at the time of a pulse generator or electrode insertion, replacement, or repositioning. When skin pocket relocation is performed as part of an explant of an existing generator followed by replacement with a new generator, the pocket relocation is reported separately. Skin pocket relocation includes all work associated with the initial pocket (eg, opening the pocket, incision and drainage of hematoma or abscess if performed, and any closure performed), in addition to the creation of a new pocket for the new generator to be placed.

Repositioning of a pacemaker electrode, implantable defibrillator electrode(s), or a left ventricular pacing electrode is reported using 33215, 33226, or 33273, as appropriate.

▶Device evaluation codes 93260, 93261, 93279-93299 for pacemaker system with lead(s) may not be reported in conjunction with pulse generator and lead insertion or revision codes 33206-33249, 33262, 33263, 33264, 33270, 33271, 33272, 33273. For leadless pacemaker systems, device evaluation codes 93279, 93286, 93288, 93294, 93296 may not be reported in conjunction with leadless pacemaker insertion and removal codes 33274, 33275. Defibrillator threshold testing (DFT) during transvenous implantable defibrillator insertion or replacement may be separately reported using 93640, 93641. DFT testing during subcutaneous implantable defibrillator system insertion is not separately reportable. DFT testing for transvenous or subcutaneous implantable defibrillator in follow-up or at the time of replacement may be separately reported using 93642 or 93644.

Radiological supervision and interpretation related to the pacemaker or implantable defibrillator procedure is included in 33206-33249, 33262, 33263, 33264, 33270, 33271, 33272, 33273, 33274, 33275. Fluoroscopy (76000, 77002), ultrasound guidance for vascular access (76937), right ventriculography (93566), and femoral venography (75820) are included in 33274, 33275, when

performed). To report fluoroscopic guidance for diagnostic lead evaluation without lead insertion, replacement, or revision procedures, use 76000.◄

The following definitions apply to 33206-33249, 33262, 33263, 33264, 33270, 33271, 33272, 33273.

Single lead: a pacemaker or implantable defibrillator with pacing and sensing function in only one chamber of the heart or a subcutaneous electrode.

Dual lead: a pacemaker or implantable defibrillator with pacing and sensing function in only two chambers of the heart.

Multiple lead: a pacemaker or implantable defibrillator with pacing and sensing function in three or more chambers of the heart.

Rationale

In support of new codes 33274 and 33275 (leadless pacemaker), the pacemaker table in the Pacemaker or Implantable Defibrillator subsection has been revised to include these codes.

Refer to the codebook and the Rationale for codes 33274 and 33275 for a full discussion of these changes.

 # 33271   Insertion of subcutaneous implantable defibrillator electrode

(Do not report 33271 in conjunction with 33240, 33262, 33270, 93260, 93261)

(For insertion or replacement of a cardiac venous system lead, see 33224, 33225)

 # 33272   Removal of subcutaneous implantable defibrillator electrode

 # 33273   Repositioning of previously implanted subcutaneous implantable defibrillator electrode

(Do not report 33272, 33273 in conjunction with 93260, 93261)

#● 33274   Transcatheter insertion or replacement of permanent leadless pacemaker, right ventricular, including imaging guidance (eg, fluoroscopy, venous ultrasound, ventriculography, femoral venography) and device evaluation (eg, interrogation or programming), when performed

#● 33275   Transcatheter removal of permanent leadless pacemaker, right ventricular

▶(Do not report 33275 in conjunction with 33274)◀

▶(Do not report 33274, 33275 in conjunction with femoral venography [75820], fluoroscopy [76000, 77002], ultrasound guidance for vascular access [76937], right ventriculography [93566])◀

▶(Do not report 33274, 33275 in conjunction with 93451, 93453, 93456, 93457, 93460, 93461, 93530, 93531, 93532, 93533, unless complete right heart catheterization is performed for indications distinct from the leadless pacemaker procedure)◀

▶(For subsequent leadless pacemaker device evaluation, see 93279, 93286, 93288, 93294, 93296)◀

▶(For insertion, replacement, repositioning, and removal of pacemaker systems with leads, see 33202, 33203, 33206, 33207, 33208, 33212, 33213, 33214, 33215, 33216, 33217, 33218, 33220, 33221, 33227, 33228, 33229, 33233, 33234, 33235, 33236, 33237)◀

Rationale

Category III codes 0387T, *Transcatheter insertion or replacement of permanent leadless pacemaker, ventricular,* and 0388T, *Transcatheter removal of permanent leadless pacemaker, ventricular,* have been deleted for 2019. In their place, two new Category I codes (33274, 33275) in the Pacemaker and Implantable Defibrillator subsection have been established. The pacemaker and implantable defibrillator guidelines have been revised and parenthetical notes have been revised and added to provide instructions on the appropriate reporting of these procedures.

Codes 0387T and 0388T included fluoroscopy, right ventriculography, and femoral venography intrinsic to the procedure, when performed. Code 0387T included device evaluation. Guidelines were provided in the Category III section that explained these services were included; however, the code descriptors of 0387T and 0388T did not state that they were included. Therefore, for 2019, these services are included in the new codes' descriptors for clarity. Code 33274 includes device evaluation when performed during the same session. Device evaluation that is performed subsequent to the insertion or replacement procedure is reported with codes 93279, 93286, 93288, 93294, and 93296, as appropriate. Refer to the codebook and the Rationale for codes 93279, 93286, 93288, 93294, and 93296 for a full discussion of these changes. Codes 0387T and 0388T only referred to the anatomic site as "ventricular." Codes 33274 and 33275 specify anatomic site as "right ventricular" for clarity.

When a leadless pacemaker is replaced, the removal of the original pacemaker is included in code 33274. Therefore, the removal code 33275 should not be reported in conjunction with code 33274. Code 33275 is reported

when the leadless pacemaker is removed at a session subsequent to the insertion procedure. Catheter insertion into the right ventricle for the purpose of insertion, replacement, or removal is included in codes 33274 and 33275. Therefore, right heart catheterization codes 93451, 93453, 93456, 93457, 93460, 93461, 93530, 93531, 93532, and 93533 should not be reported with codes 33274 and 33275, when catheterization is performed for the purpose of inserting, replacing, or removing the leadless pacemaker. However, right heart catheterization may be reported separately, as appropriate, if complete right heart catheterization is performed for indications distinct from the leadless pacemaker procedure during the same session.

Clinical Example (33274)

A 72-year-old male presents with persistent dizziness and shortness of breath. On work-up, the patient is diagnosed with bradycardia–tachycardia syndrome and a leadless pacemaker is recommended.

Description of Procedure (33274)

In the electrophysiology laboratory, depending on the leadless pacemaker system, place surface electrocardiogram (ECG) electrodes on the patient's chest and connect to the pacemaker programmer. After obtaining access via puncture of the femoral vein using ultrasound guidance, perform femoral venography to identify the anatomy. Advance a guidewire via the femoral vein into the heart. After sequential dilation and upsizing the femoral sheath, including a small incision if needed, insert the leadless pacemaker introducer into the femoral vein and remove the guidewire. Under fluoroscopic guidance, then insert the leadless pacemaker delivery catheter into the femoral vein through the introducer. Using steering and deflection, advance the delivery catheter through the inferior vena cava (IVC) to the right atrium and through the tricuspid valve into the right ventricle. Ventriculography may be performed to identify the anatomy. Then fix the leadless pacemaker to the endocardium, for example, by rotating a screw-in helix or retracting an outer sheath to deploy tines. After fixation, undock the pacemaker from the delivery system but it is still connected via tethers. Place a programming head over the pacemaker, allowing communication with an external programmer. Measure pacing capture threshold, sensing amplitude, and impedance without applying force on the device. When values are interpreted as inappropriate, re-engage and reposition the pacemaker within the right ventricle under fluoroscopic guidance. Confirm fixation of the pacemaker to the endocardium by performing a gentle "tug test" via the delivery system under fluoroscopic visualization. As needed, re-engage and reposition the pacemaker within the right ventricle under fluoroscopic

Surgery / Cardiovascular System 33010-39599

guidance. Once appropriate parameters and adequate fixation are confirmed, cut the tether and release the pacemaker from the delivery catheter. Remove the tether, delivery catheter, and sheath, and close the access site with a nonabsorbable, single figure-8 stitch around the vein that is placed prior to sheath pull.

Clinical Example (33275)

A 72-year-old male had a leadless pacemaker system placed two years ago. He has developed significantly worsening congestive heart failure (CHF). The decision is made to remove the leadless pacemaker in favor of placing a cardiac resynchronization therapy device to simultaneously treat both the arrhythmia and the CHF.

Description of Procedure (33275)

In the electrophysiology laboratory, after obtaining access via puncture of the femoral vein, femoral venography may be performed to identify the anatomy. Advance a guidewire via the femoral vein into the heart. After sequential dilation and upsizing the femoral sheath, including a small incision if needed, insert the leadless pacemaker retrieval introducer into the femoral vein and remove the guidewire. Then insert the leadless pacemaker retrieval catheter into the femoral vein through the introducer. Using steering and deflection, advance the retrieval catheter under fluoroscopic guidance through the IVC to the right atrium and through the tricuspid valve into the right ventricle. Then engage the leadless pacemaker by the retrieval catheter, for example, by snare. After confirming under fluoroscopy that the retrieval mechanism is engaged and secure, remove the coupled retrieval catheter and leadless pacemaker, and close the access site with a non-absorbable, single figure-8 stitch around the vein.

►Subcutaneous Cardiac Rhythm Monitor◄

►A subcutaneous cardiac rhythm monitor, also known as a cardiac event recorder or implantable/insertable loop recorder (ILR), is a subcutaneously placed device that continuously records the electrocardiographic rhythm, triggered automatically by rapid, irregular and/or slow heart rates or by the patient during a symptomatic episode. A subcutaneous cardiac rhythm monitor is placed using a small parasternal incision followed by insertion of the monitor into a small subcutaneous pre-pectoral pocket, followed by closure of the incision.◄

►(33282, 33284 have been deleted. To report, see 33285, 33286)◄

● **33285**   Insertion, subcutaneous cardiac rhythm monitor, including programming

● **33286**   Removal, subcutaneous cardiac rhythm monitor

►(Initial insertion includes programming. For subsequent electronic analysis and/or reprogramming, see 93285, 93291, 93298, 93299)◄

Rationale

Patient-activated cardiac event recorder implantation and removal codes (33282, 33284) have been deleted and two new codes (33285, 33286) have been added to report insertion and removal of a subcutaneous cardiac rhythm monitor. Guidelines have been added and parenthetical notes have been revised and added throughout the code set regarding the reporting of subcutaneous cardiac rhythm monitor services. The "Patient-Activated Event Recorder" subheading was replaced with a new subheading titled "Subcutaneous Cardiac Rhythm Monitor."

In the years following the addition of codes 33282 and 33284 to the code set, smaller models of cardiac rhythm monitors came into use. The work involved in implanting and removing the smaller models varies significantly enough from that of the models used in the services described by codes 33282 and 33284 to warrant separate codes. Further, the use of the older, larger models has decreased to a low enough utilization that the deletion of codes 33282 and 33284 was warranted.

The term "patient-activated cardiac event recorder" has been updated with the term "subcutaneous cardiac rhythm monitor" in codes 33285 and 33286, in order to reflect current practice and terminology for these devices. As with deleted codes 33282 and 33284, programming is included in code 33285 (implantation).

Clinical Example (33285)

A 42-year-old female presents with a history of syncopal spells with inconclusive results using various investigations. The patient continues to have distressing symptoms every three to four months. A history and physical examination were performed. She was referred for insertion of a subcutaneous cardiac rhythm monitor.

Description of Procedure (33285)

Using blunt dissection, create a subcutaneous pocket the size and shape of the cardiac rhythm monitor using a specifically designed insertion tool or surgical instrument. Maintain hemostasis using standard techniques. Then insert the cardiac rhythm monitor into the pocket with an insertion tool or manually. Verify the ECG signal quality and amplitude by placing the programmer head in a sterile sleeve over the device, establishing telemetry. Evaluate the waveform on the programmer screen and adjust the gain to optimize waveform amplitude. Then close the incision with adhesive strips, surgical glue, staples, or subcuticular absorbable sutures, as needed. Dress the wound, program the cardiac rhythm monitor using a pacemaker programmer, and initiate recording.

Clinical Example (33286)

A 44-year-old female presents with a history of syncopal spells, the cause of which was recently diagnosed using a subcutaneous cardiac rhythm monitor. A history and physical examination were performed. The procedure, indications, potential complications, and alternatives were explained to the patient who appeared to understand and indicated the same. An opportunity for questions was provided and informed consent obtained.

Description of Procedure (33286)

Make a 1- to 2-cm incision through the previous implant incision. The operator tunnels under the skin to locate the device which typically migrates significantly from the site of original implant. Once located, debride extensive adhesions to free the device for removal. Cut any sutures anchoring the recorder to the subcutaneous tissue and remove the device from the pocket. Achieve hemostasis of the pocket and tunnel. Flush the pocket and tunnel and close with adhesive strips, surgical glue, staples, or subcuticular sutures as needed. Dress the wound.

▶Implantable Hemodynamic Monitors◀

▶Transcatheter implantation of a wireless pulmonary artery pressure sensor (33289) establishes an intravascular device used for long-term remote monitoring of pulmonary artery pressures (93264). The hemodynamic data derived from this device is used to guide management of patients with heart failure. Code 33289 includes deployment and calibration of the sensor, right heart catheterization, selective pulmonary artery catheterization, radiological supervision and interpretation, and pulmonary artery angiography, when performed.◀

● **33289**   Transcatheter implantation of wireless pulmonary artery pressure sensor for long-term hemodynamic monitoring, including deployment and calibration of the sensor, right heart catheterization, selective pulmonary catheterization, radiological supervision and interpretation, and pulmonary artery angiography, when performed

▶(For remote monitoring of an implantable wireless pulmonary artery pressure sensor, use 93264)◀

▶(Do not report 33289 in conjunction with 36013, 36014, 36015, 75741, 75743, 75746, 76000, 93451, 93453, 93456, 93457, 93460, 93461, 93530, 93531, 93532, 93533, 93568)◀

Rationale

A new subsection, "Implantable Hemodynamic Monitors," has been added to the Cardiovascular System. This subsection includes guidelines and the addition of code 33289 to report implantation of a wireless pulmonary artery pressure sensor.

Code 93264 describes the remote care management of a patient with an implanted wireless hemodynamic pulmonary artery sensor. This implanted pulmonary artery sensor provides pulmonary artery (PA) pressure (PAP) and heart rate measuring and monitoring. The device is indicated for patients with New York Heart Association (NYHA) Class III heart failure, who have been hospitalized for heart failure in the previous year. The hemodynamic data are used by physicians or other qualified health care professionals for heart failure treatment with the goal of reducing heart failure hospitalizations.

The patients who receive this implant typically have a diagnosis of congestive heart failure (eg, chronic, acute, or acute on chronic, diastolic, or systolic or combined heart failure). Patients with this implanted pulmonary artery pressure monitor are expected to be monitored weekly for the life of the patient. The monitoring of the patient may be reported using code 93264, which includes remote monitoring of a wireless pulmonary artery pressure sensor for up to 30 days. Refer to the codebook and the Rationale for code 93264 for a full discussion of these changes.

Clinical Example (33289)

A 67-year-old male, who had previous multiple hospitalizations for decompensated heart failure and had persistent New York Heart Association (NYHA) functional classification III symptoms, was identified as a patient who could benefit from remote monitoring of PA pressure measurements.

Description of Procedure (33289)

In the catheterization laboratory, position the implantable (PA) measuring device on the left side of the patient. If needed, administer conscious sedation and verify adequate conscious sedation monitoring. Obtain percutaneous venous access through the right femoral vein with a 12-Fr vessel introducer sheath over an access guidewire; remove the dilator and guidewire. Insert a 7-Fr thermodilution pulmonary artery catheter (PAC) through the introducer sheath, inflate the balloon, and advance the tip to the right atrium. Confirm the external pressure transducer setup height to be at the mid-axillary line and perform baseline zeroing. Record right atrial and right ventricular pressure measurements. Advance the PAC tip, with the balloon inflated, to the descending branch of the left PA, within the lower lobe of the left lung. Record PA pressure, PA occlusion pressure, and thermodilution cardiac output measurements. Perform an anterior/posterior and left anterior oblique angiogram of the target implant site using approximately 5 cc of radiopaque contrast, hand injected through the PAC, in order to examine the target implant site for the sensor device. Review of the angiogram identified an acceptable implant site for the sensor where the vessel is of the appropriate diameter. Insert guidewire through the PAC, across the target implant site, and into the distal pulmonary artery. Carefully remove the PAC while the guidewire position is maintained. Introduce the sensor delivery catheter over the guidewire, through the sheath, and into the deployment position at the target implant site. Once appropriate sensor placement is confirmed, unscrew the cap on the delivery catheter hub and remove the wire which retained the sensor from the catheter, releasing the sensor. Slowly withdraw the delivery system and remove while the sensor position is monitored under fluoroscopy. Re-insert the PAC over the guidewire into the main PA. While monitoring the sensor position on fluoroscope, remove the guidewire. Perform sensor measurements by placing the antenna under the appropriate location using fluoroscopic guidance. The sensor signal is detected with optimal signal strength. Once the implanted PA monitor and invasive PA pressure displays both show stable, and PA pressure waveforms are valid, the baseline is set on the implanted PA device. Re-zero the PAC and record the mean PA pressure from the PAC in the entry blank on the implantable system. After the baseline value is established for the implanted sensor, the mean PA pressure should match the PAC mean PA pressure within acceptable limits. Multiple baseline wireless PA pressure readings are taken simultaneously with PAC measurements to ensure appropriate calibration. Remove the PAC and introducer sheath. Obtain hemostasis per standard of care.

Cardiac Valves

Aortic Valve

#● **33440**   Replacement, aortic valve; by translocation of autologous pulmonary valve and transventricular aortic annulus enlargement of the left ventricular outflow tract with valved conduit replacement of pulmonary valve (Ross-Konno procedure)

►(Do not report 33440 in conjunction with 33405, 33406, 33410, 33411, 33412, 33413, 33414, 33416, 33417, 33475, 33608, 33920)◄

33411   with aortic annulus enlargement, noncoronary sinus

33412   with transventricular aortic annulus enlargement (Konno procedure)

►(Do not report 33412 in conjunction with 33413, 33440)◄

►(For replacement of aortic valve with transventricular aortic annulus enlargement [Konno procedure] in conjunction with translocation of autologous pulmonary valve with allograft replacement of pulmonary valve [Ross procedure], use 33440)◄

33413   by translocation of autologous pulmonary valve with allograft replacement of pulmonary valve (Ross procedure)

►(Do not report 33413 in conjunction with 33412, 33440)◄

►(For replacement of aortic valve with transventricular aortic annulus enlargement [Konno procedure] in conjunction with translocation of autologous pulmonary valve with allograft replacement of pulmonary valve [Ross procedure], use 33440)◄

Rationale

A new code (33440) and new parenthetical notes have been added to the Cardiac Valves/Aortic Valves subsection to identify the combined services of aortic valve and root replacement with subvalvular left ventricular outflow tract enlargement to allow for an unobstructed left ventricular outflow tract. The new code replaces code 33411 as the parent code for aortic valve replacement procedures.

Code 33440 combines the services identified by two separate Category I codes into a single code. The descriptor for this new code includes language and components from the Ross procedure (33413) and the Konno procedure (33412). Ordinarily, the physician providing an aortic valve replacement service would only perform one of these procedures. As is true for other procedures in this subsection, the procedure requires cardiopulmonary bypass. As a result, cardiopulmonary bypass is inherently included as part of the service and should not be reported separately.

The parenthetical notes listed with the code for this procedure and with the associated codes direct users to the correct code to report the combined Ross-Konno procedure. They also restrict use of code 33440 in conjunction with codes 33412 and 33413, or any other aortic valve, aortic root, pulmonary valve, or ventricular reconstruction procedure to eliminate reporting overlapping services.

Clinical Example (33440)

A 4-year-old girl presents with chest pain and syncope. Echocardiography documents mixed aortic valvar stenosis and regurgitation with a transvalvar gradient of 90 mmHg and an aortic valve annulus diameter of 10 mm with tunnel-like left ventricular outflow tract obstruction. The family chooses a Ross procedure (autologous pulmonary valve replacement of the aortic valve). However, due to the multilevel left ventricular outflow tract obstruction, a Konno aortovenetriculoplasty is also performed to enlarge the left ventricular outflow tract at the time of the Ross procedure.

Description of Procedure (33440)

Under general endotracheal anesthesia, make a skin incision via a standard median sternotomy. Divide the sternum at the midline. Harvest an autologous pericardial patch for potential use. Place cardiac cannulae. Initiate cardiopulmonary bypass. Snares are snugged down on the caval cannulae allowing for complete heart bypass. Administer cardioplegia and achieve diastolic arrest of the heart. Insert a left heart vent via the right superior pulmonary vein. Make a vertical aortotomy incision extending down to the commissure between the right and left coronary cusps. Excise the thickened aortic valve leaflets. Separate the left and right coronary buttons from the aortic root with a cuff of aortic wall. Size the aortic annulus to confirm the necessity of aortic annular enlargement and enlargement of the subvalvar left ventricular outflow tract. Open the pulmonary artery and inspect the pulmonary valve. Remove the entire root of the pulmonary artery and valve taking special care to avoid injury to the septal perforator artery. Identify and protect interventricular septum. Prepare and trim the pulmonary autograft, avoiding injury to valve leaflets. Make an incision in the ascending aorta across the aortic annulus opening the ventricular septum, creating a ventricular septal defect (VSD). Excise subaortic fibrous tissue and muscular hypertrophy with care taken to avoid the area of the conduction tissue. Suture a prosthetic patch to the newly created ventricular septal defect enlarging the left ventricular outflow tract and the aortic annulus. Sew the pulmonary autograft into the newly enlarged left ventricular outflow tract. Re-implant the left and right coronary buttons into the openings created in the pulmonary autograft. Anastomose the distal autograft to the distal ascending aorta. Establish right ventricular to pulmonary artery continuity with a valved conduit that is sewn to the distal pulmonary artery orifice and to the right ventricular outflow tract,

which is augmented with a patch (autologous pericardium or other prosthetic material). Evacuate air from the cardiac chambers and release the cross-clamp. After satisfactory rewarming and resuscitation, remove the left heart vent and then wean the child from cardiopulmonary bypass. A transesophageal echocardiogram (if done) is reviewed with the cardiologist or anesthesiologist looking for right or left ventricular outflow tract obstruction, autograft valve function, and residual intracardiac shunts. Remove the cannulae and secure the sites. Place chest tubes and temporary pacing wires. Close the sternum with wires. Close the abdominal fascia, skin, and subcutaneous tissue in layers.

Mitral Valve

33440   Code is out of numerical sequence. See 33406-33412

Pulmonary Valve

Code 33477 is used to report transcatheter pulmonary valve implantation (TPVI). Code 33477 should only be reported once per session.

Code 33477 includes the work, when performed, of percutaneous access, placing the access sheath, advancing the repair device delivery system into position, repositioning the device as needed, and deploying the device(s). Angiography, radiological supervision, and interpretation performed to guide TPVI (eg, guiding device placement and documenting completion of the intervention) are included in the code.

▶Code 33477 includes all cardiac catheterization(s), intraprocedural contrast injection(s), fluoroscopic radiological supervision and interpretation, and imaging guidance performed to complete the pulmonary valve procedure. Do not report 33477 in conjunction with 76000, 93451, 93453, 93454, 93455, 93456, 93457, 93458, 93459, 93460, 93461, 93530, 93531, 93532, 93533, 93563, 93566, 93567, 93568 for angiography intrinsic to the procedure.◀

Code 33477 includes percutaneous balloon angioplasty of the conduit/treatment zone, valvuloplasty of the pulmonary valve conduit, and stent deployment within the pulmonary conduit or an existing bioprosthetic pulmonary valve, when performed. Do not report 33477 in conjunction with 37236, 37237, 92997, 92998 for pulmonary artery angioplasty/valvuloplasty or stenting within the prosthetic valve delivery site.

Rationale

In accordance with the deletion of code 76001, the guidelines in the Pulmonary Valve subsection have been revised with the removal of this code.

Refer to the codebook and the Rationale for code 76001 for a full discussion of these changes.

Thoracic Aortic Aneurysm

►When ascending aortic disease involves the aortic arch, an aortic hemiarch graft may be necessary in conjunction with the ascending aortic graft and may be reported with add-on code 33866 in conjunction with the appropriate ascending aortic graft code (33860, 33863, 33864). Aortic hemiarch graft requires all of the following components:

1. Either total circulatory arrest or isolated cerebral perfusion (retrograde or antegrade);

2. Incision into the transverse arch extending under one or more of the arch vessels (eg, innominate, left common carotid, or left subclavian arteries); and

3. Extension of the ascending aortic graft under the aortic arch by construction of a beveled anastomosis to the distal ascending aorta and aortic arch without a cross-clamp (an open anastomosis).

An ascending aortic repair with a beveled anastomosis into the arch with a cross-clamp cannot be reported separately as a hemiarch graft using 33866. Use 33866 for aortic hemiarch graft when performed in conjunction with the ascending aortic graft codes 33860, 33863, 33864.◄

33860 Ascending aorta graft, with cardiopulmonary bypass, includes valve suspension, when performed

►(Do not report 33860 in conjunction with 33870)◄

33863 Ascending aorta graft, with cardiopulmonary bypass, with aortic root replacement using valved conduit and coronary reconstruction (eg, Bentall)

►(Do not report 33863 in conjunction with 33405, 33406, 33410, 33411, 33412, 33413, 33860, 33870)◄

33864 Ascending aorta graft, with cardiopulmonary bypass with valve suspension, with coronary reconstruction and valve-sparing aortic root remodeling (eg, David Procedure, Yacoub Procedure)

►(Do not report 33864 in conjunction with 33860, 33863, 33870)◄

+● 33866 Aortic hemiarch graft including isolation and control of the arch vessels, beveled open distal aortic anastomosis extending under one or more of the arch vessels, and total circulatory arrest or isolated cerebral perfusion (List separately in addition to code for primary procedure)

►(Use 33866 in conjunction with 33860, 33863, 33864)◄

►(Do not report 33866 in conjunction with 33870)◄

33870 Transverse arch graft, with cardiopulmonary bypass

►(Do not report 33870 in conjunction with 33860, 33863, 33864, 33866)◄

►(Use 33866 for aortic hemiarch graft when performed in conjunction with ascending aortic graft [33860, 33863, 33864])◄

33875 Descending thoracic aorta graft, with or without bypass

Rationale

Code 33866 has been added to the Thoracic Aortic Aneurysm subsection to report the use of aortic hemiarch graft. New guidelines and parenthetical notes have been added to provide instruction on appropriate reporting of code 33866. In addition, parenthetical notes have been revised and added to provide instruction on the appropriate reporting of existing code 33870, *Transverse arch graft, with cardiopulmonary bypass.*

Prior to 2019, there was no code to report an aortic hemiarch graft procedure. A review of claims data revealed that code 33870 was often used to report this procedure. However, code 33870 describes a more complex procedure that includes replacement of the *entire* aortic arch (also known as transverse arch or transverse aortic arch) and *reimplantation* of the arch vessels. The hemiarch graft procedure involves anastomosis of only a portion of the aortic arch (ie, hemiarch) using a graft with *management* (not reimplantation) of the arch vessels. It was determined that a code to specifically describe aortic hemiarch graft was needed, as well as instructions that code 33870 should not be reported for aortic hemiarch graft were necessary.

The aortic hemiarch graft procedure is not typically performed on its own but may be performed in conjunction with ascending aortic graft procedures (33860, 33863, 33864). Therefore, code 33866 is designated as an add-on code to be reported with codes 33860, 33863, and 33864, when hemiarch graft is performed with ascending aortic graft procedures. There are required components that must be present in order to report code 33866, which are outlined in the new guidelines. In addition, the new guidelines explain when an aortic hemiarch graft is necessary and clarify that code 33866 is not reported for ascending aortic repair with a beveled anastomosis into the arch using a cross-clamp. Parenthetical notes have been revised and added to clarify that code 33870 is not reported for the hemiarch graft procedure.

Clinical Example (33866)

A 58-year-old male with aortic disease extending from the sino-tubular junction of the aorta to the transverse aortic arch undergoes an ascending aortic graft repair (reported separately). Since the aortic disease extends into the transverse aortic arch, a hemiarch graft repair is also indicated.

Description of Procedure (33866)

Circumferentially dissect around the base of both the innominate and left common carotid arteries and place tapes around both arteries. Initiate hypothermia; once target temperature is obtained, discontinue cardiopulmonary bypass and tighten the tapes around the innominate and common carotid arteries. Hypothermic circulatory arrest is initiated and cerebral perfusion is performed. Remove the cross-clamp and transect the aorta. Inspect the inside of the aorta and determine the extent of the intimal tear. Resect the entirety of the intimal tear. Prepare the distal end of the cut aorta for anastomosis employing additional reinforcing techniques if necessary. Perform anastomosis of the open distal aortic anastomosis to the cut end of the aorta utilizing synthetic graft with a running suture at the origin of the transverse aortic arch superiorly. Inferiorly, the suture line extends obliquely across the lesser curvature of the transverse arch of the aorta. After ensuring hemostasis of this distal anastomosis, a cross-clamp is placed on the aortic graft and full cardiopulmonary bypass is reinstituted. An extended period of re-warming is required.

Arteries and Veins

Endovascular Repair of Abdominal Aorta and/or Iliac Arteries

+ 34713   Percutaneous access and closure of femoral artery for delivery of endograft through a large sheath (12 French or larger), including ultrasound guidance, when performed, unilateral (List separately in addition to code for primary procedure)

▶(Use 34713 in conjunction with 33880, 33881, 33883, 33884, 33886, 34701, 34702, 34703, 34704, 34705, 34706, 34707, 34708, 34710, 34841, 34842, 34843, 34844, 34845, 34846, 34847, 34848, as appropriate. Do not report 34713 in conjunction with 33880, 33881, 33883, 33884, 33886, 34701, 34702, 34703, 34704, 34705, 34706, 34707, 34708, 34710, 34841, 34842, 34843, 34844, 34845, 34846, 34847, 34848, for percutaneous closure of femoral artery after delivery of endovascular prosthesis if a sheath smaller than 12 French was used)◀

Rationale

The first parenthetical note following code 34713 has been revised to include code 34710 in both the inclusionary and exclusionary portions of the parenthetical note to parallel a parenthetical note following code 34710. This parenthetical note has also been editorially revised to remove the word "However" to conform to CPT convention.

Vascular Injection Procedures

Venous

36468   Injection(s) of sclerosant for spider veins (telangiectasia), limb or trunk

(For ultrasound imaging guidance performed in conjunction with 36468, use 76942)

▶(Do not report 36468 in conjunction with 29520, 29530, 29540, 29550, 29580, 29581, 29584, for the same extremity)◀

(Do not report 36468 more than once per extremity)

(Do not report 36468 in conjunction with 37241 in the same surgical field)

36470   Injection of sclerosant; single incompetent vein (other than telangiectasia)

36471   multiple incompetent veins (other than telangiectasia), same leg

(For ultrasound imaging guidance performed in conjunction with 36470, 36471, use 76942)

▶(Do not report 36470, 36471 in conjunction with 29520, 29530, 29540, 29550, 29580, 29581, 29584, for the same extremity)◀

(Do not report 36471 more than once per extremity)

(If the targeted vein is an extremity truncal vein and injection of non-compounded foam sclerosant with ultrasound guided compression maneuvers to guide dispersion of the injectate is performed, see 36465, 36466)

(Do not report 36470, 36471 in conjunction with 37241 in the same surgical field)

 # 36465 Injection of non-compounded foam sclerosant with ultrasound compression maneuvers to guide dispersion of the injectate, inclusive of all imaging guidance and monitoring; single incompetent extremity truncal vein (eg, great saphenous vein, accessory saphenous vein)

 # 36466 multiple incompetent truncal veins (eg, great saphenous vein, accessory saphenous vein), same leg

▶(Do not report 36465, 36466 in conjunction with 29520, 29530, 29540, 29550, 29580, 29581, 29584, for the same extremity)◀

(Do not report 36465, 36466 in conjunction with 37241 in the same surgical field)

(For extremity truncal vein injection of compounded foam sclerosant[s], see 36470, 36471)

(For injection of a sclerosant into an incompetent vein without compression maneuvers to guide dispersion of the injectate, see 36470, 36471)

(For endovenous ablation therapy of incompetent vein[s] by transcatheter delivery of a chemical adhesive, see 36482, 36483)

(For vascular embolization and occlusion procedures, see 37241, 37242, 37243, 37244)

36473 Endovenous ablation therapy of incompetent vein, extremity, inclusive of all imaging guidance and monitoring, percutaneous, mechanochemical; first vein treated

+ 36474 subsequent vein(s) treated in a single extremity, each through separate access sites (List separately in addition to code for primary procedure)

(Use 36474 in conjunction with 36473)

(Do not report 36474 more than once per extremity)

▶(Do not report 36473, 36474 in conjunction with 29520, 29530, 29540, 29550, 29580, 29581, 29584, for the same extremity)◀

▶(Do not report 36473, 36474 in conjunction with 36000, 36002, 36005, 36410, 36425, 36475, 36476, 36478, 36479, 37241, 75894, 76000, 76937, 76942, 76998, 77022, 93970, 93971, in the same surgical field)◀

36475 Endovenous ablation therapy of incompetent vein, extremity, inclusive of all imaging guidance and monitoring, percutaneous, radiofrequency; first vein treated

+ 36476 subsequent vein(s) treated in a single extremity, each through separate access sites (List separately in addition to code for primary procedure)

(Use 36476 in conjunction with 36475)

(Do not report 36476 more than once per extremity)

▶(Do not report 36475, 36476 in conjunction with 29520, 29530, 29540, 29550, 29580, 29581, 29584, for the same extremity)◀

▶(Do not report 36475, 36476 in conjunction with 36000, 36002, 36005, 36410, 36425, 36478, 36479, 36482, 36483, 37241-37244, 75894, 76000, 76937, 76942, 76998, 77022, 93970, 93971, in the same surgical field)◀

36478 Endovenous ablation therapy of incompetent vein, extremity, inclusive of all imaging guidance and monitoring, percutaneous, laser; first vein treated

+ 36479 subsequent vein(s) treated in a single extremity, each through separate access sites (List separately in addition to code for primary procedure)

(Use 36479 in conjunction with 36478)

(Do not report 36479 more than once per extremity)

▶(Do not report 36478, 36479 in conjunction with 29520, 29530, 29540, 29550, 29580, 29581, 29584, for the same extremity)◀

▶(Do not report 36478, 36479 in conjunction with 36000, 36002, 36005, 36410, 36425, 36475, 36476, 36482, 36483, 37241, 75894, 76000, 76937, 76942, 76998, 77022, 93970, 93971, in the same surgical field)◀

 # 36482 Endovenous ablation therapy of incompetent vein, extremity, by transcatheter delivery of a chemical adhesive (eg, cyanoacrylate) remote from the access site, inclusive of all imaging guidance and monitoring, percutaneous; first vein treated

#+ 36483 subsequent vein(s) treated in a single extremity, each through separate access sites (List separately in addition to code for primary procedure)

(Use 36483 in conjunction with 36482)

(Do not report 36483 more than once per extremity)

▶(Do not report 36482, 36483 in conjunction with 29520, 29530, 29540, 29550, 29580, 29581, 29584, for the same extremity)◀

▶(Do not report 36482, 36483 in conjunction with 36000, 36002, 36005, 36410, 36425, 36475, 36476, 36478, 36479, 37241, 75894, 76000, 76937, 76942, 76998, 77022, 93970, 93971, in the same surgical field)◀

36481 Percutaneous portal vein catheterization by any method

★=Telemedicine ✚=Add-on code ✗=FDA approval pending #=Resequenced code ⊘=Modifier 51 exempt

Rationale

Several parenthetical notes under the "Vascular Injection Procedures" heading have been revised in the 2019 CPT code set. In accordance with the deletion of code 76001, the parenthetical notes following codes 36473, 36474, 36475, 36476, 36478, 36479, 36482, and 36483 have been revised with the removal of this code. Refer to the codebook and the Rationale for code 76001 for a full discussion of these changes.

Other changes have also been made to clarify the intended use of "for the same extremity" in the instructions. The changes that have been made reflect the intent to prevent reporting of the referenced services when they are performed on the same extremity. In accordance with these changes, exclusionary parenthetical notes following codes 36466, 36468, 36471, 36474, 36476, 36479, and 36483 have been revised and/or new exclusionary parenthetical notes have been added to preclude the use of codes 29520, 29530, 29540, 29550, 29580, 29581, and 29584.

Central Venous Access Procedures

▶To qualify as a central venous access catheter or device, the tip of the catheter/device must terminate in the subclavian, brachiocephalic (innominate) or iliac veins, the superior or inferior vena cava, or the right atrium. The venous access device may be either centrally inserted (jugular, subclavian, femoral vein or inferior vena cava catheter entry site) or peripherally inserted (eg, basilic, cephalic, or saphenous vein entry site). The device may be accessed for use either via exposed catheter (external to the skin), via a subcutaneous port or via a subcutaneous pump.◀

The procedures involving these types of devices fall into five categories:

1. ***Insertion*** (placement of catheter through a newly established venous access)

2. ***Repair*** (fixing device without replacement of either catheter or port/pump, other than pharmacologic or mechanical correction of intracatheter or pericatheter occlusion [see 36595 or 36596])

3. ***Partial replacement*** of only the catheter component associated with a port/pump device, but not entire device

4. ***Complete replacement*** of entire device via same venous access site (complete exchange)

5. ***Removal*** of entire device.

There is no coding distinction between venous access achieved percutaneously versus by cutdown or based on catheter size.

For the repair, partial (catheter only) replacement, complete replacement, or removal of both catheters (placed from separate venous access sites) of a multi-catheter device, with or without subcutaneous ports/pumps, use the appropriate code describing the service with a frequency of two.

If an existing central venous access device is removed and a new one placed via a separate venous access site, appropriate codes for both procedures (removal of old, if code exists, and insertion of new device) should be reported.

▶When imaging guidance is used for centrally inserted central venous catheters, for gaining access to the venous entry site and/or for manipulating the catheter into final central position, imaging guidance codes (eg, 76937, 77001) may be reported separately. Do not use 76937, 77001 in conjunction with 36568, 36569, 36572, 36573, 36584.◀

(For refilling and maintenance of an implantable pump or reservoir for intravenous or intra-arterial drug delivery, use 96522)

Rationale

In support of new codes 36572 and 36573 (peripherally inserted central venous catheter [PICC]) and revised codes 36568, 36569, and 36584, the guidelines for central venous access procedure have been revised to include the saphenous vein (as an example of an entry site for a PICC) and to clarify the instructions for reporting imaging guidance used for centrally inserted central venous catheters.

Refer to the codebook and the Rationale for codes 36568, 36569, 36572, 36573, and 36584 for a full discussion of these changes.

Insertion of Central Venous Access Device

36555   Insertion of non-tunneled centrally inserted central venous catheter; younger than 5 years of age

(For peripherally inserted non-tunneled central venous catheter, younger than 5 years of age, use 36568)

36565   Insertion of tunneled centrally inserted central venous access device, requiring 2 catheters via 2 separate venous access sites; without subcutaneous port or pump (eg, Tesio type catheter)

36566   with subcutaneous port(s)

The Central Venous Access Procedures Table

	Non-tunneled	Tunneled Without Port or Pump (w/out port or pump)	Central Tunneled	Tunneled With Port (w/port)	Tunneled With Pump (w/pump)	Peripheral	<5 years	≥5 years	Any Age
Insertion									
Catheter (without imaging guidance)	36555							36555	
	36556								36556	
		36557	36557				36557		
		36558	36558					36558	
	36568 (w/o port or pump)					36568 (w/o port or pump)	36568 (w/o port or pump)		
	36569 (w/o port or pump)					36569 (w/o port or pump)		36569 (w/o port or pump)	
Catheter (with bundled imaging guidance)						36572 (w/o port or pump)	36572 (w/o port or pump)		
						36573 (w/o port or pump)		36573 (w/o port or pump)	
Device			36560	36560			36560		
			36561	36561				36561	
			36563		36563				36563
		36565	36565						36565
			36566	36566					
	36570 (w/port)			36570 (w/port)		36570 (w/port)	36570 (w/port)		
	36571 (w/port)			36571 (w/port)		36571 (w/port)		36571 (w/port)	
Repair									
Catheter	36575 (w/o port or pump)	36575 (w/o port or pump)	36575 (w/o port or pump)			36575 (w/o port or pump)			36575
Device	36576 (w/port or pump)					36576 (w/port or pump)			36576
Partial Replacement - Central Venous Access Device (Catheter only)									
			36578	36578	36578	36578			36578
Complete Replacement - Central Venous Access Device (Through Same Venous Access Site)									
Catheter (without imaging guidance)	36580 (w/o port or pump)								36580
		36581	36581						36581
Catheter (with bundled imaging guidance)	36584 (w/o port or pump)					36584 (w/o port or pump)			36584 (w/o port or pump)
Device			36582	36582					36582
			36583		36583				36583
				36585 (w/port)		36585 (w/port)			36585
Removal									
Catheter		36589							36589
Device			36590	36590	36590	36590			36590
Removal of Obstructive Material from Device									
	36595 (pericatheter)	36595 (pericatheter)	36595 (pericatheter)	36595 (pericatheter)	36595 (pericatheter)	36595 (pericatheter)			36595 (pericatheter)
	36596 (intraluminal)	36596 (intraluminal)	36596 (intraluminal)	36596 (intraluminal)	36596 (intraluminal)	36596 (intraluminal)			36596 (intraluminal)
Repositioning of Catheter									
	36597	36597	36597	36597	36597	36597	36597	36597	36597

★ = Telemedicine   ✦ = Add-on code   ✚ = FDA approval pending   # = Resequenced code   ⊘ = Modifier 51 exempt

Surgery / Cardiovascular System 33010-39599

►Peripherally inserted central venous catheters (PICCs) may be placed or replaced with or without imaging guidance. When performed without imaging guidance, report using 36568 or 36569. When imaging guidance (eg, ultrasound, fluoroscopy) is used for PICC placement or repositioning, bundled service codes 36572, 36573, 36584 include all imaging necessary to complete the procedure, image documentation (representative images from all modalities used are stored to patient's permanent record), associated radiological supervision and interpretation, venography performed through the same venous puncture, and documentation of final central position of the catheter with imaging. Ultrasound guidance for PICC placement should include documentation of evaluation of the potential puncture sites, patency of the entry vein, and real-time ultrasound visualization of needle entry into the vein.

Codes 71045, 71046, 71047, 71048 should not be reported for the purpose of documenting the final catheter position on the same day of service as 36572, 36573, 36584. Codes 36572, 36573, 36584 include confirmation of catheter tip location. The physician or other qualified health care professional reporting image-guided PICC insertion cannot report confirmation of catheter tip location separately (eg, via X ray, ultrasound). Report 36572, 36573, 36584 with modifier 52 when performed without confirmation of catheter tip location.

"Midline" catheters by definition terminate in the peripheral venous system. They are **not** central venous access devices and may not be reported as a PICC service. Midline catheter placement may be reported with 36400, 36405, 36406, or 36410. PICCs placed using magnetic guidance or any other guidance modality that does not include imaging or image documentation are reported with 36568, 36569.◄

▲ **36568**   Insertion of peripherally inserted central venous catheter (PICC), without subcutaneous port or pump, without imaging guidance; younger than 5 years of age

(For placement of centrally inserted non-tunneled central venous catheter, without subcutaneous port or pump, younger than 5 years of age, use 36555)

►(For placement of peripherally inserted non-tunneled central venous catheter, without subcutaneous port or pump, with imaging guidance, younger than 5 years of age, use 36572)◄

▲ **36569**   age 5 years or older

►(Do not report 36568, 36569 in conjunction with 76937, 77001)◄

(For placement of centrally inserted non-tunneled central venous catheter, without subcutaneous port or pump, age 5 years or older, use 36556)

►(For placement of peripherally inserted non-tunneled central venous catheter, without subcutaneous port or pump, with imaging guidance, age 5 years or older, use 36573)◄

#● **36572**   Insertion of peripherally inserted central venous catheter (PICC), without subcutaneous port or pump, including all imaging guidance, image documentation, and all associated radiological supervision and interpretation required to perform the insertion; younger than 5 years of age

Peripherally Inserted Central Catheter
36572

A peripherally inserted central catheter, which is non-tunneled and without a subcutaneous port/pump, is placed in a child younger than 5 years of age.

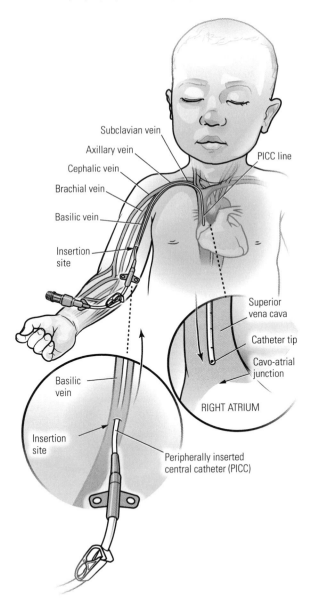

Subclavian vein
Axillary vein
Cephalic vein
Brachial vein
Basilic vein
Insertion site
PICC line
Superior vena cava
Catheter tip
Cavo-atrial junction
Basilic vein
Insertion site
RIGHT ATRIUM
Peripherally inserted central catheter (PICC)

Surgery / Cardiovascular System 33010-39599

▶(For placement of centrally inserted non-tunneled central venous catheter, without subcutaneous port or pump, younger than 5 years of age, use 36555)◀

▶(For placement of peripherally inserted non-tunneled central venous catheter, without subcutaneous port or pump, without imaging guidance, younger than 5 years of age, use 36568)◀

#● 36573   age 5 years or older

▶(For placement of centrally inserted non-tunneled central venous catheter, without subcutaneous port or pump, age 5 years or older, use 36556)◀

▶(For placement of peripherally inserted non-tunneled central venous catheter, without subcutaneous port or pump, without imaging guidance, age 5 years or older, use 36569)◀

▶(Do not report 36572, 36573 in conjunction with 76937, 77001)◀

36570   Insertion of peripherally inserted central venous access device, with subcutaneous port; younger than 5 years of age

(For insertion of tunneled centrally inserted central venous access device with subcutaneous port, younger than 5 years of age, use 36560)

36571   age 5 years or older

(For insertion of tunneled centrally inserted central venous access device with subcutaneous port, age 5 years or older, use 36561)

36572   Code is out of numerical sequence. See 36568-36571

36573   Code is out of numerical sequence. See 36568-36571

Complete Replacement of Central Venous Access Device Through Same Venous Access Site

▲ 36584   Replacement, complete, of a peripherally inserted central venous catheter (PICC), without subcutaneous port or pump, through same venous access, including all imaging guidance, image documentation, and all associated radiological supervision and interpretation required to perform the replacement

▶(For replacement of a peripherally inserted central venous catheter [PICC] without subcutaneous port or pump, through same venous access, without imaging guidance, use 37799)◀

▶(Do not report 36584 in conjunction with 76937, 77001)◀

Rationale

Changes regarding PICC procedures have been made in two subsections within Central Venous Access Procedures subsection: Insertion of Central Venous Access Device and Complete Replacement of Central Venous Access Device Through Same Venous Access Site. In the Insertion of Central Venous Access Device subsection, codes 36568 and 36569 have been revised and codes 36572 and 36573 have been added. New guidelines and parenthetical notes have been added as well. In the Complete Replacement of Central Venous Access Device Through Same Venous Access Site subsection, code 36584 has been revised and parenthetical notes have been added. The Central Venous Access Procedures Table has also been updated to reflect these code changes for PICC procedures.

Codes 36568 and 36569 described PICC insertion, but they have been revised to describe PICC insertion performed *without* imaging guidance. Conversely, codes 36572 and 36573 have been added to report PICC insertion performed *with* imaging guidance. Code 36572 is reported for patients who are younger than five years of age, while code 36573 is reported for patients who are five years of age or older. Code 36584 described PICC replacement, but it has been revised to describe PICC replacement performed with imaging guidance and regardless of the patient's age, which means it is not age-specific. Codes 36572, 36573, and 36584 include all image documentation and radiological supervision and interpretation required to perform the procedures described therein. When ultrasound guidance is performed, evaluation of the potential puncture sites, patency of the entry vein, and real-time ultrasound visualization of needle entry into the vein should be documented. Imaging to document the final catheter position or to confirm location of the catheter tip is not reported separately, as codes 36572, 36573, and 36584 include this imaging. If confirmation of catheter-tip location is not performed by the physician or other qualified health care professional performing the PICC insertion or replacement, then codes 36572, 36573, and 36584 are reported with modifier 52 appended to reflect reduction in service. Guidelines and parenthetical notes have been added to the Insertion of Central Venous Access Device subsection to provide instruction on the appropriate reporting of codes 36572, 36573, and 36584. In addition, parenthetical notes have been added following code 36584 to provide instruction on the appropriate reporting of this code.

Clinical Example (36568)

A neonatal male requires intravenous fluid management. A peripherally inserted central venous catheter (PICC) is placed without imaging guidance.

Description of Procedure (36568)

Locate the adjacent artery to avoid arterial puncture. Measure desired length of catheter insertion and cut catheter as necessary. Irrigate catheter with normal saline (NS). Upon application of tourniquet, puncture vein with insertion needle. Guide catheter through insertion needle to desired length. Fasten catheter in position and dress in standard fashion and flush or attach to IV infusion fluids.

Clinical Example (36569)

A 13-year-old male requires long-term IV antimicrobial therapy. A PICC is inserted without imaging guidance.

Description of Procedure (36569)

Locate the adjacent artery to avoid arterial puncture. Measure desired length of catheter insertion and cut catheter as necessary. Irrigate catheter with NS. Upon application of tourniquet, puncture vein with insertion needle. Guide catheter through insertion needle to desired length. Fasten the catheter in position and dress in standard fashion and flush or attach to IV infusion fluids.

Clinical Example (36572)

A 3-year-old male requires long-term IV antimicrobial therapy. A PICC is placed with imaging guidance.

Description of Procedure (36572)

Perform sterile US of the right upper extremity to assess brachial and basilic patency. Puncture the basilic vein with direct US guidance and introduce a wire fluoroscopically and centrally to the right atrium. Place the peel away sheath. Measure the peripherally inserted central venous catheter, cut to length, and position centrally within the superior vena cava (SVC) using fluoroscopic guidance. Test the catheter and flush to ensure function. Fasten catheter in position and dress in standard fashion.

Clinical Example (36573)

A 72-year-old male requires long-term IV antimicrobial therapy. He has had several prior central venous catheters and has known subclavian vein stenosis associated with an automatic implantable cardioverter-defibrillator (AICD) device. A PICC is inserted with imaging guidance.

Description of Procedure (36573)

Perform sterile US of the right upper extremity to assess brachial and basilic patency. Puncture the basilic vein using direct US guidance and pass a guidewire centrally to the right atrium using fluoroscopy. Place peel away sheath. Measure and then cut the peripherally inserted CV catheter to appropriate length and then advance to the SVC using fluoroscopy. Test the catheter and flush to ensure function. Secure the catheter in position, dress in standard fashion.

Clinical Example (36584)

A 37-year-old female is referred for dysfunction of a previously placed PICC. The catheter is completely replaced with imaging guidance.

Description of Procedure (36584)

Evaluate current catheter position and integrity under fluoroscopy. Cut existing catheter and partially withdraw. Advance a wire fluoroscopically and centrally and remove the existing catheter. Place a peel away sheath over the wire. Measure the new catheter and then cut to appropriate length. Advance the new PICC line centrally and position within the SVC using fluoroscopic guidance. Test the catheter and flush to ensure function. Fasten the catheter in position and dress and flush in standard fashion.

Transcatheter Procedures

Arterial Mechanical Thrombectomy

▶Arterial mechanical thrombectomy may be performed as a "primary" transcatheter procedure with pretreatment planning, performance of the procedure, and postprocedure evaluation focused on providing this service. Typically, the diagnosis of thrombus has been made prior to the procedure, and a mechanical thrombectomy is planned preoperatively. Primary mechanical thrombectomy is reported per vascular family using 37184 for the initial vessel treated and 37185 for second or all subsequent vessel(s) within the same vascular family. To report mechanical thrombectomy of an additional vascular family treated through a separate access site, use modifier 59 in conjunction with the primary service code (37184) for the mechanical transluminal thrombectomy.◀

Primary mechanical thrombectomy may precede or follow another percutaneous intervention. Most commonly primary mechanical thrombectomy will precede another percutaneous intervention with the decision regarding the need for other services not made until after mechanical thrombectomy has been performed. Occasionally, the performance of primary mechanical thrombectomy may follow another percutaneous intervention.

Do **NOT** report 37184-37185 for mechanical thrombectomy performed for the retrieval of short segments of thrombus or embolus evident during other percutaneous interventional procedures. See 37186 for these procedures.

Arterial mechanical thrombectomy is considered a "secondary" transcatheter procedure for removal or retrieval of short segments of thrombus or embolus when performed either before or after another percutaneous intervention (eg, percutaneous transluminal balloon angioplasty, stent placement). Secondary mechanical thrombectomy is reported using 37186. Do **NOT** report 37186 in conjunction with 37184-37185.

Rationale

Instructional guidelines on the use of codes 37184 and 37185 have been revised to comply with CPT code convention. Previously, the guidelines stated that code 37185 should be used with modifier 51 to report mechanical thrombectomy of an additional vascular family treated through a separate access site. However, because reporting an additional vascular family treated through a separate access site represents an additional distinct procedure, code 37185 should not be reported. Code 37185 is intended to report second and all subsequent vessels within the same vascular family, and it is reported without a modifier when subsequent vessels of the same family are treated. Instead, service to additional vessels from a separate access represents a distinct procedure that should be additionally reported with code 37184 to identify the additional primary percutaneous thrombectomy being done. In addition, modifier 59 should be appended to identify the additional primary thrombectomy as a distinct procedure.

Arterial Mechanical Thrombectomy

37184   Primary percutaneous transluminal mechanical thrombectomy, noncoronary, non-intracranial, arterial or arterial bypass graft, including fluoroscopic guidance and intraprocedural pharmacological thrombolytic injection(s); initial vessel

►(Do not report 37184 in conjunction with 61645, 76000, 96374)◄

+ 37185   second and all subsequent vessel(s) within the same vascular family (List separately in addition to code for primary mechanical thrombectomy procedure)

►(Do not report 37185 in conjunction with 76000, 96375)◄

(Do not report 37185 in conjunction with 61645 for treatment of the same vascular territory. See Nervous System Endovascular Therapy)

+ 37186   Secondary percutaneous transluminal thrombectomy (eg, nonprimary mechanical, snare basket, suction technique), noncoronary, non-intracranial, arterial or arterial bypass graft, including fluoroscopic guidance and intraprocedural pharmacological thrombolytic injections, provided in conjunction with another percutaneous intervention other than primary mechanical thrombectomy (List separately in addition to code for primary procedure)

►(Do not report 37186 in conjunction with 76000, 96375)◄

(Do not report 37186 in conjunction with 61645 for treatment of the same vascular territory. See Nervous System Endovascular Therapy)

Rationale

In accordance with the deletion of code 76001, the parenthetical note following code 37186 has been revised with the removal of this code.

Refer to the codebook and the Rationale for code 76001 for a full discussion of these changes.

Venous Mechanical Thrombectomy

37187   Percutaneous transluminal mechanical thrombectomy, vein(s), including intraprocedural pharmacological thrombolytic injections and fluoroscopic guidance

►(Do not report 37187 in conjunction with 76000, 96375)◄

37188   Percutaneous transluminal mechanical thrombectomy, vein(s), including intraprocedural pharmacological thrombolytic injections and fluoroscopic guidance, repeat treatment on subsequent day during course of thrombolytic therapy

►(Do not report 37188 in conjunction with 76000, 96375)◄

Rationale

In accordance with the deletion of code 76001, the parenthetical notes following codes 37187 and 37188 have been revised with the removal of this code.

Refer to the codebook and the Rationale for code 76001 for a full discussion of these changes.

Other Procedures

37197   Transcatheter retrieval, percutaneous, of intravascular foreign body (eg, fractured venous or arterial catheter), includes radiological supervision and interpretation, and imaging guidance (ultrasound or fluoroscopy), when performed

(For percutaneous retrieval of a vena cava filter, use 37193)

▶(For transcatheter removal of permanent leadless pacemaker, use 33275)◀

Rationale

In support of the establishment of code 33275 (leadless pacemaker) and the deletion of code 0388T, the cross-reference parenthetical note that follows code 37197 has been revised to direct users to code 33275.

Refer to the codebook and the Rationale for code 33275 for a full discussion of these changes.

Endovascular Revascularization (Open or Percutaneous, Transcatheter)

37224   Revascularization, endovascular, open or percutaneous, femoral, popliteal artery(s), unilateral; with transluminal angioplasty

37225   with atherectomy, includes angioplasty within the same vessel, when performed

37226   with transluminal stent placement(s), includes angioplasty within the same vessel, when performed

37227   with transluminal stent placement(s) and atherectomy, includes angioplasty within the same vessel, when performed

▶(Do not report 37224, 37225, 37226, 37227 in conjunction with 0505T, within the femoral-popliteal segment)◀

 # 37248   Transluminal balloon angioplasty (except dialysis circuit), open or percutaneous, including all imaging and radiological supervision and interpretation necessary to perform the angioplasty within the same vein; initial vein

#+ 37249   each additional vein (List separately in addition to code for primary procedure)

(Use 37249 in conjunction with 37248)

(Do not report 37248, 37249 in conjunction with 37238, 37239 when performed in the same vein during the same operative session)

▶(Do not report 37248, 37249 in conjunction with 0505T, within the femoral-popliteal segment)◀

(For transluminal balloon angioplasty in aorta/visceral artery[ies] in conjunction with fenestrated endovascular repair, see 34841, 34842, 34843, 34844, 34845, 34846, 34847, 34848)

(For transluminal balloon angioplasty in iliac, femoral, popliteal, or tibial/peroneal artery[ies] for occlusive disease, see 37220-37235)

(For transluminal balloon angioplasty in a dialysis circuit performed through the circuit, see 36902, 36903, 36904, 36905, 36906, 36907, 36908)

(For transluminal balloon angioplasty in an intracranial artery, see 61630, 61635)

(For transluminal balloon angioplasty in a coronary artery, see 92920-92944)

(For transluminal balloon angioplasty in a pulmonary artery, see 92997, 92998)

37238   Transcatheter placement of an intravascular stent(s), open or percutaneous, including radiological supervision and interpretation and including angioplasty within the same vessel, when performed; initial vein

+ 37239   each additional vein (List separately in addition to code for primary procedure)

(Use 37239 in conjunction with 37238)

▶(Do not report 37238, 37239 in conjunction with 0505T, within the femoral-popliteal segment)◀

(For placement of a stent[s] within the peripheral segment of the dialysis circuit, see 36903, 36906)

(For transcatheter placement of an intravascular stent[s] within central dialysis segment when performed through the dialysis circuit, use 36908)

Rationale

In support of the establishment of Category III code 0505T, new exclusionary parenthetical notes have been added following codes 37227, 37239, and 37249. Refer to the codebook and the Rationale for code 0505T for a full discussion of these changes.

Hemic and Lymphatic Systems

Lymph Nodes and Lymphatic Channels

Excision

(For injection for sentinel node identification, use 38792)

38500   Biopsy or excision of lymph node(s); open, superficial

(Do not report 38500 with 38700-38780)

38505   by needle, superficial (eg, cervical, inguinal, axillary)

(If imaging guidance is performed, see 76942, 77002, 77012, 77021)

▶(For fine needle aspiration biopsy, see 10004, 10005, 10006, 10007, 10008, 10009, 10010, 10011, 10012, 10021)◀

(For evaluation of fine needle aspirate, see 88172, 88173)

38510   open, deep cervical node(s)

38520   open, deep cervical node(s) with excision scalene fat pad

38525   open, deep axillary node(s)

38530   open, internal mammary node(s)

(Do not report 38530 with 38720-38746)

▶(For percutaneous needle biopsy, retroperitoneal lymph node or mass, use 49180)◀

▶(For fine needle aspiration biopsy, retroperitoneal lymph node or mass, see 10005, 10006, 10007, 10008, 10009, 10010, 10011, 10012)◀

Rationale

Parenthetical notes following codes 38505 and 38530 (lymph nodes biopsy) within the Excision subsection have been revised to direct users to codes 10004-10012 and 10021 for FNA biopsy procedures.

Refer to the codebook and the Rationale for codes 10004-10012 and 10021 for a full discussion of these changes.

● **38531**   open, inguinofemoral node(s)

▶(For bilateral procedure, report 38531 with modifier 50)◀

Rationale

Code 38531 has been established in the Hemic and Lymphatic Systems, Lymph Nodes and Lymphatic Channels, Excision subsection for open biopsy or excision of inguinofemoral nodes. Because the procedure may be performed bilaterally, instruction has been provided to use code 38531 with modifier 50 appended, in order to identify the bilateral procedure when performed. In an effort to provide further guidance regarding the intended use of this code, instruction has been added to the parenthetical note following code 38900 by adding code 38531 to the list of codes to indicate that it may be reported, when appropriate.

Clinical Example (38531)

A 65-year-old has a previously confirmed squamous cell carcinoma of the vulva that is distant (more than 2 cm) from the midline. An inguinofemoral lymph node(s) excision is performed. (**Note:** Intraoperative mapping is reported separately.)

Description of Procedure (38531)

Make a skin incision parallel to the inguinal ligament and dissect the subcutaneous fat down to and through Campers fascia. Continue the dissection both superiorly and inferiorly below Campers fascia to expose the superficial inguinal nodes. Remove any concerning superficial inguinal lymph nodes. Carry the dissection down to the cribriform fascia, identifying the Sartorius and adductor longus muscles. Ligate small veins in the process. Divide the cribriform fascia so that the deep inguinal lymph nodes can be visualized, palpated, and removed, if concerning. Remove additional lymph nodes based on intraoperative pathologic assessment. Then place a subcutaneous drain and suture and secure to the skin. Re-approximate the subcutaneous fat in layers and then close the skin with staples or sutures.

Other Procedures

+ 38900   Intraoperative identification (eg, mapping) of sentinel lymph node(s) includes injection of non-radioactive dye, when performed (List separately in addition to code for primary procedure)

▶(Use 38900 in conjunction with 19302, 19307, 38500, 38510, 38520, 38525, 38530, 38531, 38542, 38562, 38564, 38570, 38571, 38572, 38740, 38745, 38760, 38765, 38770, 38780, 56630, 56631, 56632, 56633, 56634, 56637, 56640)◀

(For injection of radioactive tracer for identification of sentinel node, use 38792)

★ = Telemedicine   ✚ = Add-on code   ✘ = FDA approval pending   # = Resequenced code   ⊘ = Modifier 51 exempt

Rationale

Sentinel lymph node biopsy can be used for staging various gynecological cancers. The parenthetical note following add-on code 38900 has been revised to include codes for pelvic and vulvar procedures as codes that may be reported in conjunction with code 38900 (intraoperative identification of sentinel lymph nodes).

Refer to the codebook and the Rationale for code 38531 for a full discussion of these changes.

Digestive System

Tongue and Floor of Mouth

Other Procedures

▶(41500 has been deleted)◀

41510   Suture of tongue to lip for micrognathia (Douglas type procedure)

41512   Tongue base suspension, permanent suture technique

(For suture of tongue to lip for micrognathia, use 41510)

Rationale

To ensure that the CPT code set reflects current clinical practice, code 41500, *Fixation of tongue, mechanical, other than suture (eg, K-wire),* has been deleted due to low utilization.

Salivary Gland and Ducts

Excision

42400   Biopsy of salivary gland; needle

▶(For fine needle aspiration biopsy, see 10004, 10005, 10006, 10007, 10008, 10009, 10010, 10011, 10012, 10021)◀

(For evaluation of fine needle aspirate, see 88172, 88173)

(If imaging guidance is performed, see 76942, 77002, 77012, 77021)

Rationale

A parenthetical note following code 42400 (salivary gland biopsy) within the Excision subsection has been revised to direct users to codes 10004-10012 and 10021 for FNA biopsy procedures. Refer to the codebook and the Rationale for codes 10004-10012 and 10021 for a full discussion of these changes.

Esophagus

Endoscopy

Esophagoscopy

43200   Esophagoscopy, flexible, transoral; diagnostic, including collection of specimen(s) by brushing or washing, when performed (separate procedure)

(Do not report 43200 in conjunction with 43197, 43198, 43201-43232)

(For diagnostic rigid transoral esophagoscopy, use 43191)

(For diagnostic flexible transnasal esophagoscopy, use 43197)

(For diagnostic flexible esophagogastroduodenoscopy, use 43235)

 # 43213   with dilation of esophagus, by balloon or dilator, retrograde (includes fluoroscopic guidance, when performed)

▶(Do not report 43213 in conjunction with 43197, 43198, 43200, 74360, 76000)◀

(For transendoscopic balloon dilation of multiple strictures during the same session, report 43213 with modifier 59 for each additional stricture dilated)

 # 43214   with dilation of esophagus with balloon (30 mm diameter or larger) (includes fluoroscopic guidance, when performed)

▶(Do not report 43214 in conjunction with 43197, 43198, 43200, 74360, 76000)◀

Rationale

In accordance with the deletion of code 76001, the parenthetical notes following codes 43213 and 43214 have been revised.

Refer to the codebook and the Rationale for code 76001 for a full discussion of these changes.

Esophagogastroduodenoscopy

43235   Esophagogastroduodenoscopy, flexible, transoral; diagnostic, including collection of specimen(s) by brushing or washing, when performed (separate procedure)

(Do not report 43235 in conjunction with 43197, 43198, 43210, 43236-43259, 43266, 43270, 44360, 44361, 44363, 44364, 44365, 44366, 44369, 44370, 44372, 44373, 44376, 44377, 44378, 44379)

43246   with directed placement of percutaneous gastrostomy tube

(Do not report 43246 in conjunction with 43197, 43198, 43235, 44360, 44361, 44363, 44364, 44365, 44366, 44369, 44370, 44372, 44376, 44377, 44378, 44379)

►(For percutaneous insertion of gastrostomy tube under fluoroscopic guidance, use 49440)◄

►(For percutaneous replacement of gastrostomy tube without imaging or endoscopy, see 43762, 43763)◄

 # 43233   with dilation of esophagus with balloon (30 mm diameter or larger) (includes fluoroscopic guidance, when performed)

►(Do not report 43233 in conjunction with 43197, 43198, 43235, 44360, 44361, 44363, 44364, 44365, 44366, 44369, 44370, 44372, 44373, 44376, 44377, 44378, 44379, 74360, 76000)◄

> ### Rationale
>
> In support of the deletion of code 43760 and the addition of codes 43762 and 43763, the existing cross-reference parenthetical note following code 43246 has been revised; the cross-reference parenthetical note directing users to code 43760 has been deleted; and a new parenthetical note has been added. The existing parenthetical note has been revised to direct users to code 49440 for percutaneous insertion of gastrostomy tube under fluoroscopic guidance. Prior to 2019, this parenthetical note directed users to code 43246 for placement of gastrostomy tube, rather than insertion, and it did not specify that the procedure is performed under fluoroscopic guidance. The new parenthetical note directs users to the new codes 43762 and 43763 for percutaneous replacement of gastrostomy tube without imaging or endoscopy. Refer to the codebook and the Rationale for codes 43760, 43762, and 43763 for a full discussion of these changes.
>
> In addition, in accordance with the deletion of code 76001, the parenthetical note following code 43233 has been revised. Refer to the codebook and the Rationale for code 76001 for a full discussion of these changes.

Stomach

Introduction

►(43760 has been deleted. To report replacement of gastrostomy tube without imaging or endoscopy, see 43762, 43763)◄

(To report fluoroscopically guided replacement of gastrostomy tube, use 49450)

(For endoscopic placement of gastrostomy tube, use 43246)

43761   Repositioning of a naso- or oro-gastric feeding tube, through the duodenum for enteric nutrition

(Do not report 43761 in conjunction with 44500, 49446)

(If imaging guidance is performed, use 76000)

(For endoscopic conversion of a gastrostomy tube to jejunostomy tube, use 44373)

(For placement of a long gastrointestinal tube into the duodenum, use 44500)

● **43762**   Replacement of gastrostomy tube, percutaneous, includes removal, when performed, without imaging or endoscopic guidance; not requiring revision of gastrostomy tract

● **43763**   requiring revision of gastrostomy tract

►(For percutaneous replacement of gastrostomy tube under fluoroscopic guidance, use 49450)◄

►(For endoscopically directed placement of gastrostomy tube, use 43246)◄

> ### Rationale
>
> Code 43760 has been deleted, codes 43762 and 43763 have been added, and three parenthetical notes have been added. The AMA RUC identified code 43760 as a result of two screens: (1) Services Surveyed by One Specialty and Now Performed by a Different Specialty screen; and (2) CMS 0-day Global Code Reported with an E/M Service More Than 50% screen. Based on further analysis by the AMA RUC, it was determined that gastrostomy tube replacement is sometimes performed in a simple, straightforward manner and in other circumstances the condition of the gastrostomy tract is such that a more complex tube replacement procedure is required. As such, it was recommended that changes be made to the CPT code set to reflect the differentiation in work.
>
> Code 43760 described percutaneous change of gastrostomy tube, performed without imaging or endoscopic guidance. In order to differentiate the work of a straightforward gastrostomy tube replacement and a tube replacement that is complicated by gastrostomy tract that requires revision, code 43760 has been deleted and

★ = Telemedicine   ✦ = Add-on code   ✗ = FDA approval pending   # = Resequenced code   ⊘ = Modifier 51 exempt

two new codes (43762, 43763) have been added. Inadvertent removal of a gastrostomy tube (eg, patient pulls the tube out) and a clogged gastrostomy tube are two typical reasons that gastrostomy tube replacement may be needed. Removal of the initial tube, when performed, is not reported separately. Code 43762 describes replacement of gastrostomy tube without the need for revision of the gastrostomy tract. Note that placement of the new gastrostomy tube, as described by code 43762, may require dilation of the gastrostomy tract without the need for an incision or other additional work to allow insertion of the dilation instrument. Code 43763 describes a more complex procedure that requires revision of the gastrostomy tract. For example, there may be broken skin in the tract that requires debridement, or the tract may require dilation but is so stenotic that an incision is required to allow insertion of the dilation instrument prior to inserting the new gastrostomy tube.

Codes 43762 and 43763 describe gastrostomy tube replacement without imaging or endoscopic guidance. If percutaneous gastrostomy tube replacement is performed under fluoroscopic guidance, then code 49450 should be reported. If percutaneous gastrostomy tube replacement is performed under endoscopic guidance, then report code 43246.

Clinical Example (43762)

A 76-year-old female suffering from significant malnutrition previously required placement of a percutaneous gastrostomy tube. The gastrostomy catheter has become clogged; attempts to establish luminal patency have been unsuccessful. The physician is requested to remove the obstructed gastrostomy catheter and replace it.

Description of Procedure (43762)

Examine existing tube site. Deflate balloon as appropriate. Remove existing gastrostomy tube by traction. Test, insert, and fill a new balloon tube to specification. Pull back the tube, and secure and check for patency.

Clinical Example (43763)

A patient with severe neurological deficit and high risk for aspiration required placement of a gastrostomy tube. The patient inadvertently dislodged the tube, but this was not recognized until the next day. The gastrostomy tube replacement requires revision of the gastrostomy tract.

Description of Procedure (43763)

Under anesthesia, as required, examine existing tube site and cleanse and debride skin at the abdominal wall as necessary. First probe the insertion site with a hemostat and/or a guidewire to assure that the stomach can be accessed. Open the strictured insertion tract using a scalpel followed by sequential dilators through the strictured tract to provide an adequate lumen to allow replacement of a new gastrostomy tube into the stomach through the original abdominal wall and gastric site openings. Once the new tube is inserted, aspiration is performed through the tube for gastric contents to confirm appropriate position in the stomach. Next, the tube balloon is inflated and pulled back to the appropriate position and secured to the abdominal wall. Final wound closure of the debrided abdominal wall is then performed as necessary. When indicated, water-soluble contrast is injected through the tube and a plain film of the abdomen is obtained and reviewed to confirm proper placement of the tube into the stomach and that no leakage into the abdominal cavity occurs.

Other Procedures

43830 Gastrostomy, open; without construction of gastric tube (eg, Stamm procedure) (separate procedure)

43831   neonatal, for feeding

▶(For percutaneous replacement of gastrostomy tube with removal when performed without imaging or endoscopy, see 43762, 43763)◀

▶(For percutaneous replacement of gastrostomy tube under fluoroscopic guidance, use 49450)◀

(Do not report modifier 63 in conjunction with 43831)

Rationale

In support of the deletion of code 43760 and the addition of codes 43762 and 43763, the cross-reference parenthetical notes following code 43831 have been revised to provide better clarity on the reporting of percutaneous gastrostomy tube replacement without imaging guidance and with imaging guidance.

Refer to the codebook and the Rationale for codes 43760, 43762, and 43763 for a full discussion of these changes.

Anus

Repair

46760   Sphincteroplasty, anal, for incontinence, adult; muscle transplant

46761   levator muscle imbrication (Park posterior anal repair)

▶(46762 has been deleted)◀

(For anoscopy with directed submucosal injection of bulking agent for fecal incontinence, use 0377T)

Rationale

Code 46762, *Sphincteroplasty, anal, for incontinence, adult; implantation artificial sphincter,* has been deleted due to low utilization and to ensure that the CPT code set reflects current clinical practice. In addition, a deletion parenthetical note to reflect this change has been added following code 46761.

Liver

Incision

47000   Biopsy of liver, needle; percutaneous

(If imaging guidance is performed, see 76942, 77002, 77012, 77021)

+ 47001   when done for indicated purpose at time of other major procedure (List separately in addition to code for primary procedure)

(If imaging guidance is performed, see 76942, 77002)

▶(For fine needle aspiration biopsy in conjunction with 47000, 47001, see 10004, 10005, 10006, 10007, 10008, 10009, 10010, 10011, 10012, 10021)◀

(For evaluation of fine needle aspirate in conjunction with 47000, 47001, see 88172, 88173)

Rationale

A parenthetical note following code 47001 (portoenterostomy) within the Incision subsection has been revised to direct users to codes 10004-10012 and 10021 for FNA biopsy procedures.

Refer to the codebook and the Rationale for codes 10004-10012 and 10021 for a full discussion of these changes.

Pancreas

Excision

48102   Biopsy of pancreas, percutaneous needle

(For radiological supervision and interpretation, see 76942, 77002, 77012, 77021)

▶(For fine needle aspiration biopsy, see 10005, 10006, 10007, 10008, 10009, 10010, 10011, 10012)◀

(For evaluation of fine needle aspirate, see 88172, 88173)

Rationale

A parenthetical note following code 48102 (pancreas biopsy) within the Excision subsection has been revised to direct users to codes 10005-10012 and 10021 for FNA biopsy procedures.

Refer to the codebook and the Rationale for codes 10004-10012 and 10021 for a full discussion of these changes.

Abdomen, Peritoneum, and Omentum

Excision, Destruction

49180   Biopsy, abdominal or retroperitoneal mass, percutaneous needle

(If imaging guidance is performed, see 76942, 77002, 77012, 77021)

▶(For fine needle aspiration biopsy, see 10004, 10005, 10006, 10007, 10008, 10009, 10010, 10011, 10012, 10021)◀

(For evaluation of fine needle aspirate, see 88172, 88173)

Rationale

A parenthetical note following code 49180 (abdominal or retroperitoneal mass biopsy) within the Excision, Destruction subsection has been revised to direct users to codes 10004-10012 and 10021 for FNA biopsy procedures.

Refer to the codebook and the Rationale for codes 10004-10012 and 10021 for a full discussion of these changes.

★ = Telemedicine   ✚ = Add-on code   ✔ = FDA approval pending   # = Resequenced code   ⊘ = Modifier 51 exempt

Introduction, Revision, Removal

Replacement

If an existing gastrostomy, duodenostomy, jejunostomy, gastro-jejunostomy, or cecostomy (or other colonic) tube is removed and a new tube is placed via a separate percutaneous access site, the placement of the new tube is not considered a replacement and would be reported using the appropriate initial placement codes 49440-49442.

49450 Replacement of gastrostomy or cecostomy (or other colonic) tube, percutaneous, under fluoroscopic guidance including contrast injection(s), image documentation and report

►(For percutaneous replacement of gastrostomy tube with removal when performed without imaging or endoscopy, see 43762, 43763)◄

Rationale

In support of the deletion of code 43760 and the addition of codes 43762 and 43763, the cross-reference parenthetical note following code 49450 has been revised to direct users to new codes 43762 and 43763 (gastrostomy tube replacement).

Refer to the codebook and the Rationale for codes 43760, 43762, and 43763 for a full discussion of these changes.

Urinary System

Kidney

Incision

50080 Percutaneous nephrostolithotomy or pyelostolithotomy, with or without dilation, endoscopy, lithotripsy, stenting, or basket extraction; up to 2 cm

50081 over 2 cm

►(For establishment of nephrostomy without nephrostolithotomy, see 50040, 50432, 50433, 52334)◄

►(For fluoroscopic guidance, use 76000)◄

►(Do not report 50080, 50081 in conjunction with 50436, 50437, when performed by the same physician or other qualified health care professional)◄

Rationale

Two parenthetical notes following code 50081 have been revised. The first note has been revised to accommodate the deletion of code 50395. In accordance with the deletion of code 76001, the second parenthetical note has been revised with the removal of this code and "see" has been replaced with "use." Finally, a third parenthetical note has been added and provides the codes that should not be reported in conjunction with codes 50080 and 50081, when performed by the same physician or other qualified health care professional.

Refer to the codebook and the Rationale for codes 50436, 50437, and 76001 for a full discussion of these changes.

Excision

50200 Renal biopsy; percutaneous, by trocar or needle

(For radiological supervision and interpretation, see 76942, 77002, 77012, 77021)

►(For fine needle aspiration biopsy, see 10005, 10006, 10007, 10008, 10009, 10010, 10011, 10012)◄

(For evaluation of fine needle aspirate, see 88172, 88173)

50205 by surgical exposure of kidney

Rationale

A parenthetical note following code 50200 (renal biopsy) within the Excision subsection has been revised to direct users to codes 10005-10012 for FNA biopsy procedures.

Refer to the codebook and the Rationale for codes 10004-10012 and 10021 for a full discussion of these changes.

Introduction

Renal Pelvis Catheter Procedures

Internally Dwelling

50384 Removal (via snare/capture) of internally dwelling ureteral stent via percutaneous approach, including radiological supervision and interpretation

(For bilateral procedure, use modifier 50)

►(Do not report 50382, 50384 in conjunction with 50436, 50437)◄

(For removal of an internally dwelling ureteral stent via a transurethral approach, use 50386)

Rationale

The parenthetical note following code 50384 has been revised to accommodate the replacement of code 50395 with codes 50436 and 50437. Refer to the codebook and the Rationale for codes 50436 and 50437 for a full discussion of these changes.

Other Introduction (Injection/Change/Removal) Procedures

▶Percutaneous genitourinary procedures are performed with imaging guidance (eg, fluoroscopy and/or ultrasound). Diagnostic nephrostogram and/or ureterogram are typically performed with percutaneous genitourinary procedures and are included in 50432, 50433, 50434, 50435, 50436, 50437, 50693, 50694, 50695.

Code 50436 describes enlargement of an existing percutaneous tract to the renal collecting system to accommodate large instruments used in an endourologic procedure. Code 50436 includes predilation urinary tract imaging, postprocedure nephrostomy tube placement, when performed, and includes all radiological supervision and interpretation and imaging guidance (eg, ultrasound, fluoroscopy). Code 50436 may not be reported with 50432, 50433, 52334 for basic dilation of a percutaneous tract during initial placement of a catheter or device.

Code 50437 includes all elements of 50436, but also includes new access into the renal collecting system performed in the same session when a pre-existing tract is not present.◀

Codes 50430 and 50431 are diagnostic procedure codes that include injection(s) of contrast material, all associated radiological supervision and interpretation, and procedural imaging guidance (eg, ultrasound and/or fluoroscopy). Code 50430 also includes accessing the collecting system and/or associated ureter with a needle and/or catheter. Codes 50430 or 50431 may not be reported together with 50432, 50433, 50434, 50435, 50693, 50694, 50695.

Codes 50432, 50433, 50434, 50435 represent therapeutic procedures describing catheter placement or exchange, and include the elements of access, drainage catheter manipulations, and imaging guidance (eg, ultra sonography and/or fluoroscopy), as well as diagnostic imaging supervision and interpretation, when performed.

Code 50433 describes percutaneous nephrostomy with the additional accessing of the ureter/bladder to ultimately place a nephroureteral catheter (a single transnephric catheter with nephrostomy and ureteral

components that allows drainage internally, externally, or both).

For codes 50430, 50431, 50432, 50433, 50434, 50435, 50606, 50693, 50694, 50695, 50705, and 50706, the renal pelvis and its associated ureter are considered a single entity for reporting purposes. Codes 50430, 50431, 50432, 50433, 50434, 50435, 50606, 50693, 50694, 50695, 50705, and 50706 may be reported once for each renal collecting system/ureter accessed (eg, two separate codes would be reported for bilateral nephrostomy tube placement or for unilateral duplicated collecting system/ureter requiring two separate procedures).

50391 Instillation(s) of therapeutic agent into renal pelvis and/or ureter through established nephrostomy, pyelostomy or ureterostomy tube (eg, anticarcinogenic or antifungal agent)

▶(50395 has been deleted. To report, see 50436, 50437)◀

#● 50436 Dilation of existing tract, percutaneous, for an endourologic procedure including imaging guidance (eg, ultrasound and/or fluoroscopy) and all associated radiological supervision and interpretation, with postprocedure tube placement, when performed

#● 50437 including new access into the renal collecting system

(For nephrostolithotomy, see 50080, 50081)

(For retrograde percutaneous nephrostomy, use 52334)

(For endoscopic surgery, see 50551-50561)

▶(Do not report 50436, 50437 in conjunction with 50080, 50081, 50382, 50384, 50430, 50431, 50432, 50433, 52334, 74485)◀

 # 50432 Placement of nephrostomy catheter, percutaneous, including diagnostic nephrostogram and/or ureterogram when performed, imaging guidance (eg, ultrasound and/or fluoroscopy) and all associated radiological supervision and interpretation

▶(Do not report 50432 in conjunction with 50430, 50431, 50433, 50436, 50437, 50694, 50695, 74425, for the same renal collecting system and/or associated ureter)◀

▶(Do not report 50432 in conjunction with 50436, 50437, for dilation of the nephrostomy tube tract)◀

 # 50433 Placement of nephroureteral catheter, percutaneous, including diagnostic nephrostogram and/or ureterogram when performed, imaging guidance (eg, ultrasound and/or fluoroscopy) and all associated radiological supervision and interpretation, new access

(Do not report 50433 in conjunction with 50430, 50431, 50432, 50693, 50694, 50695, 74425 for the same renal collecting system and/or associated ureter)

▶(Do not report 50433 in conjunction with 50436, 50437, for dilation of the nephroureteral catheter tract)◀

(For nephroureteral catheter removal and replacement, use 50387)

Rationale

Code 50395 has been deleted and codes 50436 and 50437 have been added to describe dilation of an existing urinary tract. A number of guidelines and parenthetical notes have been revised, deleted, and added to accommodate the replacement of deleted code 50395 with the two new codes (50436, 50437).

Previously, code 50395 was intended to identify accessing an existing tract to dilate the opening to accommodate devices that will be used beyond the dilated tract. Code 50432 is intended to identify an initial placement of a catheter or device within the urinary tract. Because code 50395 could be misconstrued to include establishing an initial nephrostomy tract, this code has been deleted and the two new codes (50436, 50437) established to differentiate dilation of an existing tract from initiating a new tract.

As a result, guidelines have now been added before the listing of codes 50436 and 50437 to provide instructions regarding the intended use for them. Existing guidelines following the "Other Introduction (Injection/Change/Removal) Procedures" section have also been revised to list codes 50436, 50437 as genitourinary procedures that include diagnostic nephrostogram/ureterogram. In addition, the new guidelines also list other services that are inherently included as part of each new code. For code 50436, this includes predilation urinary tract imaging, postprocedure nephrostomy tube placement, all radiologic supervision and interpretation, and imaging guidance to accomplish the dilation procedure and excludes basic dilation of a percutaneous tract during the initial placement of the catheter or device. For code 50437, this includes everything identified as part of code 50436, as well as new access into the renal collecting system performed during the same session when a pre-existing tract is not present.

Numerous parenthetical notes have been added to include radiologic supervision and interpretation and to note that imaging codes (74485) should not be reported separately for either of these new codes. This also includes the addition of these codes to exclusionary parenthetical notes that restrict reporting of these codes with other genitourinary supervision and interpretation (S&I) inclusive procedures.

Because diagnostic S&I is included for codes 50436 and 50437, the language within imaging code 74485 has been revised to remove "nephrostomy." The descriptor for this code has also been editorially revised to note "ureter(s)."

An exclusionary parenthetical note has also been added following code 74485 to restrict its use in conjunction with code 50436 or 50437. An additional instructional parenthetical note directs users to code 50436 or 50437 for dilation of a nephrostomy tract for endourologic procedure.

Clinical Example (50436)

A 65-year-old male presents with a symptomatic right renal pelvic stone confirmed by prior imaging. A percutaneous right renal pelvic 8-Fr nephrostomy tube has been previously placed. Dilation of the percutaneous tract is scheduled prior to endoscopic stone removal (reported separately).

Description of Procedure (50436)

Through existing nephroureteral access, perform and interpret antegrade nephroureterogram. Fluoroscopically introduce two stiff wires into the urinary bladder. Make skin incision. Fluoroscopically position 10-mm tract dilation balloon and dilate the tract. Over the balloon, fluoroscopically advance the 30-Fr tract sheath to secure access for the distinct and separate work of the endourologic procedure in question. Following the endourologic procedure, fluoroscopically advance a post-procedure nephrostomy tube into place. Perform and interpret post-procedure nephroureterogram. Connect catheter to a gravity drainage bag. Apply sterile dressings.

Clinical Example (50437)

A 57-year-old female presents with symptomatic chronic right renal pelvic calculi. Access to the right renal collecting system and dilation of the urinary tract is scheduled prior to endoscopic stone removal (reported separately).

Description of Procedure (50437)

Make a small skin incision. Using US and fluoroscopy to target the area of stone disease within the collecting system, insert a needle through a calyceal approach. Confirm needle placement by performing and interpreting an antegrade nephrostogram. Place a 0.018-in wire fluoroscopically down the ureter. Introduce a dilator system so that a larger, stiff 0.035-in wire can be placed in the urinary bladder. Place an 8-Fr sheath so that an additional stiff 0.035-in wire can be placed in the urinary bladder. Expand skin incision. Fluoroscopically position a 10-mm tract dilation balloon and dilate the tract. Over the balloon, fluoroscopically advance the 30-Fr tract sheath to secure access for the distinct and separate work of the endourologic procedure in question. Following the endourologic procedure, fluoroscopically advance a post-procedure nephrostomy tube into place.

Perform and interpret post-procedure nephroureterogram. Connect the catheter to a gravity drainage bag. Apply sterile dressings.

Repair

50436   Code is out of numerical sequence. See 50390-50405

50437   Code is out of numerical sequence. See 50390-50405

Bladder

Transurethral Surgery

Ureter and Pelvis

52334   Cystourethroscopy with insertion of ureteral guide wire through kidney to establish a percutaneous nephrostomy, retrograde

►(For percutaneous nephrostolithotomy, see 50080, 50081; for establishment of percutaneous nephrostomy, see 50432, 50433)◄

(For cystourethroscopy, with ureteroscopy and/or pyeloscopy, see 52351-52356)

(For cystourethroscopy with incision, fulguration, or resection of congenital posterior urethral valves or obstructive hypertrophic mucosal folds, use 52400)

►(Do not report 52334 in conjunction with 50437, 52000, 52351)◄

Rationale

In accordance with the addition of codes 50436 and 50437 and the deletion of code 50395, two parenthetical notes following code 52334 have been revised. The first parenthetical note replaced deleted code 50395 with code 50433 and provides specificity by adding the term "percutaneous." The second revised parenthetical note added new code 50437 to the list of codes that should not be reported with code 52334.

Refer to the codebook and the Rationale for codes 50436 and 50437 for a full discussion of these changes.

Urethra

Other Procedures

53850   Transurethral destruction of prostate tissue; by microwave thermotherapy

53852   by radiofrequency thermotherapy

● **53854**   by radiofrequency generated water vapor thermotherapy

53855   Insertion of a temporary prostatic urethral stent, including urethral measurement

(For insertion of permanent urethral stent, use 52282)

Rationale

Code 53854 has been established to report water vapor thermotherapy for the destruction of prostate tissue.

Prior to 2019, there was no code that specifically described destruction of prostate tissue using thermotherapy in the form of water vapor or steam, created by the indirect application of radiofrequency (RF)-generated current to ablate prostate tissue in the treatment of benign prostatic hyperplasia (BPH).

The difference between codes 53852 and 53854 is the way in which RF is applied (direct vs indirect) to create and deliver the thermotherapy energy to the prostate tissue for destruction. Code 53854 includes indirect application of RF energy to create thermotherapy in the form of water vapor or steam applied to the prostate tissue to cause tissue destruction.

Clinical Example (53854)

A 66-year-old male presents with BPH and has difficulty urinating. After discussion of treatment options, he has elected surgical treatment and has decided to proceed with transurethral destruction of prostate tissue using RF-generated water vapor thermotherapy.

Description of Procedure (53854)

Insert water vapor device through urethra under direct vision. Then perform a cystoscopy as the cystoscopy lens is inserted within the thermotherapy device sheath. Evaluate anatomy including that of the urethra, bladder, and prostatic urethra. Position the retractable treatment needle and deploy from the tip of the device through the urethral wall into prostate tissue. Turn on the RF generator to generate thermal energy in the form of water vapor to destroy prostate tissue. After completion of treatment of the first area, retract the treatment needle and reposition for the next application (an average of five treatments are needed depending on the size of the prostate). Pass a catheter and drain the bladder.

Male Genital System

Testis

Excision

(For abdominal perineal gangrene debridement, see 11004-11006)

54500 Biopsy of testis, needle (separate procedure)

▶(For fine needle aspiration biopsy, see 10004, 10005, 10006, 10007, 10008, 10009, 10010, 10011, 10012, 10021)◀

(For evaluation of fine needle aspirate, see 88172, 88173)

Rationale

A parenthetical note following code 54500 (testis biopsy) within the Excision subsection has been revised to direct users to codes 10004-10012 and 10021 for FNA biopsy procedures.

Refer to the codebook and the Rationale for codes 10004-10012 and 10021 for a full discussion of these changes.

Epididymis

Excision

54800 Biopsy of epididymis, needle

▶(For fine needle aspiration biopsy, see 10004, 10005, 10006, 10007, 10008, 10009, 10010, 10011, 10012, 10021)◀

(For evaluation of fine needle aspirate, see 88172, 88173)

54830 Excision of local lesion of epididymis

Rationale

A parenthetical note following code 54800 (epididymis biopsy) within the Excision subsection has been revised to direct users to codes 10004-10012 and 10021 for FNA biopsy procedures.

Refer to the codebook and the Rationale for codes 10004-10012 and 10021 for a full discussion of these changes.

Prostate

Incision

55700 Biopsy, prostate; needle or punch, single or multiple, any approach

(If imaging guidance is performed, see 76942, 77002, 77012, 77021)

▶(For fine needle aspiration biopsy, see 10004, 10005, 10006, 10007, 10008, 10009, 10010, 10011, 10012, 10021)◀

(For evaluation of fine needle aspirate, see 88172, 88173)

(For transperineal stereotactic template guided saturation prostate biopsies, use 55706)

55705 incisional, any approach

Rationale

A parenthetical note following code 55700 (prostate biopsy) within the Incision subsection has been revised to direct users to codes 10004-10012 and 10021 for FNA biopsy procedures.

Refer to the codebook and the Rationale for codes 10004-10012 and 10021 for a full discussion of these changes.

Female Genital System

Vulva, Perineum, and Introitus

Excision

56630 Vulvectomy, radical, partial;

(For skin graft, if used, see 15004-15005, 15120, 15121, 15240, 15241)

56631 with unilateral inguinofemoral lymphadenectomy

56632 with bilateral inguinofemoral lymphadenectomy

▶(For partial radical vulvectomy with inguinofemoral lymph node biopsy without complete inguinofemoral lymphadenectomy, use 56630 in conjunction with 38531)◀

56633 Vulvectomy, radical, complete;

56634 with unilateral inguinofemoral lymphadenectomy

56637 with bilateral inguinofemoral lymphadenectomy

▶(For complete radical vulvectomy with inguinofemoral lymph node biopsy without complete inguinofemoral lymphadenectomy, use 56633 in conjunction with 38531)◀

Surgery / Female Genital System 54000-55980

Rationale

In support of the establishment of the new Category I code 38531, parenthetical notes following codes 56632 and 56637 have been added to direct users to report codes 56630 and 56633 in conjunction with code 38531 for partial and complete radical vulvectomy with inguinofemoral lymph node biopsy without complete inguinofemoral lymphadenectomy.

Refer to the codebook and the Rationale for code 38531 and for a full discussion of these changes.

Endocrine System

Thyroid Gland

Excision

60100   Biopsy thyroid, percutaneous core needle

(If imaging guidance is performed, see 76942, 77002, 77012, 77021)

▶(For fine needle aspiration biopsy, see 10004, 10005, 10006, 10007, 10008, 10009, 10010, 10011, 10012, 10021)◀

(For evaluation of fine needle aspirate, see 88172, 88173)

Rationale

A parenthetical note following code 60100 (thyroid biopsy) within the Excision subsection has been revised to direct users to codes 10004-10012 and 10021 for FNA biopsy procedures.

Refer to the codebook and the Rationale for codes 10004-10012 and 10021 for a full discussion of these changes.

Removal

60300   Aspiration and/or injection, thyroid cyst

▶(For fine needle aspiration biopsy, see 10004, 10005, 10006, 10007, 10008, 10009, 10010, 10011, 10012, 10021)◀

(If imaging guidance is performed, see 76942, 77012)

Rationale

A parenthetical note following code 60300 (aspiration and/or injection of thyroid cyst) within the Removal subsection has been revised to direct users to codes 10004-10012 and 10021 for FNA biopsy procedures.

Refer to the codebook and the Rationale for codes 10004-10012 and 10021 for a full discussion of these changes.

Nervous System

Skull, Meninges, and Brain

Craniectomy or Craniotomy

▶(61332 has been deleted)◀

61333   Exploration of orbit (transcranial approach), with removal of lesion

61340   Subtemporal cranial decompression (pseudotumor cerebri, slit ventricle syndrome)

(For bilateral procedure, report 61340 with modifier 50)

(For decompressive craniotomy or craniectomy for intracranial hypertension, without hematoma evacuation, see 61322, 61323)

61343   Craniectomy, suboccipital with cervical laminectomy for decompression of medulla and spinal cord, with or without dural graft (eg, Arnold-Chiari malformation)

61345   Other cranial decompression, posterior fossa

(For orbital decompression by lateral wall approach, Kroenlein type, use 67445)

61450   Craniectomy, subtemporal, for section, compression, or decompression of sensory root of gasserian ganglion

61458   Craniectomy, suboccipital; for exploration or decompression of cranial nerves

61460   for section of 1 or more cranial nerves

▶(61480 has been deleted)◀

Rationale

To ensure that the CPT code set reflects current clinical practice, codes 61332, *Exploration of orbit (transcranial approach); with biopsy,* and 61480, *Craniectomy, suboccipital; for mesencephalic tractotomy or pedunculotomy,* have been deleted due to low utilization.

Surgery of Skull Base

Definitive Procedures

Base of Middle Cranial Fossa

▶Code 61611 is reported in addition to code(s) for primary procedure(s) 61605-61608. Report only one transection or ligation of carotid artery code per operative session.◀

▶(61610 has been deleted)◀

+ **61611**   Transection or ligation, carotid artery in petrous canal; without repair (List separately in addition to code for primary procedure)

▶(61612 has been deleted)◀

61613   Obliteration of carotid aneurysm, arteriovenous malformation, or carotid-cavernous fistula by dissection within cavernous sinus

Rationale

To ensure that the CPT code set reflects current clinical practice, codes 61610, *Transection or ligation, carotid artery in cavernous sinus, with repair by anastomosis or graft (List separately in addition to code for primary procedure)*, and 61612, *Transection or ligation, carotid artery in petrous canal; with repair by anastomosis or graft (List separately in addition to code for primary procedure)*, have been deleted due to low utilization. In support of the deletion of codes 61610 and 61612, these codes have been removed from the instruction in the guidelines for surgery of skull base/definitive procedures/base of middle cranial fossa.

Endovascular Therapy

61630   Balloon angioplasty, intracranial (eg, atherosclerotic stenosis), percutaneous

61635   Transcatheter placement of intravascular stent(s), intracranial (eg, atherosclerotic stenosis), including balloon angioplasty, if performed

▶(61630 and 61635 include all selective vascular catheterization of the target vascular territory, all diagnostic imaging for arteriography of the target vascular territory, and all related radiological supervision and interpretation. When diagnostic arteriogram (including imaging and selective catheterization) confirms the need for angioplasty or stent placement, 61630 and 61635 are inclusive of these services. If angioplasty or stenting are not indicated, then the appropriate codes for selective catheterization and imaging should be reported in lieu of 61630 and 61635)◀

(Do not report 61630 or 61635 in conjunction with 61645 for the same vascular territory)

(For definition of vascular territory, see the Nervous System Endovascular Therapy guidelines)

61640   Balloon dilatation of intracranial vasospasm, percutaneous; initial vessel

+▲ **61641**   each additional vessel in same vascular territory (List separately in addition to code for primary procedure)

+▲ **61642**   each additional vessel in different vascular territory (List separately in addition to code for primary procedure)

(Use 61641 and 61642 in conjunction with 61640)

(61640, 61641, 61642 include all selective vascular catheterization of the target vessel, contrast injection[s], vessel measurement, roadmapping, postdilatation angiography, and fluoroscopic guidance for the balloon dilatation)

(Do not report 61640, 61642 in conjunction with 61650 or 61651 for the same vascular territory)

(For definition of vascular territory, see the Nervous System Endovascular Therapy guidelines)

Rationale

An editorial revision has been made to two descriptors for codes within the Nervous System/Endovascular Therapy subsection. The term "family" in codes 61641 and 61642 has been replaced with "territory" for accuracy and to better describe the area of attention for the service. In addition, the parenthetical note following code 61635 has been similarly revised to reflect "territory" instead of "family."

Refer to the codebook and the Rationale within Appendix L for a full description of these changes regarding vascular branching.

Neurostimulators (Intracranial)

▶For electronic analysis with programming, when performed, of cranial nerve and brain neurostimulator pulse generator/transmitters, see codes 95970, 95976, 95977, 95983, 95984. Test stimulation to confirm correct target site placement of the electrode array(s) and/or to confirm the functional status of the system is inherent to placement and is not separately reported as electronic analysis or programming of the neurostimulator system. Electronic analysis (95970) at the time of implantation is not separately reported.◄

Microelectrode recording, when performed by the operating surgeon in association with implantation of neurostimulator electrode arrays, is an inclusive service and should not be reported separately. If another individual participates in neurophysiological mapping during a deep brain stimulator implantation procedure, this service may be reported by the second individual with codes 95961-95962.

61850   Twist drill or burr hole(s) for implantation of neurostimulator electrodes, cortical

Rationale

The guidelines listed within the Neurostimulators (Intracranial) subsection have been revised in conjunction with changes made for neurostimulator services. This includes the addition of language that electronic analysis (95970) performed at the time that the device is implanted is not reported separately in conjunction with the placement procedure because the test stimulation to confirm correct target site placement of electrode array(s) and/or to confirm the functional status of the system is inherent to placement.

Refer to the codebook and the Rationale for codes 95970-95972 and 95976-95984 for a full discussion of these changes.

Spine and Spinal Cord

Injection, Drainage, or Aspiration

62267   Percutaneous aspiration within the nucleus pulposus, intervertebral disc, or paravertebral tissue for diagnostic purposes

(For imaging, use 77003)

▶(Do not report 62267 in conjunction with 10005, 10006, 10007, 10008, 10009, 10010, 10011, 10012, 20225, 62287, 62290, 62291)◄

62268   Percutaneous aspiration, spinal cord cyst or syrinx

(For radiological supervision and interpretation, see 76942, 77002, 77012)

62269   Biopsy of spinal cord, percutaneous needle

(For radiological supervision and interpretation, see 76942, 77002, 77012)

▶(For fine needle aspiration biopsy, see 10004, 10005, 10006, 10007, 10008, 10009, 10010, 10011, 10012, 10021)◄

(For evaluation of fine needle aspirate, see 88172, 88173)

Rationale

Parenthetical notes following codes 62267 and 62269 (spine and spinal cord procedures) within the Injection, Drainage, or Aspiration subsection have been revised to direct users to codes 10004-10012 and 10021 for FNA biopsy procedures.

Refer to the codebook and the Rationale for codes 10004-10012 and 10021 for a full discussion of these changes.

Stereotaxis

63610   Stereotactic stimulation of spinal cord, percutaneous, separate procedure not followed by other surgery

▶(63615 has been deleted)◄

Rationale

To ensure that the CPT code set reflects current clinical practice, code 63615, *Stereotactic biopsy, aspiration, or excision of lesion, spinal cord,* has been deleted due to low utilization.

Neurostimulators (Spinal)

▶For electronic analysis with programming, when performed, of spinal cord neurostimulator pulse generator/transmitters, see codes 95970, 95971, 95972. Test stimulation to confirm correct target site placement of the electrode array(s) and/or to confirm the functional status of the system is inherent to placement, and is not separately reported as electronic analysis or programming of the neurostimulator system. Electronic analysis (95970) at the time of implantation is not separately reported.◄

Codes 63650, 63655, and 63661-63664 describe the operative placement, revision, replacement, or removal of the spinal neurostimulator system components to provide spinal electrical stimulation. A neurostimulator system includes an implanted neurostimulator, external controller, extension, and collection of contacts. Multiple contacts or electrodes (4 or more) provide the actual electrical stimulation in the epidural space.

For percutaneously placed neurostimulator systems (63650, 63661, 63663), the contacts are on a catheter-like lead. An array defines the collection of contacts that are on one catheter.

For systems placed via an open surgical exposure (63655, 63662, 63664), the contacts are on a plate or paddle-shaped surface.

Do not report 63661 or 63663 when removing or replacing a temporary percutaneously placed array for an external generator.

63650 Percutaneous implantation of neurostimulator electrode array, epidural

63688 Revision or removal of implanted spinal neurostimulator pulse generator or receiver

►(For electronic analysis with programming, when performed, of implanted spinal cord neurostimulator pulse generator/transmitter, see 95970, 95971, 95972)◄

Rationale

The guidelines within the Neurostimulators (Spinal) subsection of the Nervous System (Spine and Spinal Cord) listing have been revised in conjunction with changes made to neurostimulator services. This includes the addition of language that notes that electronic analysis (95970) performed at the time that the device is implanted is not reported separately in conjunction with the placement procedure because test stimulation to confirm correct target site placement of electrode array(s) and/or to confirm the functional status of the system is inherent to placement. It also includes revision to the guideline language and parenthetical note that follows code 63688 to more specifically reference "programming when performed" and "spinal cord." In addition, "system" has been changed to "transmitter" in the revised parenthetical note so that it is congruent with other neurostimulator codes.

Refer to the codebook and the Rationale for codes 95970-95972 and 95976-95984 for a full discussion of these changes.

Extracranial Nerves, Peripheral Nerves, and Autonomic Nervous System

Introduction/Injection of Anesthetic Agent (Nerve Block), Diagnostic or Therapeutic

Autonomic Nerves

64505 Injection, anesthetic agent; sphenopalatine ganglion

►(64508 has been deleted)◄

64510 stellate ganglion (cervical sympathetic)

Rationale

To ensure that the CPT code set reflects current clinical practice, code 64508, *Injection, anesthetic agent; carotid sinus (separate procedure),* has been deleted due to low utilization.

Neurostimulators (Peripheral Nerve)

►For electronic analysis with programming, when performed, of peripheral nerve neurostimulator pulse generator/transmitters, see codes 95970, 95971, 95972. An electrode array is a catheter or other device with more than one contact. The function of each contact may be capable of being adjusted during programming services. Test stimulation to confirm correct target site placement of the electrode array(s) and/or to confirm the functional status of the system is inherent to placement, and is not separately reported as electronic analysis or programming of the neurostimulator system. Electronic analysis (95970) at the time of implantation is not separately reported.◄

Rationale

The guidelines within the Neurostimulators (Peripheral Nerve) subsection have been revised in conjunction with changes made to neurostimulator services. This includes addition of language that notes that electronic analysis (95970) performed at the time that the device is implanted is not reported separately in conjunction with the placement procedure because test stimulation to confirm correct target site placement of electrode array(s) and/or to confirm the functional status of the system is inherent to placement. It also includes revision to the guidelines to specify "peripheral nerve," addition of codes 95971 and 95972 as codes that are used for reporting peripheral nerve programming, and removal of deleted code 95975 from the guidelines.

Refer to the codebook and the Rationale for codes 95970-95972 and 95976-95984 for a full discussion of these changes.

▶Codes 64553, 64555, and 64561 may be used to report both temporary and permanent placement of percutaneous electrode arrays.◀

▶(64550 has been deleted)◀

▶(For transcutaneous nerve stimulation [TENS], use 97014 for electrical stimulation requiring supervision only or use 97032 for electrical stimulation requiring constant attendance)◀

64553 Percutaneous implantation of neurostimulator electrode array; cranial nerve

(For percutaneous electrical stimulation of a cranial nerve using needle[s] or needle electrode[s] [eg, PENS, PNT], use 64999)

(For open placement of cranial nerve (eg, vagus, trigeminal) neurostimulator pulse generator or receiver, see 61885, 61886, as appropriate)

Rationale

Code 64550, which describes application of surface (transcutaneous) neurostimulator, has been deleted and a deletion parenthetical note has been added, as a result.

To ensure that the CPT code set reflects current practice, code 64550 has been deleted due to misreporting. In addition, two instructional parenthetical notes have been added: one note in the Surgery section and another in the Medicine section—both of which directs users to report code 97014 for supervision of electrical stimulation or code 97032 for electrical stimulation requiring constant attendance.

Eye and Ocular Adnexa

Anterior Segment

Anterior Sclera

Repair or Revision

(For scleral procedures in retinal surgery, see 67101 et seq)

▶(66220 has been deleted)◀

66225 Repair of scleral staphyloma with graft

(For scleral reinforcement, see 67250, 67255)

Rationale

To ensure that the CPT code set reflects current clinical practice, code 66220, *Repair of scleral staphyloma; without graft,* has been deleted due to low utilization. Because of the deletion of code 66220, its child code 66225, *Repair of scleral staphyloma with graft,* has become a parent code and now states "with graft."

Posterior Segment

Posterior Sclera

Repair

(For excision lesion sclera, use 66130)

67250 Scleral reinforcement (separate procedure); without graft

67255 with graft

(Do not report 67255 in conjunction with 66180, 66185)

▶(For repair scleral staphyloma, use 66225)◀

Ocular Adnexa

Orbit

Exploration, Excision, Decompression

67420 Orbitotomy with bone flap or window, lateral approach (eg, Kroenlein); with removal of lesion

67430 with removal of foreign body

67440 with drainage

67445 with removal of bone for decompression

(For optic nerve sheath decompression, use 67570)

★=Telemedicine   ╋=Add-on code   ✎=FDA approval pending   #=Resequenced code   ⊘=Modifier 51 exempt

67450   for exploration, with or without biopsy

▶(For orbitotomy, transcranial approach, see 61330, 61333)◀

(For orbital implant, see 67550, 67560)

(For removal of eyeball or for repair after removal, see 65091-65175)

Rationale

In support of the deletion of code 61332, the cross-reference parenthetical note following code 67450 regarding transcranial approach orbitotomy has been revised with the removal of code 61332.

Refer to the codebook and the Rationale for code 61332 for a full discussion of these changes.

Eyelids

Incision

 # 67810   Incisional biopsy of eyelid skin including lid margin

▶(For biopsy of skin of the eyelid, see 11102, 11103, 11104, 11105, 11106, 11107)◀

Rationale

In support of the establishment of codes for tangential, punch, and incisional biopsies (11102, 11103, 11104, 11105, 11106, 11107), the parenthetical note following code 67810 has been revised.

Refer to the codebook and the Rationale for codes 11102, 11103, 11104, 11105, 11106, and 11107 for a full discussion of these changes.

Surgery / Eye and Ocular Adnexa 65091-68899

Notes

Radiology

The most substantial change to the Radiology section is the addition of new codes and reporting instructions for various X-ray services. Significant changes to the Diagnostic Radiology subsection include deletion of code 76001 (fluoroscopy) due to low utilization. Five new codes (76978, 76979, 76981, 76982, 76983) have been added for reporting ultrasound examinations. In addition, two codes (77058, 77059 [magnetic resonance imaging]) have been deleted due to the addition of codes 77046, 77047, 77048, 77049 (magnetic resonance imaging of the breast). Furthermore, revisions of parenthetical notes to accommodate the use of the new codes have been made.

In support of the revisions made to other Imaging Guidance sections throughout the code set, the "Supervision and Interpretation" heading has been revised to "Supervision and Interpretation, Imaging Guidance." To clarify the appropriate use of imaging guidance, as well as radiological supervision and interpretation (RS&I) codes, new guidelines have been added to the Supervision and Interpretation section as well. The other revision in the Radiology section involves the revision of the guidelines for written reports, which now includes imaging services.

Overall, many changes have been made to the exclusionary parenthetical notes and cross-references to include reporting instructions for various guidance services in the Diagnostic Ultrasound section.

Summary of Additions, Deletions, and Revisions

The summary of changes shows the actual changes that have been made to the code descriptors.

New codes appear with a bullet (●) and are indicated as "Code added." Revised codes are preceded with a triangle (▲). Within revised codes, or if a code symbol has been deleted, the deleted language and code symbol appears with a strikethrough (⊖), while new text appears underlined.

The ✗ symbol is used to identify codes for vaccines that are pending FDA approval. The # symbol is used to identify codes that have been resequenced. CPT add-on codes are annotated by the + symbol. The ⊘ symbol is used to identify codes that are exempt from the use of modifier 51. The ★ symbol is used to identify codes that may be used for reporting telemedicine services. The ✕ is used to identify proprietary laboratory analyses (PLA) test that has an identical descriptor as another PLA test.

Code	Description
▲74485	Dilation of ~~nephrostomy, ureters,~~ ureter(s) or urethra, radiological supervision and interpretation
~~76001~~	~~Fluoroscopy, physician or other qualified health care professional time more than 1 hour, assisting a nonradiologic physician or other qualified health care professional (eg, nephrostolithotomy, ERCP, bronchoscopy, transbronchial biopsy)~~
●76391	Code added
●76978	Code added
+●76979	Code added
●76981	Code added
●76982	Code added
+●76983	Code added

▲ = Revised code   ● = New code   ▶ ◀ = Contains new or revised text   ✕ = Duplicate PLA test

Code	Description
▲77021	Magnetic resonance <u>imaging</u> guidance for needle placement (eg, for biopsy, needle aspiration, injection, or placement of localization device) radiological supervision and interpretation
▲77022	Magnetic resonance <u>imaging</u> guidance for, and monitoring of, parenchymal tissue ablation
●77046	Code added
●77047	Code added
●77048	Code added
●77049	Code added
~~77058~~	~~Magnetic resonance imaging, breast, without and/or with contrast material(s); unilateral~~
~~77059~~	~~bilateral~~
#▲77387	Guidance for localization of target volume for delivery of radiation treatment ~~delivery~~, includes intrafraction tracking, when performed
~~78270~~	~~Vitamin B-12 absorption study (eg, Schilling test); without intrinsic factor~~
~~78271~~	~~with intrinsic factor~~
~~78272~~	~~Vitamin B-12 absorption studies combined, with and without intrinsic factor~~

★=Telemedicine   ✚=Add-on code   ✔=FDA approval pending   #=Resequenced code   ⊘=Modifier 51 exempt

Radiology Guidelines (Including Nuclear Medicine and Diagnostic Ultrasound)

Guidelines to direct general reporting of services are presented in the **Introduction.** Some of the commonalities are repeated here for the convenience of those referring to this section on **Radiology (Including Nuclear Medicine and Diagnostic Ultrasound).** Other definitions and items unique to Radiology are also listed.

▶Supervision and Interpretation, Imaging Guidance◀

▶Imaging may be required during the performance of certain procedures or certain imaging procedures may require surgical procedures to access the imaged area. Many services include image guidance, and imaging guidance is not separately reportable when it is included in the base service. CPT typically defines in descriptors and/or guidelines when imaging guidance is included. When imaging is not included in a surgical procedure or procedure from the **Medicine** section, image guidance codes or codes labeled "radiological supervision and interpretation" (RS&I) may be reported for the portion of the service that requires imaging. All imaging guidance codes require: (1) image documentation in the patient record and (2) description of imaging guidance in the procedure report. All RS&I codes require: (1) image documentation in the patient's permanent record and (2) a procedure report or separate imaging report that includes written documentation of interpretive findings of information contained in the images and radiologic supervision of the service.

(The RS&I codes are not applicable to the Radiation Oncology subsection.)◀

Written Report(s)

A written report (eg, handwritten or electronic) signed by the interpreting individual should be considered an integral part of a radiologic procedure or interpretation.

▶With regard to CPT descriptors for imaging services, "images" must contain anatomic information unique to the patient for which the imaging service is provided. "Images" refer to those acquired in either an analog (ie, film) or digital (ie, electronic) manner.◀

Radiology

Diagnostic Radiology (Diagnostic Imaging)

Chest

(For fluoroscopic or ultrasonic guidance for needle placement procedures (eg, biopsy, aspiration, injection, localization device) of the thorax, see 76942, 77002)

►(71023 has been deleted. To report, see 71046, 76000)◄

(71030 has been deleted. To report, use 71048)

►(71034 has been deleted. To report, see 71048, 76000)◄

(71035 has been deleted. To report, see 71046, 71047, 71048)

Rationale

In accordance with the deletion of code 76001, the parenthetical notes in the Diagnostic Radiology subsection have been revised to reflect the removal of code 76001.

Refer to the codebook and the Rationale for code 76001 for a full discussion of these changes.

71550 Magnetic resonance (eg, proton) imaging, chest (eg, for evaluation of hilar and mediastinal lymphadenopathy); without contrast material(s)

71551 with contrast material(s)

71552 without contrast material(s), followed by contrast material(s) and further sequences

►(For breast MRI, see 77046, 77047, 77048, 77049)◄

Rationale

In support of the establishment of four new codes (77046, 77047, 77048, 77049) to report magnetic resonance imaging of the breast, the parenthetical note following code 71552 has been revised.

Refer to the codebook and the Rationale for codes 77046, 77047, 77048, and 77049 for a full discussion of these changes.

Spine and Pelvis

72275 Epidurography, radiological supervision and interpretation

(72275 includes 77003)

(For injection procedure, see 62280, 62281, 62282, 62320, 62321, 62322, 62323, 62324, 62325, 62326, 62327, 64479, 64480, 64483, 64484)

(Use 72275 only when an epidurogram is performed, images documented, and a formal radiologic report is issued)

►(Do not report 72275 in conjunction with 22586)◄

Rationale

In accordance with the deletion of Category III codes 0195T and 0196T, the parenthetical note referencing these codes following code 72275 has been updated to reflect these deletions.

Refer to the codebook and the Rationale for codes 0195T and 0196T for a full discussion of these changes.

Urinary Tract

▲ **74485** Dilation of ureter(s) or urethra, radiological supervision and interpretation

►(Do not report 74485 in conjunction with 50436, 50437)◄

(For dilation of ureter without radiologic guidance, use 52341, 52344)

(For change of nephrostomy or pyelostomy tube, use 50435)

►(For dilation of a nephrostomy tract for endourologic procedure, see 50436, 50437)◄

Rationale

Code 74485 has been revised with the deletion of "nephrostomy" from the descriptor and revision of "ureter" to "ureter(s)." In addition, two parenthetical notes have been added following code 74485: (1) to restrict reporting of code 74485 in conjunction with procedures that include dilation of a tract; and (2) to direct users to the appropriate codes to report dilation of the nephrostomy tract (50436, 50437).

Refer to the codebook and the Rationale for codes 50436 and 50437 for a full discussion of these changes.

Clinical Example (74485)

A 66-year-old male with a ureteral stricture undergoes dilation of the ureter with imaging. Radiologic supervision and interpretation (RS&I) of images is done during and immediately following dilation.

Description of Procedure (74485)

Interpret pre- and post-dilation imaging, making note of response to treatment, potential complications, and fluoroscopy time.

Other Procedures

(For computed tomography cerebral perfusion analysis, see Category III code 0042T)

(For arthrography of shoulder, use 73040; elbow, use 73085; wrist, use 73115; hip, use 73525; knee, use 73580; ankle, use 73615)

76000 Fluoroscopy (separate procedure), up to 1 hour physician or other qualified health care professional time

▶(Do not report 76000 in conjunction with 33274, 33275, 33957, 33958, 33959, 33962, 33963, 33964, 0515T, 0516T, 0517T, 0518T, 0519T, 0520T)◀

Rationale

In support of the development of codes 33274, 33275 (transcatheter insertion or replacement of a permanent leadless pacemaker) and codes 0515T-0520T (insertion, removal, and/or replacement of wireless cardiac stimulation components), these new codes have been added to the exclusionary cross-reference note that follows code 76000. The note restricts reporting fluoroscopy in conjunction with the new codes because the new services include image guidance required to complete a transcatheter pacemaker placement and wireless cardiac stimulator procedures.

Refer to the codebook and the Rationale for codes 33274, 33275, and 0515T-0520T for a full discussion of these changes.

▶(76001 has been deleted)◀

76010 Radiologic examination from nose to rectum for foreign body, single view, child

Rationale

Code 76001 has been deleted due to low utilization. The deletion of 76001 ensures that the CPT code set reflects current clinical practice.

76376 3D rendering with interpretation and reporting of computed tomography, magnetic resonance imaging, ultrasound, or other tomographic modality with image postprocessing under concurrent supervision; not requiring image postprocessing on an independent workstation

(Use 76376 in conjunction with code[s] for base imaging procedure[s])

▶(Do not report 76376 in conjunction with 31627, 34839, 70496, 70498, 70544, 70545, 70546, 70547, 70548, 70549, 71275, 71555, 72159, 72191, 72198, 73206, 73225, 73706, 73725, 74174, 74175, 74185, 74261, 74262, 74263, 75557, 75559, 75561, 75563, 75565, 75571, 75572, 75573, 75574, 75635, 76377, 77046, 77047, 77048, 77049, 77061, 77062, 77063, 78012-78999, 93355, 0523T)◀

76377 requiring image postprocessing on an independent workstation

(Use 76377 in conjunction with code[s] for base imaging procedure[s])

▶(Do not report 76377 in conjunction with 34839, 70496, 70498, 70544, 70545, 70546, 70547, 70548, 70549, 71275, 71555, 72159, 72191, 72198, 73206, 73225, 73706, 73725, 74174, 74175, 74185, 74261, 74262, 74263, 75557, 75559, 75561, 75563, 75565, 75571, 75572, 75573, 75574, 75635, 76376, 77046, 77047, 77048, 77049, 77061, 77062, 77063, 78012-78999, 93355, 0523T)◀

(76376, 76377 require concurrent supervision of image postprocessing 3D manipulation of volumetric data set and image rendering)

Rationale

Three codes (77058, 77059, 0159T) have been deleted and replaced with four new codes (77046, 77047, 77048, 77049) to report magnetic resonance imaging of the breast. As part of these revisions, the parenthetical notes following codes 76376 and 76377 have been revised to reflect the deletion of code 0159T and the addition of codes 77046, 77047, 77048, 77049. A new code to report noninvasive intraprocedural coronary fractional flow reserve (FFR) derived from angiogram data (0523T) has also been added to the parenthetical notes.

Refer to the codebook and the Rationale for codes 77046, 77047, 77048, 77049, and 0523T for a full discussion of these changes.

76390   Magnetic resonance spectroscopy

(For magnetic resonance imaging, use appropriate MRI body site code)

● **76391**   Magnetic resonance (eg, vibration) elastography

Rationale

Code 76391 has been established to report magnetic resonance elastography (MRE). MRE is a new diagnostic imaging technology that uses propagating mechanical shear waves to quantitatively image the mechanical properties of tissue and provides a quantitative counterpart to the traditional diagnostic technique of palpation. MRE requires the use of a magnetic resonance imaging (MRI) scanner, with specially modified hardware and software, to generate and image micron-level vibrations.

MRE requires (1) a mechanical driver system for generating propagating shear waves in the region of the body to be evaluated; (2) special phase-contrast MRE pulse sequences to allow the micron-level vibrations to be imaged; and (3) specialized processing software to analyze the wave patterns. Diagnostic MRE images (elastograms) quantitatively map the shear modulus of tissue in kilopascals. While MRE shares some of the technical principles of ultrasonography-based quantitative shear wave elastography, MRE technology is not limited by the requirement of an acoustic window and can evaluate tissues of large regions in all parts of the body, including those enclosed by bone, such as the intracranial region. MRE is applied to assess a variety of tissues, ranging from stiffness from lung to cartilage, to quantitatively imaging the mechanical properties of skeletal muscle, and gray and white matter in the brain, thyroid, kidney, and skin.

Clinical Example (76391)

A 55-year-old male with a body mass index (BMI) of 38 presents with fatigue. Lab testing shows elevated lipids and alanine aminotransferase (ALT). Recent abdominal ultrasonography showed evidence of hepatic steatosis. The patient's qualified health care professional is concerned that the patient may have progressed to non-alcoholic steatohepatitis and magnetic resonance (MR) elastography is performed as a noninvasive measure of liver fibrosis.

Description of Procedure (76391)

Review obtained scout views of area to image; select appropriate field of view; and confirm adequate position of passive driver relative to the organ to be evaluated. Review obtained MR elastography sequences for position of passive driver, adequacy of wave propagation, and artifacts, and repeat sequences and passive driver positioning as needed. Manually postprocess the elastogram images. Interpret all sequences resulting from the study and postprocessed data including any additional anatomy imaged that is not the organ of interest. Compare to all pertinent available prior examinations. Dictate report for medical record.

Diagnostic Ultrasound

Ultrasonic Guidance Procedures

+ **76937**   Ultrasound guidance for vascular access requiring ultrasound evaluation of potential access sites, documentation of selected vessel patency, concurrent realtime ultrasound visualization of vascular needle entry, with permanent recording and reporting (List separately in addition to code for primary procedure)

▶(Do not report 76937 in conjunction with 33274, 33275, 36568, 36569, 36572, 36573, 36584, 37191, 37192, 37193, 37760, 37761, 76942)◀

Rationale

In support of the establishment of codes 33274, 33275, 36572, and 36573, and the revision of codes 36568, 36569, and 36584, the first exclusionary parenthetical note following code 76937 has been revised to include these codes.

Refer to the codebook and the Rationale for codes 33274, 33275, 36568, 36569, 36572, 36573, and 36584 for a full discussion of these changes.

★ = Telemedicine   ✚ = Add-on code   ✗ = FDA approval pending   # = Resequenced code   ⊘ = Modifier 51 exempt

▶(Do not report 76937 in conjunction with 0505T for ultrasound guidance for vascular access)◀

(If extremity venous non-invasive vascular diagnostic study is performed separate from venous access guidance, see 93970, 93971)

Rationale

In support of the establishment of code 0505T, a new exclusionary parenthetical note has been added following code 76937 precluding its use with 0505T for ultrasound guidance for vascular access.

Refer to the codebook and the Rationale for code 0505T for a full discussion of these changes.

76942   Ultrasonic guidance for needle placement (eg, biopsy, aspiration, injection, localization device), imaging supervision and interpretation

▶(Do not report 76942 in conjunction with 10004, 10005, 10006, 10021, 10030, 19083, 19285, 20604, 20606, 20611, 27096, 32554, 32555, 32556, 32557, 37760, 37761, 43232, 43237, 43242, 45341, 45342, 55874, 64479, 64480, 64483, 64484, 64490, 64491, 64493, 64494, 64495, 76975, 0213T, 0214T, 0215T, 0216T, 0217T, 0218T, 0228T, 0229T, 0230T, 0231T, 0232T, 0249T, 0481T)◀

(For harvesting, preparation, and injection[s] of platelet rich plasma, use 0232T)

Rationale

A parenthetical note has been revised within the Ultrasonic Guidance Procedures subsection for radiology (diagnostic ultrasound) procedures following code 76942 to direct users to the new and revised codes to report fine needle aspiration (FNA) biopsy procedures (10004-10006, 10021).

Refer to the codebook and the Rationale for codes 10004-10012 and 10021 for a full discussion of these changes.

Other Procedures

76977   Ultrasound bone density measurement and interpretation, peripheral site(s), any method

● **76978**   Ultrasound, targeted dynamic microbubble sonographic contrast characterization (non-cardiac); initial lesion

+● **76979**   each additional lesion with separate injection (List separately in addition to code for primary procedure)

▶(Use 76979 in conjunction with 76978)◀

▶(Do not report 76978, 76979 in conjunction with 96374)◀

Rationale

Two new codes (76978, 76979) have been established to report noncardiac ultrasound, targeted dynamic microbubble sonographic contrast characterization. In addition, new parenthetical notes have been added to clarify the reporting of these services. Dynamic microbubble sonographic contrast using targeted ultrasound is an ultrasound procedure that allows accurate reporting of the procedure used for dynamic evaluation and enhancement of a lesion with the use of microbubble technology.

Microbubble sonographic contrast agents enhance sonographic reflection and allow vascularity of masses/organs to be assessed. The contrast agents break down and are exhaled through the lungs rather than the kidneys, as is the case with iodinated compound. Hence, there is no risk of renal toxicity. They are chemically unrelated to either gadolinium compounds or iodinated contrast.

Code 76978 describes targeted dynamic microbubble sonographic contrast evaluation performed of a lesion previously demonstrated on a diagnostic imaging study. Code 76979 is an add-on code, so it should not be reported as a stand-alone code. Code 76979 describes targeted dynamic microbubble sonographic contrast evaluation of each additional lesion previously demonstrated on a diagnostic imaging study. In addition, it can only be reported if a separate injection is performed during evaluation of each additional lesion.

A parenthetical note has been added precluding the use of codes 76978 and 76979 with 96374. Code 96374, *Therapeutic, prophylactic, or diagnostic injection (specify substance or drug); intravenous push, single or initial substance/drug,* is not reported separately because it is inherently included as part of microbubble sonographic contrast evaluation (76978, 76979).

Clinical Example (76978)

A 27-year-old female has abnormal liver enzymes. An abdominal ultrasound performed several days earlier demonstrated a fatty liver and a 2-cm hypoechoic mass in the right hepatic lobe. Targeted dynamic ultrasound microbubble sonographic contrast evaluation is performed for lesion characterization.

Description of Procedure (76978)

Position patient and prepare with physician guidance. Perform a targeted ultrasound to identify the lesion previously demonstrated on a diagnostic imaging study.

Radiology 70010-79999

Under physician direction, activate the contrast imaging mode on the ultrasound machine. Physician injects an appropriate bolus of microbubble sonographic contrast followed by a rapid saline flush. Physician performs concurrent ultrasound evaluation of the lesion while scanning or while the ultrasound technologist scans the patient. Additional contrast injection and scanning is performed as needed for initial lesion characterization (typically, lesion characterization requires two or three injections). Obtain permanent static ultrasound images and cine clips during the wash-in, equilibrium, and wash-out phases. Review and interpret saved images and cine clips with comparison to prior imaging studies. Dictate a report.

Clinical Example (76979)

A 42-year-old female with abnormal liver enzymes is found to have two separate solid-appearing liver lesions with different sonographic features in the right and left hepatic lobes on recent abdominal ultrasound. After evaluation and characterization of the right lobe lesion (reported separately), an additional targeted dynamic microbubble sonographic contrast evaluation is performed for lesion characterization of the left lobe lesion. (**Note:** This is an add-on service. Only consider the additional work related to targeted dynamic microbubble sonographic contrast evaluation.)

Description of Procedure (76979)

Review prior diagnostic ultrasound or other imaging study on which an additional lesion has been found. If needed, reposition patient and prepare with physician guidance for the additional lesion. Perform a targeted ultrasound to identify the lesion previously demonstrated on a diagnostic imaging study. Under physician direction, activate the contrast imaging mode on the ultrasound machine. Physician injects an appropriate bolus of microbubble sonographic contrast followed by a rapid saline flush. Physician performs concurrent ultrasound evaluation of the lesion while scanning or while the ultrasound technologist scans the patient. Additional contrast injection and scanning is performed as needed for initial lesion characterization (typically, lesion characterization requires two or three injections). Obtain permanent static ultrasound images and cine clips during the wash-in, equilibrium, and wash-out phases. Review and interpret saved images and cine clips with comparison to prior imaging studies. Dictate a report.

● **76981** Ultrasound, elastography; parenchyma (eg, organ)

● **76982** first target lesion

+● **76983** each additional target lesion (List separately in addition to code for primary procedure)

▶(Use 76983 in conjunction with 76982)◀

▶(Report 76981 only once per session for evaluation of the same parenchymal organ)◀

▶(To report shear wave liver elastography without imaging, use 91200)◀

▶(For evaluation of a parenchymal organ and lesion[s] in the same parenchymal organ at the same session, report only 76981)◀

▶(Do not report 76983 more than two times per organ)◀

Rationale

Three new Category I codes (76981, 76982, 76983) have been established to report ultrasound elastography. These new Category I codes have been created because of an increase in usage frequency of code 0346T. Therefore, these new Category I codes are now appropriate to report ultrasound elastography.

Instructional parenthetical notes have been established to instruct the use of these three new codes as well. Category III code 0346T, which was previously used to report ultrasound elastography, has been deleted along with all related cross-references. A parenthetical note following code 91200 has been added to indicate that code 91200 cannot be reported with the new ultrasound elastography codes, as code 91200 is intended to be reported for liver elastography without imaging.

Clinical Example (76981)

A 45-year-old male has a history of chronic hepatitis C for 15 years. The patient has had no significant complications secondary to portal hypertension and routine ultrasounds of the liver has been normal, with no imaging evidence of cirrhosis. The patient is being considered for definitive treatment for the hepatitis C and undergoes an ultrasound elastogram of the liver to determine the existing, baseline degree of hepatic fibrosis.

Description of Procedure (76981)

Review obtained ultrasound elastography images at the picture archiving and communication system (PACS) workstation. The anatomic images and elastography images are analyzed by the radiologist. If additional images are required, this is communicated to the technologist. The radiologist interprets all images and evaluates stiffness measurements of the parenchyma of interest. The current examination is compared to any prior examinations to evaluate for stability or interval changes. The radiologist dictates the examination report.

Clinical Example (76982)

A 45-year-old female undergoes mammography for a right breast mass. A diagnostic ultrasound demonstrates a solid hypoechoic mass at 10:00 location. Ultrasound elastography of the right breast mass is performed (reported separately) to characterize the lesion.

Description of Procedure (76982)

Review obtained ultrasound elastography images at the PACS workstation. The anatomic images and elastography images are analyzed by the radiologist. If additional images of the first target lesion are required, this is communicated to the technologist. The radiologist interprets all images and evaluates stiffness measurements of the lesion of interest. The current examination is compared to any prior examinations to evaluate for stability or interval changes. The radiologist dictates the examination report.

Clinical Example (76983)

A 52-year-old female undergoes mammography for bilateral breast masses. A diagnostic ultrasound demonstrates bilateral solid hypoechoic masses. Ultrasound elastography of the left breast mass is performed after prior ultrasound elastography of the right breast mass (reported separately) to characterize the additional lesion. (List separately in addition to code for primary procedure.)

Description of Procedure (76983)

Review the request for appropriateness and discuss with ordering physician. Review clinical history. Review prior diagnostic ultrasound or other imaging study on which additional lesion of interest is found. Communicate with ultrasound technologist to delineate additional lesion to be interrogated and any structures to be avoided. The obtained ultrasound elastography images are reviewed at the PACS workstation. The anatomic images and elastography images are analyzed by the radiologist. If additional images of the additional target lesion are required, this is communicated to the technologist. The radiologist interprets all images and evaluates stiffness measurements of the lesion of interest. The current examination is compared to any prior examinations to evaluate for stability or interval changes. The radiologist dictates the examination report. Review, edit, and sign report for the medical record. Communicate the findings with referring provider and/or patient as needed.

76998   Ultrasonic guidance, intraoperative

▶(Do not report 76998 in conjunction with 36475, 36479, 37760, 37761, 47370, 47371, 47380, 47381, 47382, 0249T, 0515T, 0516T, 0517T, 0518T, 0519T, 0520T)◀

(For ultrasound guidance for open and laparoscopic radiofrequency tissue ablation, use 76940)

Rationale

In support of development of codes 0515T-0520T (insertion, removal, and/or replacement of wireless cardiac stimulation components), these codes have been added to the exclusionary cross-reference note that follows code 76998. The note restricts the reporting of ultrasonic guidance in conjunction with codes 0515T-0520T because these new codes include image guidance required to complete a wireless cardiac stimulator procedure.

Refer to the codebook and the Rationale for codes 0515T-0520T for a full discussion of these changes.

Radiologic Guidance

Fluoroscopic Guidance

(Do not report guidance codes 77001, 77002, 77003 for services in which fluoroscopic guidance is included in the descriptor)

+ **77001**   Fluoroscopic guidance for central venous access device placement, replacement (catheter only or complete), or removal (includes fluoroscopic guidance for vascular access and catheter manipulation, any necessary contrast injections through access site or catheter with related venography radiologic supervision and interpretation, and radiographic documentation of final catheter position) (List separately in addition to code for primary procedure)

▶(Do not report 77001 in conjunction with 33957, 33958, 33959, 33962, 33963, 33964, 36568, 36569, 36572, 36573, 36584, 77002)◀

(If formal extremity venography is performed from separate venous access and separately interpreted, use 36005 and 75820, 75822, 75825, or 75827)

Rationale

In support of the addition of codes 36572 and 36573, and the revision of codes 36568, 36569, and 36584, the exclusionary parenthetical note following code 77001 has been revised to include these codes.

Refer to the codebook and the Rationale for codes 36568, 36569, 36572, 36573, and 36584 for a full discussion of these changes.

+ 77002 Fluoroscopic guidance for needle placement (eg, biopsy, aspiration, injection, localization device) (List separately in addition to code for primary procedure)

(See appropriate surgical code for procedure and anatomic location)

▶(Use 77002 in conjunction with 10160, 20206, 20220, 20225, 20520, 20525, 20526, 20550, 20551, 20552, 20553, 20555, 20600, 20605, 20610, 20612, 20615, 21116, 21550, 23350, 24220, 25246, 27093, 27095, 27369, 27648, 32400, 32405, 32553, 36002, 38220, 38221, 38222, 38505, 38794, 41019, 42400, 42405, 47000, 47001, 48102, 49180, 49411, 50200, 50390, 51100, 51101, 51102, 55700, 55876, 60100, 62268, 62269, 64505, 64600, 64605)◀

(77002 is included in all arthrography radiological supervision and interpretation codes. See **Administration of Contrast Material[s]** introductory guidelines for reporting of arthrography procedures)

Rationale

In accordance with the deletion of codes 10022, 27370, and 64508, the parenthetical note following code 77002 has been revised with the removal of these codes and the addition of 27369. Refer to the codebook and the Rationale for codes 10004-10012, 10021, 27369, and 64508 for a full discussion of these changes.

The parenthetical note following code 77002 has also been revised to indicate that code 38222 may be reported in conjunction with code 77002. The procedure identified by code 38222 does not inherently include fluoroscopic guidance for needle placement. As a result, if fluoroscopic guidance is used for this biopsy service, it should be reported with code 77002 in addition to code 38222. To reflect this, code 38222 has been included within the instructional parenthetical note following that code.

Computed Tomography Guidance

77011 Computed tomography guidance for stereotactic localization

77012 Computed tomography guidance for needle placement (eg, biopsy, aspiration, injection, localization device), radiological supervision and interpretation

▶(Do not report 77011, 77012 in conjunction with 22586)◀

Rationale

In accordance with the deletion of Category III codes 0195T and 0196T, the parenthetical note referencing these codes following code 77012 has been updated to reflect these deletions.

Refer to the codebook and the Rationale for codes 0195T and 0196T for a full discussion of these changes.

▶(Do not report 77012 in conjunction with 10009, 10010, 10030, 27096, 32554, 32555, 32556, 32557, 64479, 64480, 64483, 64484, 64490, 64491, 64492, 64493, 64494, 64495, 64633, 64634, 64635, 64636, 0232T, 0481T)◀

(For harvesting, preparation, and injection[s] of platelet-rich plasma, use 0232T)

Rationale

Parenthetical notes within the Computed Tomography Guidance subsection for radiological guidance procedures have been revised following code 77012 to direct users to the new codes (10009, 10010) to report FNA biopsy procedures.

Refer to the codebook and the Rationale for codes 10004-10012 and 10021 for a full discussion of these changes.

▶Magnetic Resonance Imaging Guidance◀

▲ **77021** Magnetic resonance imaging guidance for needle placement (eg, for biopsy, needle aspiration, injection, or placement of localization device) radiological supervision and interpretation

(For procedure, see appropriate organ or site)

▶(Do not report 77021 in conjunction with 10011, 10012, 10030, 19085, 19287, 32554, 32555, 32556, 32557, 0232T, 0481T)◀

(For harvesting, preparation, and injection[s] of platelet-rich plasma, use 0232T)

▲ **77022** Magnetic resonance imaging guidance for, and monitoring of, parenchymal tissue ablation

(Do not report 77022 in conjunction with 20982, 20983, 32994, 32998, 0071T, 0072T)

(For percutaneous ablation, see 47382, 47383, 50592, 50593)

(For focused ultrasound ablation treatment of uterine leiomyomata, see Category III codes 0071T, 0072T)

★ = Telemedicine   ✚ = Add-on code   ✗ = FDA approval pending   # = Resequenced code   ⊘ = Modifier 51 exempt

(To report stereotactic localization guidance for breast biopsy or for placement of breast localization device[s], see 19081, 19283)

(To report mammographic guidance for placement of breast localization device[s], use 19281)

Rationale

Codes 77021 and 77022 have been editorially revised with the addition of "imaging" following "magnetic resonance" in the code descriptors in order to clarify that these are imaging guidance codes. In support of the revision of codes 77021 and 77022, the "Magnetic Resonance" heading has also been revised to "Magnetic Resonance Imaging Guidance."

In addition, the parenthetical note following code 77021 has been revised to include codes 10011 and 10012 for FNA biopsy procedures. Refer to the codebook and the Rationale for codes 10004-10012 and 10021 for a full discussion of these changes.

Breast, Mammography

● **77046**   Magnetic resonance imaging, breast, without contrast material; unilateral

● **77047**   bilateral

● **77048**   Magnetic resonance imaging, breast, without and with contrast material(s), including computer-aided detection (CAD real-time lesion detection, characterization and pharmacokinetic analysis), when performed; unilateral

● **77049**   bilateral

▶(77058 has been deleted. To report, see 77046, 77048)◀

▶(77059 has been deleted. To report, see 77047, 77049)◀

77061   Digital breast tomosynthesis; unilateral

Rationale

Codes 77058 and 77059 have been deleted and replaced with four new codes (77046, 77047, 77048, 77049) to report magnetic resonance imaging of the breast. The revisions have been made to align with the structure of other breast imaging families. With changes in clinical practice, these four new magnetic resonance codes that specify the use of contrast materials and "include computer-aided detection (CAD), when performed" will enable accurate reporting of the specific breast imaging performed.

Clinical Example (77046)

A 67-year-old female who is status post right mastectomy with implant reconstruction and suspected implant rupture.

Description of Procedure (77046)

Interpret images, evaluating implant integrity and for evidence of intra- or extra-capsular implant rupture. Evaluate for etiology of clinical examination findings or abnormalities questioned on previous imaging. Assess the breast tissue for any abnormalities. Evaluate remainder of structures in the visualized anatomy, including axilla, internal mammary lymph node chain, skin, pectoral muscles and chest wall, bones, visualized mediastinum, and upper abdomen. Compare the current imaging to all pertinent available prior studies. Dictate a report, utilizing standardized lexicon to describe findings and formulating a final recommendation according to standardized reporting system (Breast Imaging Reporting and Data System [BIRADS]).

Clinical Example (77047)

A 53-year-old female with bilateral breast implants and suspected implant rupture.

Description of Procedure (77047)

Interpret images, evaluating implant integrity and for evidence of intra- or extra-capsular implant rupture. Evaluate for etiology of clinical examination findings or abnormalities questioned on previous imaging. Assess the breast tissue for any abnormalities. Evaluate remainder of structures in the visualized anatomy, including axilla, internal mammary lymph node chain, skin, pectoral muscles and chest wall, bones, visualized mediastinum, and upper abdomen. Compare the current imaging to all pertinent available prior studies. Dictate a report, utilizing standardized lexicon to describe findings and formulating a final recommendation according to standardized reporting system (BIRADS).

Clinical Example (77048)

A 54-year-old female presents who is status post left mastectomy for previous breast cancer and at high risk for breast cancer based on genetic mutation.

Description of Procedure (77048)

Interpret images, evaluating background parenchymal enhancement, biopsy sites, and any cystic or solid masses or nonmass enhancement. Characterize lesions with respect to margins, enhancement pattern, associated features (including architectural distortion, edema, skin or nipple retraction), location, and depth from the nipple. Activate computer-aided detection (CAD).

Review CAD images to determine if there are lesions that enhance to a greater extent than normal background parenchymal enhancement. Use CAD software to acquire kinetic enhancement curves to determine temporal pattern of enhancement. If multiple lesions are present, establish whether there is multifocal or multicentric disease. Determine if any findings require further imaging or intervention (eg, second look ultrasound and/or MR-guided biopsy). Evaluate remainder of structures in the visualized anatomy, including axilla, internal mammary lymph node chain, skin, pectoral muscles and chest wall, bones, visualized mediastinum, and upper abdomen. Compare the current imaging to all pertinent available prior studies. Correlate biopsy results with imaging findings. Dictate a report, utilizing standardized lexicon to describe findings and formulating a final recommendation according to standardized reporting system (BIRADS).

Clinical Example (77049)

A 46-year-old female with recently diagnosed invasive lobular breast carcinoma undergoing evaluation for extent of disease, including unsuspected contralateral synchronous breast carcinoma, before undergoing preoperative (neoadjuvant) chemotherapy.

Description of Procedure (77049)

Interpret images, evaluating background parenchymal enhancement, biopsy sites, and any cystic or solid masses or nonmass enhancement. Characterize lesions with respect to margins, enhancement pattern, associated features (including architectural distortion, edema, skin or nipple retraction), location, and depth from the nipple. Activate CAD. Review CAD images to determine if there are lesions that enhance to a greater extent than normal background parenchymal enhancement. Use CAD software to acquire kinetic enhancement curves to determine temporal pattern of enhancement. If multiple lesions are present, establish whether there is multifocal, multicentric, or contralateral disease. Determine if any findings require further imaging or intervention (eg, second look ultrasound and/or MR-guided biopsy). Evaluate remainder of structures in the visualized anatomy, including axilla, internal mammary lymph node chain, skin, pectoral muscles and chest wall, bones, visualized mediastinum, and upper abdomen. Compare the current imaging to all pertinent available prior studies. Correlate biopsy results with imaging findings. Dictate a report, utilizing standardized lexicon to describe findings and formulating a final recommendation according to standardized reporting system (BIRADS).

Radiation Oncology

Radiation Treatment Delivery

#▲ **77387**   Guidance for localization of target volume for delivery of radiation treatment, includes intrafraction tracking, when performed

(Do not report technical component [TC] with 77385, 77386, 77371, 77372, 77373)

(For placement of interstitial device[s] for radiation therapy guidance, see 31627, 32553, 49411, 55876)

Rationale

Code 77387 has been editorially revised with the removal of the second reference "delivery" within the code descriptor because it was repetitive.

Nuclear Medicine

Diagnostic

Gastrointestinal System

78267   Urea breath test, C-14 (isotopic); acquisition for analysis

78268   analysis

(For breath hydrogen or methane testing and analysis, use 91065)

▶(78270, 78271, 78272 have been deleted)◀

Rationale

To ensure that the CPT code set reflects current clinical practice, codes 78270, *Vitamin B-12 absorption study (eg, Schilling test); without intrinsic factor;* 78271, *Vitamin B-12 absorption study (eg, Schilling test); with intrinsic factor;* and 78272, *Vitamin B-12 absorption studies combined, with and without intrinsic factor,* have been deleted due to low utilization.

Pathology and Laboratory

In the Pathology and Laboratory section, 95 new codes have been added, of which 44 are new PLA codes (0018U-0061U) and 45 are tier 1 molecular pathology codes; five codes have been deleted, of which two are deleted PLA codes (0004U, 0015U) and three are tier 1 molecular pathology codes (81211, 81213, 81214); and 11 are revised tier 1 and tier 2 molecular pathology codes (81216, 81244, 81287, 81237, 81400-81405, 81407). The Tier 1 Molecular Pathology Procedures subsection changes include the addition of 45 new codes (81163-81167, 81171-81174, 81177-81190, 81204, 81233, 81234, 81236, 81237, 81239, 81271, 81274, 81284-81286, 81289, 81305, 81306, 81312, 81320, 81333, 81336, 81337, 81343-81345) and revision of code 81162 to conform to the parent code structure. As for the Tier 2 Molecular Pathology Procedures subsection, the changes include revisions in the code descriptors for six codes (81400-81405, 81407).

As indicated, the Molecular Pathology subsection has substantial changes, which include deletions, additions, and revisions.

Finally, numerous changes have been made in the Multianalyte Assays with Algorithmic Analyses (MAAA) section, which include:

- Addition of two new Category I MAAA codes: 81518 (prognostic ability of breast cancer) and 81596 (replacement of deleted code 0001M [administrative MAAA]); and

- Three new administrative MAAA codes that are located in Appendix O.

Summary of Additions, Deletions, and Revisions

The summary of changes shows the actual changes that have been made to the code descriptors.

New codes appear with a bullet (●) and are indicated as "Code added." Revised codes are preceded with a triangle (▲). Within revised codes, or if a code symbol has been deleted, the deleted language and code symbol appears with a ~~strikethrough~~ (⊖), while new text appears <u>underlined</u>.

The ⊁ symbol is used to identify codes for vaccines that are pending FDA approval. The # symbol is used to identify codes that have been resequenced. CPT add-on codes are annotated by the ✦ symbol. The ⊘ symbol is used to identify codes that are exempt from the use of modifier 51. The ★ symbol is used to identify codes that may be used for reporting telemedicine services. The ⊁ is used to identify proprietary laboratory analyses (PLA) test that has an identical descriptor as another PLA test.

Code	Description
●81171	Code added
●81172	Code added
#●81204	Code added
#●81173	Code added
#●81174	Code added
●81177	Code added

Code	Description
●81178	Code added
●81179	Code added
●81180	Code added
●81181	Code added
●81182	Code added
●81183	Code added
81211	~~BRCA1, BRCA2 (breast cancer 1 and 2) (eg, hereditary breast and ovarian cancer) gene analysis; full sequence analysis and common duplication/deletion variants in BRCA1 (ie, exon 13 del 3.835kb, exon 13 dup 6kb, exon 14-20 del 26kb, exon 22 del 510bp, exon 8-9 del 7.1kb)~~
#▲81162	_BRCA1 (BRCA1, DNA repair associated), BRCA2 (BRCA2, DNA repair associated)_~~(breast cancer 1 and 2)~~ (eg, hereditary breast and ovarian cancer) gene analysis; full sequence analysis and full duplication/deletion analysis _(ie, detection of large gene rearrangements)_
#●81163	Code added
#●81164	Code added
▲81212	185delAG, 5385insC, 6174delT variants
81213	~~uncommon duplication/deletion variants~~
81214	~~BRCA1 (breast cancer 1) (eg, hereditary breast and ovarian cancer) gene analysis; full sequence analysis and common duplication/deletion variants (ie, exon 13 del 3.835kb, exon 13 dup 6kb, exon 14-20 del 26kb, exon 22 del 510bp, exon 8-9 del 7.1kb)~~
#●81165	Code added
#●81166	Code added
▲81215	known familial variant
▲81216	_BRCA2_ ~~(breast cancer 2~~_BRCA2, DNA repair associated)_ (eg, hereditary breast and ovarian cancer) gene analysis; full sequence analysis
#●81167	Code added
▲81217	known familial variant
#●81233	Code added
#●81184	Code added
#●81185	Code added
#●81186	Code added
#●81187	Code added
#●81188	Code added
#●81189	Code added
#●81190	Code added
#●81234	Code added

★=Telemedicine   ✚=Add-on code   ✗=FDA approval pending   #=Resequenced code   ⊘=Modifier 51 exempt

Code	Description
#●81239	Code added
●81236	Code added
●81237	Code added
▲81244	characterization of alleles (eg, expanded size and <u>promoter</u> methylation status)
#●81284	Code added
#●81285	Code added
#●81286	Code added
#●81289	Code added
#●81271	Code added
#●81274	Code added
#▲81287	*MGMT (O-6-methylguanine-DNA methyltransferase)* (eg, glioblastoma multiforme)~~;~~ <u>promoter</u> methylation analysis
●81305	Code added
#●81306	Code added
#●81312	Code added
#●81320	Code added
#●81343	Code added
▲81327	*SEPT9 (Septin9)* (eg, colorectal cancer) <u>promoter</u> methylation analysis
●81329	Code added
#●81336	Code added
#●81337	Code added
#●81344	Code added
#●81345	Code added
●81333	Code added
▲81400	Molecular pathology procedure, Level 1 (eg, identification of single germline variant [eg, SNP] by techniques such as restriction enzyme digestion or melt curve analysis) ~~SMN1 (survival of motor neuron 1, telomeric) (eg, spinal muscular atrophy), exon 7 deletion~~

Code	Description
▲81401	Molecular pathology procedure, Level 2 (eg, 2-10 SNPs, 1 methylated variant, or 1 somatic variant [typically using nonsequencing target variant analysis], or detection of a dynamic mutation disorder/triplet repeat)
	~~AFF2 (AF4/FMR2 family, member 2 [FMR2]) (eg, fragile X mental retardation 2 [FRAXE]), evaluation to detect abnormal (eg, expanded) alleles~~
	~~AR (androgen receptor) (eg, spinal and bulbar muscular atrophy, Kennedy disease, X chromosome inactivation), characterization of alleles (eg, expanded size or methylation status)~~
	~~ATN1 (atrophin 1) (eg, dentatorubral-pallidoluysian atrophy), evaluation to detect abnormal (eg, expanded) alleles~~
	~~ATXN1 (ataxin 1) (eg, spinocerebellar ataxia), evaluation to detect abnormal (eg, expanded) alleles~~
	~~ATXN2 (ataxin 2) (eg, spinocerebellar ataxia), evaluation to detect abnormal (eg, expanded) alleles~~
	~~ATXN3 (ataxin 3) (eg, spinocerebellar ataxia, Machado-Joseph disease), evaluation to detect abnormal (eg, expanded) alleles~~
	~~ATXN7 (ataxin 7) (eg, spinocerebellar ataxia), evaluation to detect abnormal (eg, expanded) alleles~~
	~~ATXN8OS (ATXN8 opposite strand [non-protein coding]) (eg, spinocerebellar ataxia), evaluation to detect abnormal (eg, expanded) alleles~~
	~~ATXN10 (ataxin 10) (eg, spinocerebellar ataxia), evaluation to detect abnormal (eg, expanded) alleles~~
	~~CACNA1A (calcium channel, voltage-dependent, P/Q type, alpha 1A subunit) (eg, spinocerebellar ataxia), evaluation to detect abnormal (eg, expanded) alleles~~
	~~CNBP (CCHC-type zinc finger, nucleic acid binding protein) (eg, myotonic dystrophy type 2), evaluation to detect abnormal (eg, expanded) alleles~~
	~~CSTB (cystatin B [stefin B]) (eg, Unverricht-Lundborg disease), evaluation to detect abnormal (eg, expanded) alleles~~
	~~DMPK (dystrophia myotonica-protein kinase) (eg, myotonic dystrophy, type 1), evaluation to detect abnormal (eg, expanded) alleles~~
	~~FXN (frataxin) (eg, Friedreich ataxia), evaluation to detect abnormal (expanded) alleles~~
	~~HTT (huntingtin) (eg, Huntington disease), evaluation to detect abnormal (eg, expanded) alleles~~
	~~PABPN1 (poly[A] binding protein, nuclear 1) (eg, oculopharyngeal muscular dystrophy), evaluation to detect abnormal (eg, expanded) alleles~~
	~~PPP2R2B (protein phosphatase 2, regulatory subunit B, beta) (eg, spinocerebellar ataxia), evaluation to detect abnormal (eg, expanded) alleles~~
	~~SMN1/SMN2 (survival of motor neuron 1, telomeric/survival of motor neuron 2, centromeric) (eg, spinal muscular atrophy), dosage analysis (eg, carrier testing)~~
	~~TBP (TATA box binding protein) (eg, spinocerebellar ataxia), evaluation to detect abnormal (eg, expanded) alleles~~
▲81403	Molecular pathology procedure, Level 4 (eg, analysis of single exon by DNA sequence analysis, analysis of >10 amplicons using multiplex PCR in 2 or more independent reactions, mutation scanning or duplication/deletion variants of 2-5 exons)
	~~SMN1 (survival of motor neuron 1, telomeric) (eg, spinal muscular atrophy), known familial sequence variant(s)~~

★ = Telemedicine   ✚ = Add-on code   ✗ = FDA approval pending   # = Resequenced code   ⊘ = Modifier 51 exempt

Code	Description
▲81404	Molecular pathology procedure, Level 5 (eg, analysis of 2-5 exons by DNA sequence analysis, mutation scanning or duplication/deletion variants of 6-10 exons, or characterization of a dynamic mutation disorder/triplet repeat by Southern blot analysis) *AFF2 (AF4/FMR2 family, member 2 [FMR2]) (eg, fragile X mental retardation 2 [FRAXE]), characterization of alleles (eg, expanded size and methylation status)* *CSTB (cystatin B [stefin B]) (eg, Unverricht-Lundborg disease), full gene sequence* *DMPK (dystrophia myotonica-protein kinase) (eg, myotonic dystrophy type 1), characterization of abnormal (eg, expanded) alleles* *FXN (frataxin) (eg, Friedreich ataxia), full gene sequence*
▲81405	Molecular pathology procedure, Level 6 (eg, analysis of 6-10 exons by DNA sequence analysis, mutation scanning or duplication/deletion variants of 11-25 exons, regionally targeted cytogenomic array analysis) *AR (androgen receptor) (eg, androgen insensitivity syndrome), full gene sequence* *SMN1 (survival of motor neuron 1, telomeric) (eg, spinal muscular atrophy), full gene sequence*
▲81407	Molecular pathology procedure, Level 8 (eg, analysis of 26-50 exons by DNA sequence analysis, mutation scanning or duplication/deletion variants of >50 exons, sequence analysis of multiple genes on one platform) *CACNA1A (calcium channel, voltage-dependent, P/Q type, alpha 1A subunit) (eg, familial hemiplegic migraine), full gene sequence*
●81443	Code added
●81518	Code added
●81596	Code added
●82642	Code added
●83722	Code added
0004U	~~Infectious disease (bacterial), DNA, 27 resistance genes, PCR amplification and probe hybridization in microarray format (molecular detection and identification of AmpC, carbapenemase and ESBL coding genes), bacterial culture colonies, report of genes detected or not detected, per isolate~~
▲0006U	~~Prescrip~~Detec~~tion drug monitoring~~ of interacting medications, substances, supplements and foods, 120 or more ~~drugs and substances,~~ analytes, definitive ~~tandem mass spectrometry with~~ chromatography~~, urine, qualitative report of presence (including quantitative levels, when detected) or absence of each drug or substance~~ with mass spectrometry, urine, description and severity of ~~potential~~ each interactions~~, with~~ identified ~~substances~~, per date of service
0015U	~~Drug metabolism (adverse drug reactions), DNA, 22 drug metabolism and transporter genes, real-time PCR, blood or buccal swab, genotype and metabolizer status for therapeutic decision support~~
●0018U	Code added
●0019U	Code added
✕●0020U	Code added
●0021U	Code added
●0022U	Code added
●0023U	Code added
●0024U	Code added

▲ = Revised code   ● = New code   ▶ ◀ = Contains new or revised text   ✕ = Duplicate PLA test

Code	Description
●0025U	Code added
●0026U	Code added
●0027U	Code added
●0028U	Code added
●0029U	Code added
●0030U	Code added
●0031U	Code added
●0032U	Code added
●0033U	Code added
●0034U	Code added
●0035U	Code added
●0036U	Code added
●0037U	Code added
●0038U	Code added
●0039U	Code added
●0040U	Code added
●0041U	Code added
●0042U	Code added
●0043U	Code added
●0044U	Code added
●0045U	Code added
●0046U	Code added
●0047U	Code added
●0048U	Code added
●0049U	Code added
●0050U	Code added
●0051U	Code added
●0052U	Code added
●0053U	Code added
●0054U	Code added
●0055U	Code added
●0056U	Code added

★ = Telemedicine   ✚ = Add-on code   ✗ = FDA approval pending   # = Resequenced code   ⊘ = Modifier 51 exempt

Code	Description
●**0057U**	Code added
●**0058U**	Code added
●**0059U**	Code added
●**0060U**	Code added
●**0061U**	Code added

Pathology and Laboratory

Drug Assay

Definitive Drug Testing

# **80327**	Anabolic steroids; 1 or 2
# **80328**	3 or more

▶(For dihydrotestosterone analysis for endogenous hormone levels or therapeutic monitoring, use 82642)◀

Rationale

In support of development of code 82642, an instructional cross-reference has been added to direct users to code 82642 to report dihydrotestosterone analysis for endogenous hormone levels or therapeutic monitoring.

Refer to the codebook and the Rationale for code 82642 for a full discussion of these changes.

Molecular Pathology

Codes that describe tests to assess for the presence of gene variants (see definitions) use common gene variant names. Typically, all of the listed variants would be tested. However, these lists are not exclusive. If other variants are also tested in the analysis, they would be included in the procedure and not reported separately. Full gene sequencing should not be reported using codes that assess for the presence of gene variants unless specifically stated in the code descriptor.

The molecular pathology codes include all analytical services performed in the test (eg, cell lysis, nucleic acid stabilization, extraction, digestion, amplification, and detection). Any procedures required prior to cell lysis (eg, microdissection, codes 88380 and 88381) should be reported separately.

The results of the procedure may require interpretation by a physician or other qualified health care professional. When only the interpretation and report are performed, modifier 26 may be appended to the specific molecular pathology code.

All analyses are qualitative unless otherwise noted.

For microbial identification, see 87149-87153 and 87471-87801, and 87900-87904. For in situ hybridization analyses, see 88271-88275 and 88365-88368.

Molecular pathology procedures that are not specified in 81161, 81200-81383 should be reported using either the appropriate Tier 2 code (81400-81408) or the unlisted molecular pathology procedure code, 81479.

Definitions

For purposes of CPT reporting, the following definitions apply:

Abnormal allele: an alternative form of a gene that contains a disease-related variation from the normal sequence.

Cytogenomic: chromosome analysis using molecular techniques.

▶***DNA methylation:*** the process of adding methyl groups to a DNA sequence, specifically adenine and cytosine nucleotides, thereby affecting transcription of that sequence. DNA hyper-methylation in a gene promoter typically represses gene transcription. DNA methylation serves as a regulatory mechanism in numerous scenarios including development, chromosome inactivation, and carcinogenesis.

DNA methylation analysis: analytical protocols are designed to evaluate the degree of DNA methylation related to specific disease processes. This analysis has various applications, qualitative or quantitative, and could be gene specific or encompass global degrees of methylation. All assays employ specific maneuvers (eg, chemical, enzymatic) that allow for distinguishable evaluation of methylated and non-methylated sequences.◀

Duplication/Deletion (Dup/Del): terms that are usually used together with the "/" to refer to molecular testing, which assesses the dosage of a particular genomic region. The region tested is typically of modest to substantial size—from several dozen to several million or more nucleotides. Normal gene dosage is two copies per cell, except for the sex chromosomes (X and Y). Thus, zero or one copy represents a deletion, and three (or more) copies represent a duplication.

Dynamic mutation: polynucleotide (eg, trinucleotide) repeats that are in or associated with genes that can undergo disease-producing increases or decreases in the numbers of repeats within tissues and across generations.

Gene: a nucleic acid sequence that typically contains information for coding a protein as well as for the regulated expression of that protein. Human genes usually contain multiple protein coding regions (exons) separated by non-protein coding regions (introns). See also *exon*, *intron*, and *polypeptide*.

★=Telemedicine   ✚=Add-on code   ✗=FDA approval pending   #=Resequenced code   ⊘=Modifier 51 exempt

►*Gene expression:* the sequence of events that results in the production and assembly of a protein product corresponding to the information encoded in a specific gene. The process begins with the transcription of gene sequences to produce an mRNA intermediary, which is subsequently translated to produce a specific protein product.◄

Genome: The total (nuclear) human genetic content.

Heteroplasmy: The copy number of a variant within a cell; it is expressed as a percent. It reflects the varied distribution and dosage of mutant mitochondria in tissues and organs (mitotic segregation).

Polypeptide: a sequence of amino acids covalently linked in a specified order. Polypeptides alone or in combination with other polypeptide subunits are the building blocks of proteins.

►*Promoter:* a region of DNA associated with a gene (on the same strand) which regulates gene expression. Promoter regions can affect gene transcription through the binding of specific transcription factors.◄

Short Tandem Repeat (STR): a region of DNA where a pattern of two or more nucleotides are repeated. The number of repeating segments can be used as genetic markers for human identity testing.

Single-nucleotide polymorphism (SNP): a DNA sequence variation existing at a significant frequency in the population, in which a single nucleotide (A, T, C, or G) differs between individuals and/or within an individual's paired chromosomes.

Rationale

DNA methylation, DNA methylation analysis, gene expression, and promoter definitions have been added to the Molecular Pathology guidelines.

DNA methylation affects gene transcription and gene expression. Prior to 2019, codes 81244, 81287, and 81327 only described methylation analysis and did not specify methylation analysis on a gene promoter, which is the service these codes are intended to describe. This distinction is important because methylation on a gene promoter can affect gene expression differently than methylation in regions other than the promoter region. Thus, the new and more uniform nomenclature is intended to recognize similar services.

The new definitions clarify what gene expression is and the effect of DNA methylation on transcription of gene sequences and gene expression. DNA methylation analysis evaluates the impact of methylation on gene transcription. A gene promoter is DNA that regulates gene expression. When hypermethylation occurs in a gene promoter, it typically represses transcription. Analysis of methylation in a gene promoter evaluates the degree to which methylation is repressing gene transcription. The newly added definitions will help users understand the distinction of tests involving methylation analysis and to ensure the appropriate codes are reported.

Tier 1 Molecular Pathology Procedures

81163	Code is out of numerical sequence. See 81182-81220
81164	Code is out of numerical sequence. See 81182-81220
81165	Code is out of numerical sequence. See 81182-81220
81166	Code is out of numerical sequence. See 81182-81220
81167	Code is out of numerical sequence. See 81182-81220
● **81171**	*AFF2 (AF4/FMR2 family, member 2 [FMR2])* (eg, fragile X mental retardation 2 [FRAXE]) gene analysis; evaluation to detect abnormal (eg, expanded) alleles
● **81172**	characterization of alleles (eg, expanded size and methylation status)
81173	Code is out of numerical sequence. See 81171-81176
81174	Code is out of numerical sequence. See 81171-81176

Rationale

In the Molecular Pathology section, 27 gene tests have been moved from the Tier 2 Molecular Pathology Procedures subsection to the Tier 1 Molecular Pathology Procedures subsection as new codes. Since these tests were added to the Tier 2 subsection, their performance-frequency level has increased to the level that is consistent with its intended clinical use. Therefore, the tests have been assigned individual codes in the Tier 1 subsection. The conversion of code 81401 to Tier 1 code 81329 also revised the dosage analysis of the SMN1 and SMN2 genes to include deletion analysis, and to clarify that code 81329 includes analysis of the SMN2 gene, if performed.

In addition to the conversion of the following gene tests to Tier 1, six Tier 1 codes for these new gene tests have been added: AR (81174), CACNA1A (81186), CSTB (81190), FXN (81285, 81289), and HTT (81274).

See Table 1 for a crosswalk of the converted Tier 2 codes to Tier 1 codes. *Note that Table 1 does not include the complete Tier 1 code descriptors.* Refer to the CPT code set for the complete code descriptors.

Crosswalked Tier 2 Codes to Tier 1 Codes

Prior to 2019	Effective 2019		
Tier 2	Tier 1	Gene	Test
81401	●81171	AFF2	Evaluation to detect abnormal (eg, expanded) alleles
81404	●81172	AFF2	Characterization of alleles (eg, expanded size and methylation status)
81401	#●81204	AR	Characterization of alleles (eg, expanded size or methylation status)
81405	#●81173	AR	Full gene sequence
–	#●81174	AR	Known familial variant
81401	●81177	ATN1	Evaluation to detect abnormal (eg, expanded) alleles
81401	●81178	ATXN1	Evaluation to detect abnormal (eg, expanded) alleles
81401	●81179	ATXN2	Evaluation to detect abnormal (eg, expanded) alleles
81401	●81180	ATXN3	Evaluation to detect abnormal (eg, expanded) alleles
81401	●81181	ATXN7	Evaluation to detect abnormal (eg, expanded) alleles
81401	●81182	ATXN8OS	Evaluation to detect abnormal (eg, expanded) alleles
81401	●81183	ATXN10	Evaluation to detect abnormal (eg, expanded) alleles
81401	#●81184	CACNA1A	Evaluation to detect abnormal (eg, expanded) alleles
81407	#●81185	CACNA1A	Full gene sequence
–	#●81186	CACNA1A	Known familial variant
81401	#●81187	CNBP	Evaluation to detect abnormal (eg, expanded) alleles
81401	#●81188	CSTB	Evaluation to detect abnormal (eg, expanded) alleles
81404	#●81189	CSTB	Full gene sequence
–	#●81190	CSTB	Known familial variant(s)
81404	#●81234	DMPK	Evaluation to detect abnormal (expanded) alleles
81401	#●81239	DMPK	Characterization of alleles (eg, expanded size)
81401	#●81284	FXN	Evaluation to detect abnormal (expanded) alleles
–	#●81285	FXN	Characterization of alleles (eg, expanded size)
81404	#●81286	FXN	Full gene sequence
–	#●81289	FXN	Known familial variant(s)
81401	#●81271	HTT	Evaluation to detect abnormal (eg, expanded) alleles
–	#●81274	HTT	Characterization of alleles (eg, expanded size)
81401	#●81312	PABPN1	Evaluation to detect abnormal (eg, expanded) alleles
81401	#●81343	PPP2R2B	Evaluation to detect abnormal (eg, expanded) alleles
81401	●81329	SMN1	Dosage/deletion analysis (eg, carrier testing), includes SMN2 (survival of motor neuron 2, centromeric) analysis, if performed
81405	#●81336	SMN1	Full gene sequence
81403	#●81337	SMN1	Known familial sequence variant(s)
81401	#●81344	TBP	Evaluation to detect abnormal (eg, expanded) alleles

– Indicates that these tests were not previously described in Tier 2 codes. Separate rationales will be provided for codes that are not listed in this table.

★ = Telemedicine   ✚ = Add-on code   ✔ = FDA approval pending   # = Resequenced code   ⊘ = Modifier 51 exempt

Clinical Example (81171)

A 5-year-old male presents to his physician with learning disability and delayed speech, poor writing skills, hyperactivity, and a short attention span. An anticoagulated peripheral-blood sample is submitted for fragile X E (AFF2) mutation analysis.

Description of Procedure (81171)

Isolate and subject high-quality genomic DNA from whole blood to PCR and capillary electrophoresis analysis to detect expanded alleles. The pathologist or other qualified health care professional examines the size and allele calls in the AFF2 gene and composes a report that specifies the patient's mutation status. Edit and sign the report and communicate the results to the appropriate caregivers.

Clinical Example (81172)

A 5-year-old male presents to his physician with learning disability and delayed speech, poor writing skills, hyperactivity, and a short attention span. An anticoagulated peripheral-blood sample is submitted for fragile X E (AFF2) mutation analysis and a large expansion is detected. The sample is then reflexed for characterization of the expanded allele for both size and methylation status.

Description of Procedure (81172)

Isolate and subject high-quality genomic DNA from whole blood to Southern analysis. The pathologist or other qualified health care professional examines the expansion and methylation results and composes a report that specifies the patient's mutation and methylation status. Edit and sign the report and communicate the results to the appropriate caregivers.

# **81201**	*APC (adenomatous polyposis coli)* (eg, familial adenomatosis polyposis [FAP], attenuated FAP) gene analysis; full gene sequence	
# **81202**	known familial variants	
# **81203**	duplication/deletion variants	
#● **81204**	*AR (androgen receptor)* (eg, spinal and bulbar muscular atrophy, Kennedy disease, X chromosome inactivation) gene analysis; characterization of alleles (eg, expanded size or methylation status)	
#● **81173**	full gene sequence	
#● **81174**	known familial variant	

Clinical Example (81173)

A 15-year-old female presents to her physician with sparse or absent hair in the pubic area and has not had a menstrual period. An anticoagulated peripheral-blood sample is submitted for androgen-insensitivity syndrome-sequence analysis.

Description of Procedure (81173)

Isolate and subject high-quality genomic DNA from whole blood to DNA sequencing of the AR gene. The pathologist or other qualified health care professional examines the results and composes a report that specifies the patient's mutation status. Edit and sign the report and communicate the results to the appropriate caregivers.

Clinical Example (81174)

A 30-year-old female presents with a son recently diagnosed with androgen-insensitivity syndrome due to a mutation in the AR gene. An anticoagulated peripheral-blood sample is submitted for mutation analysis to assess the patient's AR genotype status.

Description of Procedure (81174)

Isolate and subject high-quality genomic DNA from whole blood to PCR and sequence analysis for the known familial variant. The pathologist or other qualified health care professional examines the sequence results for the known familial variant in the AR gene and composes a report that specifies the patient's mutation status. Edit and sign the report and communicate the results to the appropriate caregivers.

Clinical Example (81204)

A 35-year-old male presents to his physician with symptoms of muscle weakness and wasting (atrophy) and progressive problems with swallowing and speech. An anticoagulated peripheral-blood sample is submitted for spinal and bulbar muscular atrophy (AR) mutation analysis.

Description of Procedure (81204)

Isolate and subject high-quality genomic DNA from whole blood to PCR and capillary electrophoresis analysis to detect expanded alleles. The pathologist or other qualified health care professional examines the size and allele calls in the AR gene and composes a report that specifies the patient's mutation status. Edit and sign the report and communicate the results to the appropriate caregivers.

# **81200**	*ASPA (aspartoacylase)* (eg, Canavan disease) gene analysis, common variants (eg, E285A, Y231X)	

● **81177**   *ATN1 (atrophin 1)* (eg, dentatorubral-pallidoluysian atrophy) gene analysis, evaluation to detect abnormal (eg, expanded) alleles

● **81178**   *ATXN1 (ataxin 1)* (eg, spinocerebellar ataxia) gene analysis, evaluation to detect abnormal (eg, expanded) alleles

● **81179**   *ATXN2 (ataxin 2)* (eg, spinocerebellar ataxia) gene analysis, evaluation to detect abnormal (eg, expanded) alleles

● **81180**   *ATXN3 (ataxin 3)* (eg, spinocerebellar ataxia, Machado-Joseph disease) gene analysis, evaluation to detect abnormal (eg, expanded) alleles

● **81181**   *ATXN7 (ataxin 7)* (eg, spinocerebellar ataxia) gene analysis, evaluation to detect abnormal (eg, expanded) alleles

● **81182**   *ATXN8OS (ATXN8 opposite strand [non-protein coding])* (eg, spinocerebellar ataxia) gene analysis, evaluation to detect abnormal (eg, expanded) alleles

● **81183**   *ATXN10 (ataxin 10)* (eg, spinocerebellar ataxia) gene analysis, evaluation to detect abnormal (eg, expanded) alleles

Clinical Example (81177)

A 30-year-old male presents to his physician with involuntary movements, mental and emotional problems, and a decline in thinking ability. An anticoagulated peripheral-blood sample is submitted for dentatorubral-pallidoluysian atrophy (ATN1) mutation analysis.

Description of Procedure (81177)

Isolate and subject high-quality genomic DNA from whole blood to PCR and capillary electrophoresis analysis to detect expanded alleles. The pathologist or other qualified health care professional examines the size and allele calls in the ATN1 gene and composes a report that specifies the patient's mutation status. Edit and sign the report and communicate the results to the appropriate caregivers.

Clinical Example (81178)

A 35-year-old male presents to his physician with problems with coordination and balance (ataxia), speech and swallowing difficulties, muscle stiffness (spasticity), and involuntary eye movements (nystagmus). An anticoagulated peripheral-blood sample is submitted for spinocerebellar ataxia type 1 (ATXN1) mutation analysis.

Description of Procedure (81178)

Isolate and subject high-quality genomic DNA from whole blood to PCR and capillary electrophoresis

analysis to detect expanded alleles. The pathologist or other qualified health care professional examines the size and allele calls in the ATXN1 gene and composes a report that specifies the patient's mutation status. Edit and sign the report and communicate the results to the appropriate caregivers.

Clinical Example (81179)

A 35-year-old male presents to his physician with progressive problems with movement, coordination, and balance (ataxia), speech and swallowing difficulties, rigidity, tremors, and weakness in the muscles that control eye movement (ophthalmoplegia). An anticoagulated peripheral-blood sample is submitted for spinocerebellar ataxia type 2 (ATXN2) mutation analysis.

Description of Procedure (81179)

Isolate and subject high-quality genomic DNA from whole blood to PCR and capillary electrophoresis analysis to detect expanded alleles. The pathologist or other qualified health care professional examines the size and allele calls in the ATXN2 gene and composes a report that specifies the patient's mutation status. Edit and sign the report and communicate the results to the appropriate caregivers.

Clinical Example (81180)

A 35-year-old male presents to his physician with progressive problems with movement, speech difficulties, uncontrolled muscle tensing (dystonia), muscle stiffness (spasticity), rigidity, tremors, bulging eyes, and double vision. An anticoagulated peripheral-blood sample is submitted for spinocerebellar ataxia type 3 (ATXN3) mutation analysis.

Description of Procedure (81180)

Isolate and subject high-quality genomic DNA from whole blood to PCR and capillary electrophoresis analysis to detect expanded alleles. The pathologist or other qualified health care professional examines the size and allele calls in the ATXN3 gene and composes a report that specifies the patient's mutation status. Edit and sign the report and communicate the results to the appropriate caregivers.

Clinical Example (81181)

A 35-year-old male presents to his physician with progressive problems with movement, coordination, and balance (ataxia), speech and swallowing difficulties, rigidity, tremors, and weakness in the muscles that control eye movement (ophthalmoplegia). An anticoagulated peripheral-blood sample is submitted for spinocerebellar ataxia type 7 (ATXN7) mutation analysis.

Description of Procedure (81181)

Isolate and subject high-quality genomic DNA from whole blood to PCR and capillary electrophoresis analysis to detect expanded alleles. The pathologist or other qualified health care professional examines the size and allele calls in the ATXN7 gene and composes a report that specifies the patient's mutation status. Edit and sign the report and communicate the results to the appropriate caregivers.

Clinical Example (81182)

A 35-year-old male presents to his physician with progressive problems with movement, coordination, and balance (ataxia), speech and swallowing difficulties, rigidity, tremors, and weakness in the muscles that control eye movement (ophthalmoplegia). An anticoagulated peripheral-blood sample is submitted for spinocerebellar ataxia type 8 (ATXN8OS) mutation analysis.

Description of Procedure (81182)

Isolate and subject high-quality genomic DNA from whole blood to PCR and capillary electrophoresis analysis to detect expanded alleles. The pathologist or other qualified health care professional examines the size and allele calls in the ATXN8OS gene and composes a report that specifies the patient's mutation status. Edit and sign the report and communicate the results to the appropriate caregivers.

Clinical Example (81183)

A 35-year-old male presents to his physician with problems with coordination and balance (ataxia), speech and swallowing difficulties, muscle stiffness (spasticity), and involuntary eye movements (nystagmus). An anticoagulated peripheral-blood sample is submitted for spinocerebellar ataxia type 10 (ATXN10) mutation analysis.

Description of Procedure (81183)

Isolate and subject high-quality genomic DNA from whole blood to PCR and capillary electrophoresis analysis to detect expanded alleles. The pathologist or other qualified health care professional examines the size and allele calls in the ATXN10 gene and composes a report that specifies the patient's mutation status. Edit and sign the report and communicate the results to the appropriate caregivers.

Code	Description
81184	Code is out of numerical sequence. See 81182-81220
81185	Code is out of numerical sequence. See 81182-81220
81186	Code is out of numerical sequence. See 81182-81220
81187	Code is out of numerical sequence. See 81223-81226
81188	Code is out of numerical sequence. See 81223-81226
81189	Code is out of numerical sequence. See 81223-81226
81190	Code is out of numerical sequence. See 81223-81226
81200	Code is out of numerical sequence. See 81171-81176
81201	Code is out of numerical sequence. See 81171-81176
81202	Code is out of numerical sequence. See 81171-81176
81203	Code is out of numerical sequence. See 81171-81176
81204	Code is out of numerical sequence. See 81171-81176
81205	Code is out of numerical sequence. See 81182-81220
81206	Code is out of numerical sequence. See 81182-81220
81207	Code is out of numerical sequence. See 81182-81220
81208	Code is out of numerical sequence. See 81182-81220
81209	Code is out of numerical sequence. See 81182-81220
81210	Code is out of numerical sequence. See 81182-81220

\# 81205 *BCKDHB (branched-chain keto acid dehydrogenase E1, beta polypeptide)* (eg, maple syrup urine disease) gene analysis, common variants (eg, R183P, G278S, E422X)

\# 81206 *BCR/ABL1 (t(9;22))* (eg, chronic myelogenous leukemia) translocation analysis; major breakpoint, qualitative or quantitative

\# 81207 minor breakpoint, qualitative or quantitative

\# 81208 other breakpoint, qualitative or quantitative

\# 81209 *BLM (Bloom syndrome, RecQ helicase-like)* (eg, Bloom syndrome) gene analysis, 2281del6ins7 variant

\# 81210 *BRAF (B-Raf proto-oncogene, serine/threonine kinase)* (eg, colon cancer, melanoma), gene analysis, V600 variant(s)

\#▲ 81162 *BRCA1 (BRCA1, DNA repair associated), BRCA2 (BRCA2, DNA repair associated)* (eg, hereditary breast and ovarian cancer) gene analysis; full sequence analysis and full duplication/deletion analysis (ie, detection of large gene rearrangements)

►(Do not report 81162 in conjunction with 81163, 81164, 81165, 81166, 81167, 81216, 81217, 81432)◄

\#● 81163 full sequence analysis

\#● 81164 full duplication/deletion analysis (ie, detection of large gene rearrangements)

►(To report *BRCA1, BRCA2* full sequence analysis and full duplication/deletion analysis on the same date of service, use 81162)◄

▶(For analysis of common duplication/deletion variant(s) in *BRCA1* [ie, exon 13 del 3.835kb, exon 13 dup 6kb, exon 14-20 del 26kb, exon 22 del 510bp, exon 8-9 del 7.1kb], use 81479)◀

▶(Do not report 81163 in conjunction with 81162, 81164, 81165, 81216, 81432)◀

▶(Do not report 81164 in conjunction with 81162, 81163, 81166, 81167, 81217)◀

▲ 81212   185delAG, 5385insC, 6174delT variants

▶(81211, 81213 have been deleted. To report see 81162, 81163, 81164)◀

▶(81214 has been deleted. To report, see 81165, 81166)◀

#● 81165   *BRCA1 (BRCA1, DNA repair associated)* (eg, hereditary breast and ovarian cancer) gene analysis; full sequence analysis

#● 81166   full duplication/deletion analysis (ie, detection of large gene rearrangements)

▲ 81215   known familial variant

▶(For analysis of common duplication/deletion variant(s) in *BRCA1* [ie, exon 13 del 3.835kb, exon 13 dup 6kb, exon 14-20 del 26kb, exon 22 del 510bp, exon 8-9 del 7.1kb], use 81479)◀

▶(Do not report 81165 in conjunction with 81162, 81163, 81432)◀

▶(Do not report 81166 in conjunction with 81162, 81164)◀

▲ 81216   *BRCA2 (BRCA2, DNA repair associated)* (eg, hereditary breast and ovarian cancer) gene analysis; full sequence analysis

#● 81167   full duplication/deletion analysis (ie, detection of large gene rearrangements)

▲ 81217   known familial variant

▶(Do not report 81216 in conjunction with 81162, 81163, 81432)◀

▶(Do not report 81167 in conjunction with 81162, 81164, 81217)◀

▶(Do not report 81217 in conjunction with 81162, 81164, 81167)◀

Rationale

Comprehensive changes have been made to the Pathology and Laboratory codes for reporting BRCA1 and BRCA2 services. These changes have been made to address changes in clinical practice and to update the coding structure so it is more consistent with the structure of other Molecular Pathology codes. To facilitate the numerous changes, the codes have been expanded, updated, and restructured. In addition, a number of

parenthetical notes have been added and/or revised throughout the affected codes to accommodate these changes.

Because the BRCA 1 and BRCA 2 codes were restructured, codes 81211, 81213, and 81214 have been deleted and five new codes (81163, 81164, 81165, 81166, 81167) have been created.

Code 81211 (BRCA1 and BRCA2 gene analysis, full analysis, and common duplication and deletion variants in BRCA1, including specifying five specific variants that were important in the testing) has been deleted. Because of the restructure, child code 81213 has also been deleted and code 81162 has been revised and established as a parent code.

Code 81162 (full-sequence analysis and full-duplication/deletion analysis) was originally a child code to code 81211.The revision to code 81162 includes the addition of BRCA1 and BRCA2 gene analysis, full-sequence analysis, and full-duplication/deletion analysis. Because code 81162 was revised, new child codes 81163 (full-sequence analysis only) and 81164 (full-duplication/deletion analysis only) have been created.

As 81212 was a child code to 81211, it still remains a child code to the new parent code 81162 and follows code 81164.

Code 81214 (gene analysis, full analysis, and common duplication and deletion variants, but for BRCA1 only) has been deleted. Because code 81214 was deleted, codes 81165 (gene analysis full analysis) and 81166 (full-duplication/deletion analysis) have been created for BRCA1 gene analysis.

As 81215 was a child code to 81214, it still remains a child code to the new parent code 81165 and follows code 81166.

New parenthetical notes have been created to instruct users on the appropriate reporting for the new services represented by the new codes.

Code 81432 also includes BRCA1 and BRCA2, which is used for testing for hereditary breast cancer related disorders. Therefore, parenthetical notes have been added to instruct users not to use code 81432 in conjunction with codes 81162, 81163, 81165, and 81216. Similarly, a parenthetical note has been added for codes 81164 and 81165 with instructions on when to use code 81479 (unlisted molecular pathology procedure) for analysis of common duplication/deletion variant(s) in BRCA1.

In addition to the restructuring of the new BRCA1 BRCA2 codes, the HUGO gene name for BRCA1 and BRCA2 has been changed from "breast cancer" and "breast cancer 2" to "BRCA1, DNA repair associated" and "BRCA2, DNA repair associated."

★ = Telemedicine   + = Add-on code   ⊁ = FDA approval pending   # = Resequenced code   ⊘ = Modifier 51 exempt

Clinical Example (81162)

A premenopausal 36-year-old female with a family history significant for breast and ovarian cancer presents with a small left-breast lump. Biopsy reveals invasive ductal carcinoma. An anticoagulated peripheral-blood specimen is submitted for full-gene sequence analysis of BRCA1 and BRCA2 gene variants along with evaluation of both "common" and "uncommon" duplications/deletions.

Description of Procedure (81162)

Isolate high-quality DNA from whole blood. Using exon capture using a custom designed bait-tile library, followed by library creation and advanced sequencing, perform sequencing of the BRCA1 and BRCA2 genes. Perform large rearrangement analysis using multiplex ligation primer amplification (MLPA) of all exons in BRCA1 and BRCA2, with the exception of exon 1 of BRCA1.

Clinical Example (81163)

A premenopausal 36-year-old female with a family history significant for breast and ovarian cancer presents with a small left-breast lump. Biopsy reveals invasive ductal carcinoma. An anticoagulated peripheral-blood specimen is submitted for full-gene sequence analysis of BRCA1 and BRCA2 gene variants, which are associated with hereditary breast and ovarian cancer.

Description of Procedure (81163)

Isolate high-quality DNA from whole blood. Using exon capture using a custom designed bait-tile library, followed by library creation and advanced sequencing, perform sequencing of the BRCA1 and BRCA2 genes.

Clinical Example (81164)

A premenopausal 42-year-old female with a history significant for breast cancer presents with recently diagnosed ovarian cancer. The patient had undergone full sequence analysis of the BRCA1 and BRCA2 genes for common variants, which was unrevealing. An anticoagulated peripheral-blood specimen is submitted for duplication/deletion analysis of BRCA1 and BRCA2 gene to detect "uncommon" duplications/deletions.

Description of Procedure (81164)

Isolate high-quality DNA from whole blood. Perform large rearrangement analysis using multiplex ligation primer amplification (MLPA) of all exons in BRCA1 and BRCA2, with the exception of exon 1 of BRCA1.

Clinical Example (81165)

A premenopausal 36-year-old woman of Norwegian and Irish Catholic ancestry with a family history significant for breast and ovarian cancer presents with a small left-breast lump. A biopsy of the patient's left-breast lump reveals invasive ductal carcinoma. An anticoagulated peripheral-blood specimen is submitted for full-gene sequence analysis of BRCA1 gene variants associated with hereditary breast and ovarian cancer.

Description of Procedure (81165)

Isolate high-quality DNA from whole blood. Using exon capture using a custom designed bait-tile library, followed by library creation and advanced sequencing, perform sequencing of the BRCA1 and BRCA2 genes.

Clinical Example (81166)

A premenopausal 36-year-old woman of Norwegian and Irish Catholic ancestry with a history significant for breast cancer presents with recently diagnosed ovarian cancer and a small left-breast lump. A full sequence analysis of the BRCA1 gene in the past was unrevealing. An anticoagulated peripheral-blood specimen is submitted for full duplication/deletion analysis of the BRCA1 gene to identify common and uncommon large rearrangements associated with hereditary breast and ovarian cancer.

Description of Procedure (81166)

Isolate high-quality DNA from whole blood. Perform large rearrangement analysis using multiplex ligation primer amplification (MLPA) of all exons in BRCA1, with the exception of exon 1 of BRCA1.

Clinical Example (81167)

A premenopausal 36-year-old woman of Norwegian and Irish Catholic ancestry with a history significant for breast cancer presents with recently diagnosed ovarian cancer and a small left-breast lump. A full-sequence analysis of the BRCA2 gene in the past was unrevealing. An anticoagulated peripheral-blood specimen is submitted for full duplication/deletion analysis of the BRCA2 gene to identify common and uncommon large rearrangements associated with hereditary breast and ovarian cancer.

Description of Procedure (81167)

Isolate high-quality DNA from whole blood. Perform large rearrangement analysis using multiplex ligation primer amplification (MLPA) of all exons in BRCA2.

#● **81233**   *BTK (Bruton's tyrosine kinase)* (eg, chronic lymphocytic leukemia) gene analysis, common variants (eg, C481S, C481R, C481F)

Rationale

Tier 1 Molecular Pathology code 81233, which describes gene analysis, common variants of BTK, has been added to report BTK mutation gene analysis for diseases such as chronic lymphocytic leukemia. Unlisted code 81479 was previously used to report this test, however, it does not adequately describe testing for gene analysis of BTK by common variants. In addition, the usage-volume of this test warrants its own code. (Refer to code 81320 to report PLCG2 mutation gene analysis for chronic lymphocytic leukemia.)

Clinical Example (81233)

A 70-year-old patient was diagnosed with chronic lymphocytic leukemia del(l-7p) by FISH technique and IGHV-unmutated status and was started on Ibrutinib. On the high-risk genetic features, the patient initially achieved a good response to the therapy with resolution of lymphocytosis and improvement in performance status. The CLL recurred several months into therapy with increased clonal lymphocytes in the circulation. Molecular testing was requested to assess if a mutation in BTK was responsible for the development of treatment resistance.

Description of Procedure (81233)

DNA is extracted from a peripheral-blood specimen. PCR amplification is performed on DNA using bidirectional sequencing to detect BTK. An unrelated internal control gene is amplified to ensure adequacy of sample and assay conditions. The pathologist analyzes appropriate laboratory control results and patient sample results to establish mutation status. The pathologist composes a report that specifies the presence or absence of mutation in BTK in the patient's DNA sample and includes a comment on the implications of the test result for patient care. The report is edited and signed, and the results are communicated to appropriate caregivers.

#● **81184**   *CACNA1A (calcium voltage-gated channel subunit alpha1 A)* (eg, spinocerebellar ataxia) gene analysis; evaluation to detect abnormal (eg, expanded) alleles

#● **81185**   full gene sequence

#● **81186**   known familial variant

Clinical Example (81184)

A 35-year-old male presents to his physician with progressive problems with movement, coordination, and balance (ataxia), speech difficulties, involuntary eye movements (nystagmus), and double vision. An anticoagulated peripheral-blood sample is submitted for spinocerebellar ataxia type 6 (CACNA1A) mutation analysis.

Description of Procedure (81184)

Isolate and subject high-quality genomic DNA from whole blood to PCR and capillary electrophoresis analysis to detect expanded alleles. The pathologist or other qualified health care professional examines the size and allele calls in the CACNA1A gene and composes a report that specifies the patient's mutation status. Edit and sign the report and communicate the results to the appropriate caregivers.

Clinical Example (81185)

A 15-year-old female presents to her physician with symptoms of aura preceding a migraine. An anticoagulated peripheral-blood sample is submitted for familial hemiplegic migraine sequence analysis.

Description of Procedure (81185)

Isolate and subject high-quality genomic DNA from whole blood to DNA sequencing of the CACNA1A gene. The pathologist or other qualified health care professional examines the results and composes a report that specifies the patient's mutation status. Edit and sign the report and communicate the results to the appropriate caregivers.

Clinical Example (81186)

A 21-year-old female presents to her physician with migraines, whose father was recently diagnosed with familial hemiplegic migraines due to a mutation in the CACNA1A gene. An anticoagulated peripheral-blood sample is submitted for mutation analysis to assess the patient's CACNA1A genotype status.

Description of Procedure (81186)

Isolate and subject high-quality genomic DNA from whole blood to PCR and sequence analysis for the known familial variant. The pathologist or other qualified health care professional examines the sequence results for the known familial variant in the CACNA1A gene and composes a report that specifies the patient's mutation status. Edit and sign the report and communicate the results to the appropriate caregivers.

★ = Telemedicine   ✚ = Add-on code   ✒ = FDA approval pending   # = Resequenced code   ⊘ = Modifier 51 exempt

 # 81219   *CALR (calreticulin)* (eg, myeloproliferative disorders), gene analysis, common variants in exon 9

81218   *CEBPA (CCAAT/enhancer binding protein [C/EBP], alpha)* (eg, acute myeloid leukemia), gene analysis, full gene sequence

81219   Code is out of numerical sequence. See 81182-81220

 # 81267   Chimerism (engraftment) analysis, post transplantation specimen (eg, hematopoietic stem cell), includes comparison to previously performed baseline analyses; without cell selection

 # 81268   with cell selection (eg, CD3, CD33), each cell type

(If comparative STR analysis of recipient [using buccal swab or other germline tissue sample] and donor are performed after hematopoietic stem cell transplantation, report 81265, 81266 in conjunction with 81267, 81268 for chimerism testing)

#● 81187   *CNBP (CCHC-type zinc finger nucleic acid binding protein)* (eg, myotonic dystrophy type 2) gene analysis, evaluation to detect abnormal (eg, expanded) alleles

Clinical Example (81187)

A 30-year-old female presents to her physician with prolonged muscle contractions (myotonia) and slurred speech or temporary locking of the jaw. An anticoagulated peripheral-blood sample is submitted for myotonic dystrophy type 2 (CNBP) mutation analysis.

Description of Procedure (81187)

Isolate and subject high-quality genomic DNA from whole blood to PCR and capillary electrophoresis analysis to detect expanded alleles. The pathologist or other qualified health care professional examines the size and allele calls in the CNBP gene and composes a report that specifies the patient's mutation status. Edit and sign the report and communicate the results to the appropriate caregivers.

 # 81265   Comparative analysis using Short Tandem Repeat (STR) markers; patient and comparative specimen (eg, pre-transplant recipient and donor germline testing, post-transplant non-hematopoietic recipient germline [eg, buccal swab or other germline tissue sample] and donor testing, twin zygosity testing, or maternal cell contamination of fetal cells)

#+ 81266   each additional specimen (eg, additional cord blood donor, additional fetal samples from different cultures, or additional zygosity in multiple birth pregnancies) (List separately in addition to code for primary procedure)

(Use 81266 in conjunction with 81265)

#● 81188   *CSTB (cystatin B)* (eg, Unverricht-Lundborg disease) gene analysis; evaluation to detect abnormal (eg, expanded) alleles

#● 81189   full gene sequence

#● 81190   known familial variant(s)

Clinical Example (81188)

A 35-year-old male presents to his physician with episodes of involuntary muscle jerking or twitching (myoclonus). An anticoagulated peripheral-blood sample is submitted for myotonic Unverricht-Lundborg disease (CSTB) mutation analysis.

Description of Procedure (81188)

Isolate and subject high-quality genomic DNA from whole blood to PCR and capillary electrophoresis analysis to detect expanded alleles. The pathologist or other qualified health care professional examines the size and allele calls in the CSTB gene and composes a report that specifies the patient's mutation status. Edit and sign the report and communicate the results to the appropriate caregivers.

Clinical Example (81189)

A 6-year-old male presents to his physician with symptoms of episodes of involuntary muscle jerking or twitching (myoclonus), which increased in frequency and severity over time. An anticoagulated peripheral-blood sample is submitted for Unverricht-Lundborg disease sequence analysis.

Description of Procedure (81189)

Isolate and subject high-quality genomic DNA from whole blood to DNA sequencing of the CSTB gene. The pathologist or other qualified health care professional examines the results and composes a report that specifies the patient's mutation status. Edit and sign the report and communicate the results to the appropriate caregivers.

Clinical Example (81190)

A 30-year-old female whose son was recently diagnosed with Unverricht-Lundborg disease due to two different sequence mutations in the CSTB gene. An anticoagulated peripheral-blood sample is submitted for mutation analysis to assess the patient's CSTB genotype status.

Description of Procedure (81190)

Isolate and subject high-quality genomic DNA from whole blood to PCR and sequence analysis for the known familial variants. The pathologist or other qualified health care professional examines the sequence results for the known familial variants in the CSTB gene and composes a report that specifies the patient's mutation status. Edit and sign the report and communicate the results to the appropriate caregivers.

expansion results and composes a report that specifies the patient's mutation status. Edit and sign the report and communicate the results to the appropriate caregivers.

81227   CYP2C9 (cytochrome P450, family 2, subfamily C, polypeptide 9) (eg, drug metabolism), gene analysis, common variants (eg, *2, *3, *5, *6)

81225   CYP2C19 (cytochrome P450, family 2, subfamily C, polypeptide 19) (eg, drug metabolism), gene analysis, common variants (eg, *2, *3, *4, *8, *17)

81226   CYP2D6 (cytochrome P450, family 2, subfamily D, polypeptide 6) (eg, drug metabolism), gene analysis, common variants (eg, *2, *3, *4, *5, *6, *9, *10, *17, *19, *29, *35, *41, *1XN, *2XN, *4XN)

81227   Code is out of numerical sequence. See 81223-81226

#● 81234   DMPK (DM1 protein kinase) (eg, myotonic dystrophy type 1) gene analysis; evaluation to detect abnormal (expanded) alleles

#● 81239   characterization of alleles (eg, expanded size)

Clinical Example (81234)

A 30-year-old female presents to her physician with prolonged muscle contractions (myotonia) and slurred speech or temporary locking of the jaw. An anticoagulated peripheral-blood sample is submitted for myotonic dystrophy (DMPK) mutation analysis.

Description of Procedure (81234)

Isolate and subject high-quality genomic DNA from whole blood to PCR and capillary electrophoresis analysis to detect expanded alleles. The pathologist or other qualified health care professional examines the size and allele calls in the DMPK gene and composes a report that specifies the patient's mutation status. Edit and sign the report and communicate the results to the appropriate caregivers.

Clinical Example (81239)

A newborn male presents at birth with symptoms of hypotonia, clubfoot, breathing problems, delayed development, and intellectual disability. An anticoagulated peripheral-blood sample is submitted for congenital myotonic dystrophy sequence analysis and a large expansion is detected. The sample is then reflexed for characterization of the expanded allele.

Description of Procedure (81239)

Isolate and subject high-quality genomic DNA from whole blood to Southern analysis. The pathologist or other qualified health care professional examines the

81233   Code is out of numerical sequence. See 81182-81220

81234   Code is out of numerical sequence. See 81228-81235

● 81236   EZH2 (enhancer of zeste 2 polycomb repressive complex 2 subunit) (eg, myelodysplastic syndrome, myeloproliferative neoplasms) gene analysis, full gene sequence

● 81237   EZH2 (enhancer of zeste 2 polycomb repressive complex 2 subunit) (eg, diffuse large B-cell lymphoma) gene analysis, common variant(s) (eg, codon 646)

Rationale

Two new Tier 1 Molecular Pathology codes (81236, 81237) have been added to report EZH2 mutation gene analysis for diseases such as hematologic neoplasms. Code 81236 reports gene analysis, full gene sequence of EZH2 and code 81237 reports gene analysis, common variant of EZH2. Unlisted code 81479 was previously used to report these tests, however, it did not adequately describe testing for gene analysis of EZH2 by full gene sequence and common variant(s). In addition, the usage volume of these tests warrants specific codes.

Clinical Example (81236)

A 71-year-old male presents with worsening fatigue, abdominal fullness, petechia of recent onset, and splenomegaly. Peripheral-blood count shows leukocytosis due to absolute monocytosis, with anemia and mild thrombocytopenia. A bone marrow biopsy reveals a uniformly hypercellular bone marrow with increased mononuclear cells displaying morphologic features between myelocytes and monocytes, 15% blasts confirmed by flow cytometry, and no observed cytogenetic abnormalities. Molecular testing is ordered to detect the presence of an EZH2 mutation, to support the diagnosis of chronic myelomonocytic leukemia with worse clinical prognosis and evaluate clonality.

Description of Procedure (81236)

DNA is extracted from peripheral blood or bone marrow. The EZH2 gene is amplified by PCR and sequenced. An unrelated internal control gene is amplified to ensure adequacy of sample and assay conditions. Laboratory control results and patient sample results are reviewed and analyzed to establish mutation status. A report that specifies the presence or absence of mutation in EZH2

★ = Telemedicine   ✚ = Add-on code   ✒ = FDA approval pending   # = Resequenced code   ⊘ = Modifier 51 exempt

in the patient's DNA sample and includes a clinical interpretation, is generated and issued.

Clinical Example (81237)

A 75-year-old male with a history of worsening fatigue, night sweats, and fever presents with enlarged axillary lymph nodes and increased LDH levels. Biopsy of an axillary lymph node showed diffuse effacement of the lymph node architecture due to an atypical large lymphocytic infiltrate. Immunophenotyping results A were consistent with the diagnosis of diffuse large B-cell lymphoma (DLBCL). Additional immunohistochemistry studies were performed to further characterize as either germinal center B-cell (GCB) or activated B-cell (ABC) origin, but results were inconclusive. EZH2 mutation analysis was ordered, which has been shown to be specific for GCB subtype.

Description of Procedure (81237)

DNA is extracted from peripheral blood or bone marrow. The EZH2 gene is amplified by PCR and sequenced to detect commonly known variants. An unrelated internal control gene is amplified to ensure adequacy of sample and assay conditions. Laboratory control results and patient sample results are reviewed and analyzed to establish mutation status. A report that specifies the presence or absence of mutations in EZH2 in the patient's DNA sample and includes a clinical interpretation is generated and issued.

81239	Code is out of numerical sequence. See 81228-81235
# 81245	*FLT3 (fms-related tyrosine kinase 3)* (eg, acute myeloid leukemia), gene analysis; internal tandem duplication (ITD) variants (ie, exons 14, 15)
# 81246	tyrosine kinase domain (TKD) variants (eg, D835, I836)
81243	*FMR1 (fragile X mental retardation 1)* (eg, fragile X mental retardation) gene analysis; evaluation to detect abnormal (eg, expanded) alleles
	(For evaluation to detect and characterize abnormal alleles, see 81243, 81244)
	(For evaluation to detect and characterize abnormal alleles using a single assay [eg, PCR], use 81243)
▲ 81244	characterization of alleles (eg, expanded size and promoter methylation status)

Rationale

Codes 81244, 81287, and 81327 have been revised to include "promoter."

Refer to the codebook and the Rationale for the new definition for "promoter" in the molecular pathology guidelines for a full discussion of these changes.

Clinical Example (81244)

During a routine pediatric office visit, the mother of a 10-year-old girl describes what she considers to be unusual shyness leading to apparent social isolation, as well as occasional stereotypic behaviors such as hand wringing. The child attends regular school classes and her performance is somewhat below average. There is no family history of mental retardation or other neurologic problems. Both parents are healthy and of average intelligence and the patient has a 13-year-old brother who is otherwise healthy and performs well in school. The patient had a normal karyotype and array CGH study. FMR1 gene testing performed by gel-based PCR analysis revealed a single allele of normal CGG repeat size, but did not definitely show the presence of a second allele. A sample of anticoagulated peripheral blood is sent to the laboratory for Southern blot testing for fragile X syndrome using a methylation specific enzyme.

Description of Procedure (81244)

Upon receipt of the specimen, isolate a large quantity of high-quality genomic DNA. Perform gel electrophoresis of the extracted DNA to assess DNA integrity. The DNA specimen undergoes double restriction digestion with the methylation-sensitive restriction enzyme EagI and the methylation-insensitive restriction enzyme. The genomic fragments are separated by gel electrophoresis, transferred to a nylon membrane by capillary action, and hybridized to a labeled probe. The hybridization pattern is visualized on X-ray film by autoradiography. The physician examines the image, compares the observed fragments to a sizing ladder to estimate CGG repeat numbers, and analyzes the patterns generated to assess the methylation status of the promoter region of the expanded FMR1 allele. Based on this analysis, the physician determines the patient's allele status, presence of expanded allele(s), and methylation status of the FMR1 promoter. The physician composes a report that specifies the patient's allele status, approximate allele sizes, and promoter-methylation status. The report is edited, signed, and the results are communicated to the appropriate caregivers.

81245	Code is out of numerical sequence. See 81240-81248
81246	Code is out of numerical sequence. See 81240-81248
#● **81284**	*FXN (frataxin)* (eg, Friedreich ataxia) gene analysis; evaluation to detect abnormal (expanded) alleles
#● **81285**	characterization of alleles (eg, expanded size)
#● **81286**	full gene sequence
#● **81289**	known familial variant(s)

Clinical Example (81284)

A 5-year-old male presents to his physician with symptoms of impaired muscle coordination (ataxia) that is worsening over time; gradual loss of strength and sensation in the arms and legs; muscle stiffness (spasticity); and impaired speech, hearing, and vision. An anticoagulated peripheral-blood sample is submitted for Friedreich ataxia (FXN) mutation analysis.

Description of Procedure (81284)

Isolate and subject high-quality genomic DNA from whole blood to PCR and capillary electrophoresis analysis to detect expanded alleles. The pathologist or other qualified health care professional examines the size and allele calls in the FXN gene and composes a report that specifies the patient's mutation status. Edit and sign the report and communicate the results to the appropriate caregivers.

Clinical Example (81285)

A 7-year-old male presents to his physician with symptoms of ataxia that are worsening over time. Other symptoms include the gradual loss of strength and sensation in the arms and legs; spasticity; and impaired speech, hearing, and vision. An anticoagulated peripheral-blood sample is submitted for Friedreich ataxia gene analysis. An abnormal sized allele and an extremely large expansion are detected. The sample is then reflexed for characterization of the expanded allele.

Description of Procedure (81285)

Isolate and subject high-quality genomic DNA from whole blood to Southern analysis. The pathologist or other qualified health care professional examines the expansion results and composes a report that specifies the patient's mutation status. Edit and sign the report and communicate the results to the appropriate caregivers.

Clinical Example (81286)

A 7-year-old male presents to his physician with symptoms of ataxia that are worsening over time. Other symptoms include the gradual loss of strength and

sensation in the arms and legs; spasticity; and impaired speech, hearing, and vision. An anticoagulated peripheral-blood sample is submitted for Friedreich ataxia gene analysis and only one expanded allele is detected. The sample is then reflexed for full-gene sequencing of the FXN gene.

Description of Procedure (81286)

Isolate and subject high-quality genomic DNA from whole blood to DNA sequencing of the FXN gene. The pathologist or other qualified health care professional examines the results and composes a report that specifies the patient's mutation status. Edit and sign the report and communicate the results to the appropriate caregivers.

Clinical Example (81289)

A 30-year-old female whose son was recently diagnosed with Friedreich ataxia because of one abnormally expanded allele and another intragenic pathogenic variant on the other allele. An anticoagulated peripheral-blood sample is submitted for mutation analysis to assess the patient's FXN genotype status for the intragenic pathogenic variant.

Description of Procedure (81289)

Isolate and subject high-quality genomic DNA from whole blood to PCR and sequence analysis for the known familial variant. The pathologist or other qualified health care professional examines the sequence results for the known familial variant in the FXN gene and composes a report that specifies the patient's mutation status. Edit and sign the report and communicate the results to the appropriate caregivers.

# **81250**	*G6PC (glucose-6-phosphatase, catalytic subunit)* (eg, Glycogen storage disease, type 1a, von Gierke disease) gene analysis, common variants (eg, R83C, Q347X)
81247	*G6PD (glucose-6-phosphate dehydrogenase)* (eg, hemolytic anemia, jaundice), gene analysis; common variant(s) (eg, A, A-)
81248	known familial variant(s)
81249	full gene sequence
81250	Code is out of numerical sequence. See 81243-81248
# **81257**	*HBA1/HBA2 (alpha globin 1 and alpha globin 2)* (eg, alpha thalassemia, Hb Bart hydrops fetalis syndrome, HbH disease), gene analysis; common deletions or variant (eg, Southeast Asian, Thai, Filipino, Mediterranean, alpha3.7, alpha4.2, alpha20.5, Constant Spring)
# **81258**	known familial variant

★ = Telemedicine   ✚ = Add-on code   𝒩 = FDA approval pending   # = Resequenced code   ⊘ = Modifier 51 exempt

# **81259**	full gene sequence	
# **81269**	duplication/deletion variants	
# **81361**	*HBB (hemoglobin, subunit beta)* (eg, sickle cell anemia, beta thalassemia, hemoglobinopathy); common variant(s) (eg, HbS, HbC, HbE)	
# **81362**	known familial variant(s)	
# **81363**	duplication/deletion variant(s)	
# **81364**	full gene sequence	
81257	Code is out of numerical sequence. See 81253-81256	
81258	Code is out of numerical sequence. See 81253-81256	
81259	Code is out of numerical sequence. See 81253-81256	
#● **81271**	*HTT (huntingtin)* (eg, Huntington disease) gene analysis; evaluation to detect abnormal (eg, expanded) alleles	
#● **81274**	characterization of alleles (eg, expanded size)	

Clinical Example (81271)

A 35-year-old male presents to his physician with symptoms of irritability, depression, small involuntary movements, poor coordination, and trouble learning new information or making decisions. An anticoagulated peripheral-blood sample is submitted for Huntington disease (HTT) mutation analysis.

Description of Procedure (81271)

Isolate and subject high-quality genomic DNA from whole blood to PCR and capillary electrophoresis analysis to detect expanded alleles. The pathologist or other qualified health care professional examines the size and allele calls in the HTT gene and composes a report that specifies the patient's mutation status. Edit and sign the report and communicate the results to the appropriate caregivers.

Clinical Example (81274)

A 10-year-old male presents to his physician with symptoms of movement problems and mental and emotional changes. Additional symptoms include slow movements, clumsiness, frequent falling, rigidity, slurred speech, and drooling. His school performance has also been declining. An anticoagulated peripheral-blood sample is submitted for Huntington disease (HTT) mutation analysis and a large expansion is detected. The sample is then reflexed for characterization of the expanded allele for size.

Description of Procedure (81274)

Isolate and subject high-quality genomic DNA from whole blood to Southern analysis. The pathologist or other qualified health care professional examines the

expansion results and composes a report that specifies the patient's mutation status. Edit and sign the report and communicate the results to the appropriate caregivers.

# **81261**	*IGH@ (Immunoglobulin heavy chain locus)* (eg, leukemias and lymphomas, B-cell), gene rearrangement analysis to detect abnormal clonal population(s); amplified methodology (eg, polymerase chain reaction)	
# **81262**	direct probe methodology (eg, Southern blot)	
# **81263**	*IGH@ (Immunoglobulin heavy chain locus)* (eg, leukemia and lymphoma, B-cell), variable region somatic mutation analysis	
# **81264**	*IGK@ (Immunoglobulin kappa light chain locus)* (eg, leukemia and lymphoma, B-cell), gene rearrangement analysis, evaluation to detect abnormal clonal population(s)	
	(For immunoglobulin lambda gene *[IGL@]* rearrangement or immunoglobulin kappa deleting element, *[IGKDEL]* analysis, use 81479)	
81261	Code is out of numerical sequence. See 81255-81270	
81262	Code is out of numerical sequence. See 81255-81270	
81263	Code is out of numerical sequence. See 81255-81270	
81264	Code is out of numerical sequence. See 81255-81270	
81265	Code is out of numerical sequence. See 81223-81226	
81266	Code is out of numerical sequence. See 81223-81226	
81267	Code is out of numerical sequence. See 81223-81226	
81268	Code is out of numerical sequence. See 81223-81226	
81271	Code is out of numerical sequence. See 81255-81270	
81274	Code is out of numerical sequence. See 81255-81270	
81283	Code is out of numerical sequence. See 81255-81270	
81284	Code is out of numerical sequence. See 81243-81248	
81285	Code is out of numerical sequence. See 81243-81248	
81286	Code is out of numerical sequence. See 81243-81248	
81289	Code is out of numerical sequence. See 81243-81248	
# **81302**	*MECP2 (methyl CpG binding protein 2)* (eg, Rett syndrome) gene analysis; full sequence analysis	
# **81303**	known familial variant	
# **81304**	duplication/deletion variants	
#▲ **81287**	*MGMT (O-6-methylguanine-DNA methyltransferase)* (eg, glioblastoma multiforme) promoter methylation analysis	

Rationale

Codes 81244, 81287, and 81327 have been revised to include "promoter."

Refer to the codebook and the Rationale for the new definition of "promoter" in the molecular pathology guidelines for a full discussion of these changes.

Clinical Example (81287)

Patient 1: A 70-year-old male presents with glioblastoma and in otherwise good health. He is reluctant to receive temozolomide (TMZ) chemotherapy because of the toxicities of concurrent chemoradiation followed by chemotherapy. O-6-methylguanine-DNA [deoxyribonucleic acid] methyltransferase (MGMT) status testing is requested to determine if he would benefit from the addition of chemotherapy to his care.

Patient 2: A 54-year-old female has her first magnetic resonance imaging (MRI) to determine if a tumor has responded to chemotherapy. The resulting MRI shows contrast enhancement and enlargement of noncontrast T2/FLAIR hyperintense signal surrounding the enhancement, which indicates that the tumor is progressing. Examination of the tumor location during secondary surgery shows only tissue necrosis and no viable tumor area. This "false MRI" has been termed as "pseudoprogression" because of the incorrect indication by the MRI diagnostic that the tumor has regrown. Pseudoprogression is difficult to distinguish from true progression in patients undergoing chemoradiation. MGMT-positive patients frequently experience pseudoprogression because of inflammatory changes from the therapeutic response. MGMT status allows clinicians to determine whether continued treatment is beneficial or surgical intervention is needed for true progression.

For healthy adult patients who initially receive chemoradiation regardless of MGMT status (as there are currently no other approved therapeutic options beyond TMZ/RT [radiotherapy]), MGMT testing can determine whether to continue treatment when treatment-related toxicities occur.

Description of Procedure (81287)

Send formalin-fixed, paraffin-embedded (FFPE) tissue for testing (40 total microns of tissue are used and supplied as 10 micron slices mounted on glass slides). The tumor area on tissue section is removed, taking care to avoid normal tissue areas. The FFPE tumor area material is deparaffinized and treated with detergent and proteases to release deoxyribonucleic acid (DNA) from the cells. The DNA is then separated from this mixture by organic phase separation (phenol chloroform). DNA quantity is measured.

A maximum of 1.5 µg of the isolated genomic DNA (gDNA) is treated with a DNA bisulfite modification kit. In this process, the gDNA is treated with sodium hydroxide (NaOH) to denature the DNA strands and then incubated with sodium bisulfite (NaHSO$_3$). All chemicals are then removed by passing the modified DNA over a column that initially traps the DNA, thereby, allowing the bisulfite chemicals to be washed away. The DNA is then released from the column and is ready for methylation-specific polymerase chain reaction (PCR).

Two distinct quantitative PCR reactions are run on each sample. One PCR reaction has primers specific for the methylated MGMT gene; the other PCR reaction has primers specific for beta-actin (ACTB), which are designed to be methylation-nonspecific. If the ACTB copy numbers do not reach a specific value (1250 copies), the sample is considered to be inadequate for further analysis. If the sample has >1250 copies of ACTB, then the methylated MGMT PCR signal is evaluated. The normalized ratio of m_MGMT:ACTB is calculated and compared to a cutoff. Above a specific cutoff, the sample is considered methylated; below the cutoff, it is nonmethylated.

Copy numbers are derived in each of the two PCR reactions via a standard curve. Each PCR run is checked for various quality control (QC) parameters, including PCR efficiency, positive control (PC) and negative control (NC) parameters, and standard curve replicates. If the run QC is acceptable, the resulting sample interpretation is reported.

# **81301**		Microsatellite instability analysis (eg, hereditary non-polyposis colorectal cancer, Lynch syndrome) of markers for mismatch repair deficiency (eg, BAT25, BAT26), includes comparison of neoplastic and normal tissue, if performed
# **81292**		*MLH1 (mutL homolog 1, colon cancer, nonpolyposis type 2)* (eg, hereditary non-polyposis colorectal cancer, Lynch syndrome) gene analysis; full sequence analysis
# **81288**		promoter methylation analysis
# **81293**		known familial variants
# **81294**		duplication/deletion variants
# **81295**		*MSH2 (mutS homolog 2, colon cancer, nonpolyposis type 1)* (eg, hereditary non-polyposis colorectal cancer, Lynch syndrome) gene analysis; full sequence analysis

81291	Code is out of numerical sequence. See 81299-81310
81292	Code is out of numerical sequence. See 81276-81297
81293	Code is out of numerical sequence. See 81276-81297
81294	Code is out of numerical sequence. See 81276-81297
81295	Code is out of numerical sequence. See 81276-81297
81301	Code is out of numerical sequence. See 81276-81297
81302	Code is out of numerical sequence. See 81276-81297
81303	Code is out of numerical sequence. See 81276-81297
81304	Code is out of numerical sequence. See 81276-81297

 # 81291 *MTHFR (5,10-methylenetetrahydrofolate reductase)* (eg, hereditary hypercoagulability) gene analysis, common variants (eg, 677T, 1298C)

● 81305 *MYD88 (myeloid differentiation primary response 88)* (eg, Waldenstrom's macroglobulinemia, lymphoplasmacytic leukemia) gene analysis, p.Leu265Pro (L265P) variant

Rationale

Code 81305 has been added to report analysis of the MYD88 gene to identify p.Leu265Pro (L265P) variant.

Clinical Example (81305)

A 66-year-old male presents with fatigue and is found to have anemia and mildly elevated lymphocyte count with increased numbers of plasma cells in the peripheral blood. Bone-marrow biopsy demonstrated 50% involvement of small B-cell lymphoma with plasmacytic differentiation. Laboratory testing identified an IgM monoclonal gammopathy. Mutation testing for MYD88 L265P was requested.

Description of Procedure (81305)

Isolate and subject high-quality genomic DNA from the patient's specimen to targeted mutation testing of MYD88 gene to identify the L265P mutation. The pathologist or other qualified health care professional analyzes the data and composes a report specifying the patient's mutation status. Edit and sign the report and communicate the results to the appropriate caregivers.

81306	Code is out of numerical sequence. See 81310-81318
81310	*NPM1 (nucleophosmin)* (eg, acute myeloid leukemia) gene analysis, exon 12 variants
81311	*NRAS (neuroblastoma RAS viral [v-ras] oncogene homolog)* (eg, colorectal carcinoma), gene analysis, variants in exon 2 (eg, codons 12 and 13) and exon 3 (eg, codon 61)
81312	Code is out of numerical sequence. See 81310-81318

#● 81306 *NUDT15 (nudix hydrolase 15)* (eg, drug metabolism) gene analysis, common variant(s) (eg, *2, *3, *4, *5, *6)

Rationale

Code 81306 has been established to report NUDT15 (nudix hydrolase 15) (eg, drug metabolism) gene analysis. With the advances in medicine, Tier 1 code 81306 will enable better tracking of testing performed nationally and to better determine testing volumes. An NUDT15 gene analysis is typically ordered to assess a patient's metabolizer status.

Clinical Example (81306)

A 14-year-old female of Asian ancestry presents to her physician complaining of fatigue, dyspnea, and fever. She is pale with multiple petechiae. Complete blood cell count (CBC) reveals anemia, neutropenia, and thrombocytopenia with large numbers of circulating lymphoblasts and, together with bone-marrow examination, which is consistent with a diagnosis of acute lymphoblastic leukemia (ALL). A BCR-ABL1 translocation is not present. NUDT15 gene analysis is ordered to assess the patient's metabolizer status in anticipation of thiopurine drug therapy.

Description of Procedure (81306)

Isolate and subject high-quality genomic DNA from whole blood to molecular testing using real-time PCR and hydrolysis probe analysis, which determine the genotype for NUDT15 variant(s). A pathologist or other qualified health care professional examines the variant calls for the NUDT15 gene and composes a report that specifies the patient's metabolizer status according to the Clinical Pharmacogenetics Implementation Consortium (CPIC®) guidelines, and communicates the results to the ordering physician and appropriate caregivers.

#● 81312 *PABPN1 (poly[A] binding protein nuclear 1)* (eg, oculopharyngeal muscular dystrophy) gene analysis, evaluation to detect abnormal (eg, expanded) alleles

Clinical Example (81312)

A 40-year-old male presents to his physician with symptoms of muscle weakness, droopy eyelids (ptosis), followed by difficulty swallowing (dysphagia). An anticoagulated peripheral-blood sample is submitted for oculopharyngeal muscular dystrophy (PABPN1) mutation analysis.

Description of Procedure (81312)

Isolate and subject high-quality genomic DNA from whole blood to PCR and capillary electrophoresis analysis to detect expanded alleles. The pathologist or other qualified health care professional examines the size and allele calls in the PABPN1 gene and composes a report that specifies the patient's mutation status. Edit and sign the report and communicate the results to the appropriate caregivers.

#● **81320**   *PLCG2 (phospholipase C gamma 2)* (eg, chronic lymphocytic leukemia) gene analysis, common variants (eg, R665W, S707F, L845F)

Rationale

Tier 1 Molecular Pathology code 81320 has been added to report PLCG2 mutation gene analysis for diseases such as chronic lymphocytic leukemia. Code 81320 describes gene analysis, common variant of PLCG2. Unlisted code 81479 was previously used to report this test, however, it did not adequately describe testing for gene analysis of PLCG2 by common variants. In addition, the usage volume of this test warrants its own code. (Refer to code 81233 to report BTK mutation gene analysis for chronic lymphocytic leukemia.)

Clinical Example (81320)

A 70-year-old patient was diagnosed with chronic lymphocytic leukemia with del(17p) by FISH technique and IGHV-unmutated status and was started on Ibrutinib based on these high-risk genetic features. The patient initially achieved a good response to the therapy with resolution of lymphocytosis and improvement in performance status. The CLL recurred several months into therapy with increased clonal lymphocytes in the circulation. Molecular testing was requested to assess if a mutation in PLCG2 was responsible for the development of treatment resistance.

Description of Procedure (81320)

DNA is extracted from a hematologic tissue sample such as peripheral blood or bone marrow. PCR amplification is performed on DNA using bidirectional sequencing to detect PLCG2. An unrelated internal control gene is amplified to ensure adequacy of sample and assay conditions. The pathologist analyzes appropriate laboratory control results and patient sample results to establish mutation status. The pathologist composes a report that specifies the presence or absence of mutation in PLCG2 in the patient's DNA sample and includes a comment on the implications of the test result for patient

care. The report is edited and signed, and the results are communicated to appropriate caregivers.

\# **81324**   *PMP22 (peripheral myelin protein 22)* (eg, Charcot-Marie-Tooth, hereditary neuropathy with liability to pressure palsies) gene analysis; duplication/deletion analysis

\# **81325**   full sequence analysis

\# **81326**   known familial variant

81320   Code is out of numerical sequence. See 81310-81318

#● **81343**   *PPP2R2B (protein phosphatase 2 regulatory subunit Bbeta)* (eg, spinocerebellar ataxia) gene analysis, evaluation to detect abnormal (eg, expanded) alleles

Clinical Example (81343)

A 35-year-old male presents to his physician with progressive problems with movement, coordination, and balance (ataxia), speech difficulties, involuntary eye movements (nystagmus), and double vision. An anticoagulated peripheral-blood sample is submitted for spinocerebellar ataxia type 12 (PPP2R2B) mutation analysis.

Description of Procedure (81343)

Isolate and subject high-quality genomic DNA from whole blood to PCR and capillary electrophoresis analysis to detect expanded alleles. The pathologist or other qualified health care professional examines the size and allele calls in the PPP2R2B gene and composes a report that specifies the patient's mutation status. Edit and sign the report and communicate the results to the appropriate caregivers.

81324   Code is out of numerical sequence. See 81310-81318

81325   Code is out of numerical sequence. See 81310-81318

81326   Code is out of numerical sequence. See 81310-81318

▲ **81327**   *SEPT9 (Septin9)* (eg, colorectal cancer) promoter methylation analysis

Rationale

Codes 81244, 81287, and 81327 have been revised to include "promoter."

Refer to the codebook and the Rationale for the new definition of "promoter" in the molecular pathology guidelines for a full discussion of these changes.

★ = Telemedicine   ✚ = Add-on code   ✗ = FDA approval pending   \# = Resequenced code   ⊘ = Modifier 51 exempt

Clinical Example (81327)

A 61-year-old male is at average risk for colorectal cancer but he is not up to date on screening. He presents to his primary physician for an annual physical examination. He is offered various screening options and accepts the SEPT9 methylation test for colorectal cancer screening. The physician orders a blood draw for SEPT9 testing.

Description of Procedure (81327)

Extract cell-free DNA from plasma and treat with ammonium bisulfite, purify and use for polymerase chain reaction (PCR). Real-time PCR amplification is performed with primers specific for a SEPT9 promoter region and with control primers specific for ACTB in a duplex reaction. Generate a report that describes the *promoter* methylation status of the SEPT9 gene to show correlation with risk of colorectal cancer.

81332   *SERPINA1 (serpin peptidase inhibitor, clade A, alpha-1 antiproteinase, antitrypsin, member 1)* (eg, alpha-1-antitrypsin deficiency), gene analysis, common variants (eg, *S and *Z)

81328   *SLCO1B1 (solute carrier organic anion transporter family, member 1B1)* (eg, adverse drug reaction), gene analysis, common variant(s) (eg, *5)

● 81329   *SMN1 (survival of motor neuron 1, telomeric)* (eg, spinal muscular atrophy) gene analysis; dosage/deletion analysis (eg, carrier testing), includes *SMN2 (survival of motor neuron 2, centromeric)* analysis, if performed

#● 81336   full gene sequence

#● 81337   known familial sequence variant(s)

Clinical Example (81329)

A couple seeks counseling for prepregnancy planning and carrier testing for the SMN1 deletion associated with spinal muscular atrophy. A blood specimen is collected and quantitative SMN1 dosage analysis is performed.

Description of Procedure (81329)

Isolate and subject high-quality genomic DNA from whole blood to dosage testing for SMN1/SMN2. The pathologist or other qualified health care professional examines the results and composes a report that specifies the patient's dosage status. Edit and sign the report and communicate the results to the appropriate caregivers.

Clinical Example (81336)

A couple with a family history of spinal muscular atrophy presents with a pregnancy at 12 weeks gestation. One parent has a rare sequence variant in the SMN1 gene, but the familial variant is unknown. Chorionic villus biopsy is performed, and the fetus is found to carry a single copy of SMN1. The specimen is submitted for testing for full-gene sequencing.

Description of Procedure (81336)

Isolate and subject high-quality genomic DNA from whole blood to full-gene sequencing of the SMN1 gene. The pathologist or other qualified health care professional examines the results and composes a report that specifies the patient's variant status. Edit and sign the report and communicate the results to the appropriate caregivers.

Clinical Example (81337)

A couple with a family history of spinal muscular atrophy presents with a pregnancy at 12 weeks gestation. One parent has a known rare pathogenic sequence variant in the SMN1 gene. Chorionic villus biopsy is performed, and the fetus is found to carry a single copy of SMN1. The specimen is submitted for testing for the known familial variant.

Description of Procedure (81337)

Isolate and subject high-quality genomic DNA from whole blood to targeted gene sequencing of the SMN1 gene for known familial pathogenic variant. The pathologist or other qualified health care professional examines the results and composes a report that specifies the patient's status for the known familial pathogenic variant. Edit and sign the report and communicate the results to the appropriate caregivers.

81332   Code is out of numerical sequence. See 81318-81335

#● 81344   *TBP (TATA box binding protein)* (eg, spinocerebellar ataxia) gene analysis, evaluation to detect abnormal (eg, expanded) alleles

Clinical Example (81344)

A 35-year-old male presents to his physician with symptoms of irritability, depression, small involuntary movements, poor coordination, and trouble learning new information or making decisions. An anticoagulated peripheral-blood sample is submitted for Huntington disease-like 4/ spinocerebellar ataxia type 17 (TBP) mutation analysis.

Description of Procedure (81344)

Isolate and subject high-quality genomic DNA from whole blood to PCR and capillary electrophoresis analysis to detect expanded alleles. The pathologist or other qualified health care professional examines the size and allele calls in the TBP gene and composes a report that specifies the patient's mutation status. Edit and sign the report and communicate the results to the appropriate caregivers.

#● **81345**   *TERT (telomerase reverse transcriptase)* (eg, thyroid carcinoma, glioblastoma multiforme) gene analysis, targeted sequence analysis (eg, promoter region)

Rationale

Code 81345 has been added to report targeted sequence analysis of the TERT (telomerase reverse transcriptase) gene. TERT promoter mutation analysis is a clinical application that is used to diagnose diseases such as multiple malignancies, including thyroid, glioblastoma multiforme, urothelial carcinomas, and melanoma.

Clinical Example (81345)

A 45-year-old female with a single thyroid nodule undergoes fine-needle aspiration for cytologic evaluation, which reveals a Bethesda grade III atypia of undetermined significance (AUS) or follicular lesion of undetermined significance (FLUS) (Bethesda grade III). A sample of the specimen is sent for molecular pathology testing, including telomerase (TERT) promotor mutation studies.

Description of Procedure (81345)

Isolate and subject high-quality genomic DNA from the patient's specimen to sequence analysis of the TERT gene promoter region to identify mutations. The pathologist or other qualified health care professional analyzes the data and composes a report specifying the patient's mutation status. Edit and sign the report and communicate the results to the appropriate caregivers.

● **81333**   *TGFBI (transforming growth factor beta-induced)* (eg, corneal dystrophy) gene analysis, common variants (eg, R124H, R124C, R124L, R555W, R555Q)

Rationale

Code 81333 has been established to report the test that detects the mutations responsible for diseases such as the five distinct corneal dystrophies associated with mutations in the TGFBI gene. Unlisted code 81479 was previously used, however, it did not adequately describe testing that identifies mutations responsible for the five distinct corneal dystrophies associated with mutations in the TGFBI gene. In addition, the usage volume and clinical importance of this test warrant its own code.

Clinical Example (81333)

A 25-year-old female presents for refractive surgery evaluation because of contact-lens intolerance. Slit-lamp examination reveals a few small, nonspecific superficial opacities of uncertain origin in both corneas. Family history suggests corneal dystrophy. To determine if the corneal opacities are secondary to postinfectious scarring or dystrophic deposits, a buccal swab is obtained and sent for transforming growth factor beta-induced (TGFBI) genetic gene analysis.

Description of Procedure (81333)

Isolate and subject high-quality genomic DNA from epithelial cells collected by buccal swab to targeted analysis of the corneal dystrophy-associated common variants within TGFBI. The pathologist or other qualified health care professional evaluates the data and composes a report specifying the patient's TGFBI variant status. Edit and sign the report and communicate results to the appropriate caregivers.

81335	*TPMT (thiopurine S-methyltransferase)* (eg, drug metabolism), gene analysis, common variants (eg, *2, *3)
81336	Code is out of numerical sequence. See 81318-81335
81337	Code is out of numerical sequence. See 81318-81335
81343	Code is out of numerical sequence. See 81318-81335
81344	Code is out of numerical sequence. See 81318-81335
81345	Code is out of numerical sequence. See 81318-81335
81361	Code is out of numerical sequence. See 81253-81256
81362	Code is out of numerical sequence. See 81253-81256
81363	Code is out of numerical sequence. See 81253-81256
81364	Code is out of numerical sequence. See 81253-81256

★ = Telemedicine   ✚ = Add-on code   ✗ = FDA approval pending   # = Resequenced code   ⊘ = Modifier 51 exempt

Tier 2 Molecular Pathology Procedures

▲ **81400**   Molecular pathology procedure, Level 1 (eg, identification of single germline variant [eg, SNP] by techniques such as restriction enzyme digestion or melt curve analysis)

ACADM (acyl-CoA dehydrogenase, C-4 to C-12 straight chain, MCAD) (eg, medium chain acyl dehydrogenase deficiency), K304E variant

ACE (angiotensin converting enzyme) (eg, hereditary blood pressure regulation), insertion/deletion variant

AGTR1 (angiotensin II receptor, type 1) (eg, essential hypertension), 1166A>C variant

BCKDHA (branched chain keto acid dehydrogenase E1, alpha polypeptide) (eg, maple syrup urine disease, type 1A), Y438N variant

CCR5 (chemokine C-C motif receptor 5) (eg, HIV resistance), 32-bp deletion mutation/794 825del32 deletion

CLRN1 (clarin 1) (eg, Usher syndrome, type 3), N48K variant

F2 (coagulation factor 2) (eg, hereditary hypercoagulability), 1199G>A variant

F5 (coagulation factor V) (eg, hereditary hypercoagulability), HR2 variant

F7 (coagulation factor VII [serum prothrombin conversion accelerator]) (eg, hereditary hypercoagulability), R353Q variant

F13B (coagulation factor XIII, B polypeptide) (eg, hereditary hypercoagulability), V34L variant

FGB (fibrinogen beta chain) (eg, hereditary ischemic heart disease), -455G>A variant

FGFR1 (fibroblast growth factor receptor 1) (eg, Pfeiffer syndrome type 1, craniosynostosis), P252R variant

FGFR3 (fibroblast growth factor receptor 3) (eg, Muenke syndrome), P250R variant

FKTN (fukutin) (eg, Fukuyama congenital muscular dystrophy), retrotransposon insertion variant

GNE (glucosamine [UDP-N-acetyl]-2-epimerase/N-acetylmannosamine kinase) (eg, inclusion body myopathy 2 [IBM2], Nonaka myopathy), M712T variant

IVD (isovaleryl-CoA dehydrogenase) (eg, isovaleric acidemia), A282V variant

LCT (lactase-phlorizin hydrolase) (eg, lactose intolerance), 13910 C>T variant

NEB (nebulin) (eg, nemaline myopathy 2), exon 55 deletion variant

PCDH15 (protocadherin-related 15) (eg, Usher syndrome type 1F), R245X variant

SERPINE1 (serpine peptidase inhibitor clade E, member 1, plasminogen activator inhibitor -1, PAI-1) (eg, thrombophilia), 4G variant

SHOC2 (soc-2 suppressor of clear homolog) (eg, Noonan-like syndrome with loose anagen hair), S2G variant

SRY (sex determining region Y) (eg, 46,XX testicular disorder of sex development, gonadal dysgenesis), gene analysis

TOR1A (torsin family 1, member A [torsin A]) (eg, early-onset primary dystonia [DYT1]), 907_909delGAG (904_906delGAG) variant

▲ **81401**   Molecular pathology procedure, Level 2 (eg, 2-10 SNPs, 1 methylated variant, or 1 somatic variant [typically using nonsequencing target variant analysis], or detection of a dynamic mutation disorder/triplet repeat)

ABCC8 (ATP-binding cassette, sub-family C [CFTR/MRP], member 8) (eg, familial hyperinsulinism), common variants (eg, c.3898-9G>A [c.3992-9G>A], F1388del)

ABL1 (ABL proto-oncogene 1, non-receptor tyrosine kinase) (eg, acquired imatinib resistance), T315I variant

ACADM (acyl-CoA dehydrogenase, C-4 to C-12 straight chain, MCAD) (eg, medium chain acyl dehydrogenase deficiency), commons variants (eg, K304E, Y42H)

ADRB2 (adrenergic beta-2 receptor surface) (eg, drug metabolism), common variants (eg, G16R, Q27E)

APOB (apolipoprotein B) (eg, familial hypercholesterolemia type B), common variants (eg, R3500Q, R3500W)

APOE (apolipoprotein E) (eg, hyperlipoproteinemia type III, cardiovascular disease, Alzheimer disease), common variants (eg, *2, *3, *4)

CBFB/MYH11 (inv(16)) (eg, acute myeloid leukemia), qualitative, and quantitative, if performed

CBS (cystathionine-beta-synthase) (eg, homocystinuria, cystathionine beta-synthase deficiency), common variants (eg, I278T, G307S)

CCND1/IGH (BCL1/IgH, t(11;14)) (eg, mantle cell lymphoma) translocation analysis, major breakpoint, qualitative, and quantitative, if performed

CFH/ARMS2 (complement factor H/age-related maculopathy susceptibility 2) (eg, macular degeneration), common variants (eg, Y402H [CFH], A69S [ARMS2])

DEK/NUP214 (t(6;9)) (eg, acute myeloid leukemia), translocation analysis, qualitative, and quantitative, if performed

E2A/PBX1 (t(1;19)) (eg, acute lymphocytic leukemia), translocation analysis, qualitative, and quantitative, if performed

EML4/ALK (inv(2)) (eg, non-small cell lung cancer), translocation or inversion analysis

ETV6/NTRK3 (t(12;15)) (eg, congenital/infantile fibrosarcoma), translocation analysis, qualitative, and quantitative, if performed

ETV6/RUNX1 (t(12;21)) (eg, acute lymphocytic leukemia), translocation analysis, qualitative, and quantitative, if performed

EWSR1/ATF1 (t(12;22)) (eg, clear cell sarcoma), translocation analysis, qualitative, and quantitative, if performed

EWSR1/ERG (t(21;22)) (eg, Ewing sarcoma/peripheral neuroectodermal tumor), translocation analysis, qualitative, and quantitative, if performed

EWSR1/FLI1 (t(11;22)) (eg, Ewing sarcoma/peripheral neuroectodermal tumor), translocation analysis, qualitative, and quantitative, if performed

EWSR1/WT1 (t(11;22)) (eg, desmoplastic small round cell tumor), translocation analysis, qualitative, and quantitative, if performed

F11 (coagulation factor XI) (eg, coagulation disorder), common variants (eg, E117X [Type II], F283L [Type III], IVS14del14, and IVS14+1G>A [Type I])

FGFR3 (fibroblast growth factor receptor 3) (eg, achondroplasia, hypochondroplasia), common variants (eg, 1138G>A, 1138G>C, 1620C>A, 1620C>G)

FIP1L1/PDGFRA (del[4q12]) (eg, imatinib-sensitive chronic eosinophilic leukemia), qualitative, and quantitative, if performed

FLG (filaggrin) (eg, ichthyosis vulgaris), common variants (eg, R501X, 2282del4, R2447X, S3247X, 3702delG)

FOXO1/PAX3 (t(2;13)) (eg, alveolar rhabdomyosarcoma), translocation analysis, qualitative, and quantitative, if performed

FOXO1/PAX7 (t(1;13)) (eg, alveolar rhabdomyosarcoma), translocation analysis, qualitative, and quantitative, if performed

FUS/DDIT3 (t(12;16)) (eg, myxoid liposarcoma), translocation analysis, qualitative, and quantitative, if performed

GALC (galactosylceramidase) (eg, Krabbe disease), common variants (eg, c.857G>A, 30-kb deletion)

GALT (galactose-1-phosphate uridylyltransferase) (eg, galactosemia), common variants (eg, Q188R, S135L, K285N, T138M, L195P, Y209C, IVS2-2A>G, P171S, del5kb, N314D, L218L/N314D)

H19 (imprinted maternally expressed transcript [non-protein coding]) (eg, Beckwith-Wiedemann syndrome), methylation analysis

IGH@/BCL2 (t(14;18)) (eg, follicular lymphoma), translocation analysis; single breakpoint (eg, major breakpoint region [MBR] or minor cluster region [mcr]), qualitative or quantitative

(When both MBR and mcr breakpoints are performed, use 81402)

KCNQ1OT1 (KCNQ1 overlapping transcript 1 [non-protein coding]) (eg, Beckwith-Wiedemann syndrome), methylation analysis

LINC00518 (long intergenic non-protein coding RNA 518) (eg, melanoma), expression analysis

LRRK2 (leucine-rich repeat kinase 2) (eg, Parkinson disease), common variants (eg, R1441G, G2019S, I2020T)

MED12 (mediator complex subunit 12) (eg, FG syndrome type 1, Lujan syndrome), common variants (eg, R961W, N1007S)

MEG3/DLK1 (maternally expressed 3 [non-protein coding]/delta-like 1 homolog [Drosophila]) (eg, intrauterine growth retardation), methylation analysis

MLL/AFF1 (t(4;11)) (eg, acute lymphoblastic leukemia), translocation analysis, qualitative, and quantitative, if performed

MLL/MLLT3 (t(9;11)) (eg, acute myeloid leukemia), translocation analysis, qualitative, and quantitative, if performed

MT-ATP6 (mitochondrially encoded ATP synthase 6) (eg, neuropathy with ataxia and retinitis pigmentosa [NARP], Leigh syndrome), common variants (eg, m.8993T>G, m.8993T>C)

MT-ND4, MT-ND6 (mitochondrially encoded NADH dehydrogenase 4, mitochondrially encoded NADH dehydrogenase 6) (eg, Leber hereditary optic neuropathy [LHON]), common variants (eg, m.11778G>A, m.3460G>A, m.14484T>C)

MT-ND5 (mitochondrially encoded tRNA leucine 1 [UUA/G], mitochondrially encoded NADH dehydrogenase 5) (eg, mitochondrial encephalopathy with lactic acidosis and stroke-like episodes [MELAS]), common variants (eg, m.3243A>G, m.3271T>C, m.3252A>G, m.13513G>A)

MT-RNR1 (mitochondrially encoded 12S RNA) (eg, nonsyndromic hearing loss), common variants (eg, m.1555A>G, m.1494C>T)

MT-TK (mitochondrially encoded tRNA lysine) (eg, myoclonic epilepsy with ragged-red fibers [MERRF]), common variants (eg, m.8344A>G, m.8356T>C)

MT-TL1 (mitochondrially encoded tRNA leucine 1 [UUA/G]) (eg, diabetes and hearing loss), common variants (eg, m.3243A>G, m.14709 T>C) MT-TL1

MT-TS1, MT-RNR1 (mitochondrially encoded tRNA serine 1 [UCN], mitochondrially encoded 12S RNA) (eg, nonsyndromic sensorineural deafness [including aminoglycoside-induced nonsyndromic deafness]), common variants (eg, m.7445A>G, m.1555A>G)

MUTYH (mutY homolog [E. coli]) (eg, MYH-associated polyposis), common variants (eg, Y165C, G382D)

NOD2 (nucleotide-binding oligomerization domain containing 2) (eg, Crohn's disease, Blau syndrome), common variants (eg, SNP 8, SNP 12, SNP 13)

NPM1/ALK (t(2;5)) (eg, anaplastic large cell lymphoma), translocation analysis

PAX8/PPARG (t(2;3) (q13;p25)) (eg, follicular thyroid carcinoma), translocation analysis

PRAME (preferentially expressed antigen in melanoma) (eg, melanoma), expression analysis

PRSS1 (protease, serine, 1 [trypsin 1]) (eg, hereditary pancreatitis), common variants (eg, N29I, A16V, R122H)

PYGM (phosphorylase, glycogen, muscle) (eg, glycogen storage disease type V, McArdle disease), common variants (eg, R50X, G205S)

RUNX1/RUNX1T1 (t(8;21)) (eg, acute myeloid leukemia) translocation analysis, qualitative, and quantitative, if performed

SS18/SSX1 (t(X;18)) (eg, synovial sarcoma), translocation analysis, qualitative, and quantitative, if performed

SS18/SSX2 (t(X;18)) (eg, synovial sarcoma), translocation analysis, qualitative, and quantitative, if performed

VWF (von Willebrand factor) (eg, von Willebrand disease type 2N), common variants (eg, T791M, R816W, R854Q)

▲ **81403** Molecular pathology procedure, Level 4 (eg, analysis of single exon by DNA sequence analysis, analysis of >10 amplicons using multiplex PCR in 2 or more independent reactions, mutation scanning or duplication/deletion variants of 2-5 exons)

ANG (angiogenin, ribonuclease, RNase A family, 5) (eg, amyotrophic lateral sclerosis), full gene sequence

ARX (aristaless-related homeobox) (eg, X-linked lissencephaly with ambiguous genitalia, X-linked mental retardation), duplication/deletion analysis

CEL (carboxyl ester lipase [bile salt-stimulated lipase]) (eg, maturity-onset diabetes of the young [MODY]), targeted sequence analysis of exon 11 (eg, c.1785delC, c.1686delT)

CTNNB1 (catenin [cadherin-associated protein], beta 1, 88kDa) (eg, desmoid tumors), targeted sequence analysis (eg, exon 3)

DAZ/SRY (deleted in azoospermia and sex determining region Y) (eg, male infertility), common deletions (eg, AZFa, AZFb, AZFc, AZFd)

DNMT3A (DNA [cytosine-5-]-methyltransferase 3 alpha) (eg, acute myeloid leukemia), targeted sequence analysis (eg, exon 23)

EPCAM (epithelial cell adhesion molecule) (eg, Lynch syndrome), duplication/deletion analysis

F8 (coagulation factor VIII) (eg, hemophilia A), inversion analysis, intron 1 and intron 22A

F12 (coagulation factor XII [Hageman factor]) (eg, angioedema, hereditary, type III; factor XII deficiency), targeted sequence analysis of exon 9

FGFR3 (fibroblast growth factor receptor 3) (eg, isolated craniosynostosis), targeted sequence analysis (eg, exon 7)

(For targeted sequence analysis of multiple FGFR3 exons, use 81404)

GJB1 (gap junction protein, beta 1) (eg, Charcot-Marie-Tooth X-linked), full gene sequence

GNAQ (guanine nucleotide-binding protein G[q] subunit alpha) (eg, uveal melanoma), common variants (eg, R183, Q209)

Human erythrocyte antigen gene analyses (eg, SLC14A1 [Kidd blood group], BCAM [Lutheran blood group], ICAM4 [Landsteiner-Wiener blood group], SLC4A1 [Diego blood group], AQP1 [Colton blood group], ERMAP [Scianna blood group], RHCE [Rh blood group, CcEe antigens], KEL [Kell blood group], DARC [Duffy blood group], GYPA, GYPB, GYPE [MNS blood group], ART4 [Dombrock blood group]) (eg, sickle-cell disease, thalassemia, hemolytic transfusion reactions, hemolytic disease of the fetus or newborn), common variants

HRAS (v-Ha-ras Harvey rat sarcoma viral oncogene homolog) (eg, Costello syndrome), exon 2 sequence

JAK2 (Janus kinase 2) (eg, myeloproliferative disorder), exon 12 sequence and exon 13 sequence, if performed

KCNC3 (potassium voltage-gated channel, Shaw-related subfamily, member 3) (eg, spinocerebellar ataxia), targeted sequence analysis (eg, exon 2)

KCNJ2 (potassium inwardly-rectifying channel, subfamily J, member 2) (eg, Andersen-Tawil syndrome), full gene sequence

KCNJ11 (potassium inwardly-rectifying channel, subfamily J, member 11) (eg, familial hyperinsulinism), full gene sequence

Killer cell immunoglobulin-like receptor (KIR) gene family (eg, hematopoietic stem cell transplantation), genotyping of KIR family genes

Known familial variant not otherwise specified, for gene listed in Tier 1 or Tier 2, or identified during a genomic sequencing procedure, DNA sequence analysis, each variant exon

(For a known familial variant that is considered a common variant, use specific common variant Tier 1 or Tier 2 code)

MC4R (melanocortin 4 receptor) (eg, obesity), full gene sequence

MICA (MHC class I polypeptide-related sequence A) (eg, solid organ transplantation), common variants (eg, *001, *002)

Pathology and Laboratory 80047-89398, 0001U-0061U

MPL (myeloproliferative leukemia virus oncogene, thrombopoietin receptor, TPOR) (eg, myeloproliferative disorder), exon 10 sequence

MT-RNR1 (mitochondrially encoded 12S RNA) (eg, nonsyndromic hearing loss), full gene sequence

MT-TS1 (mitochondrially encoded tRNA serine 1) (eg, nonsyndromic hearing loss), full gene sequence

NDP (Norrie disease [pseudoglioma]) (eg, Norrie disease), duplication/deletion analysis

NHLRC1 (NHL repeat containing 1) (eg, progressive myoclonus epilepsy), full gene sequence

PHOX2B (paired-like homeobox 2b) (eg, congenital central hypoventilation syndrome), duplication/deletion analysis

PLN (phospholamban) (eg, dilated cardiomyopathy, hypertrophic cardiomyopathy), full gene sequence

RHD (Rh blood group, D antigen) (eg, hemolytic disease of the fetus and newborn, Rh maternal/fetal compatibility), deletion analysis (eg, exons 4, 5, and 7, pseudogene)

RHD (Rh blood group, D antigen) (eg, hemolytic disease of the fetus and newborn, Rh maternal/fetal compatibility), deletion analysis (eg, exons 4, 5, and 7, pseudogene), performed on cell-free fetal DNA in maternal blood

(For human erythrocyte gene analysis of RHD, use a separate unit of 81403)

SH2D1A (SH2 domain containing 1A) (eg, X-linked lymphoproliferative syndrome), duplication/deletion analysis

TWIST1 (twist homolog 1 [Drosophila]) (eg, Saethre-Chotzen syndrome), duplication/deletion analysis

UBA1 (ubiquitin-like modifier activating enzyme 1) (eg, spinal muscular atrophy, X-linked), targeted sequence analysis (eg, exon 15)

VHL (von Hippel-Lindau tumor suppressor) (eg, von Hippel-Lindau familial cancer syndrome), deletion/duplication analysis

VWF (von Willebrand factor) (eg, von Willebrand disease types 2A, 2B, 2M), targeted sequence analysis (eg, exon 28)

▲ **81404** Molecular pathology procedure, Level 5 (eg, analysis of 2-5 exons by DNA sequence analysis, mutation scanning or duplication/deletion variants of 6-10 exons, or characterization of a dynamic mutation disorder/triplet repeat by Southern blot analysis)

ACADS (acyl-CoA dehydrogenase, C-2 to C-3 short chain) (eg, short chain acyl-CoA dehydrogenase deficiency), targeted sequence analysis (eg, exons 5 and 6)

AQP2 (aquaporin 2 [collecting duct]) (eg, nephrogenic diabetes insipidus), full gene sequence

ARX (aristaless related homeobox) (eg, X-linked lissencephaly with ambiguous genitalia, X-linked mental retardation), full gene sequence

AVPR2 (arginine vasopressin receptor 2) (eg, nephrogenic diabetes insipidus), full gene sequence

BBS10 (Bardet-Biedl syndrome 10) (eg, Bardet-Biedl syndrome), full gene sequence

BTD (biotinidase) (eg, biotinidase deficiency), full gene sequence

C10orf2 (chromosome 10 open reading frame 2) (eg, mitochondrial DNA depletion syndrome), full gene sequence

CAV3 (caveolin 3) (eg, CAV3-related distal myopathy, limb-girdle muscular dystrophy type 1C), full gene sequence

CD40LG (CD40 ligand) (eg, X-linked hyper IgM syndrome), full gene sequence

CDKN2A (cyclin-dependent kinase inhibitor 2A) (eg, CDKN2A-related cutaneous malignant melanoma, familial atypical mole-malignant melanoma syndrome), full gene sequence

CLRN1 (clarin 1) (eg, Usher syndrome, type 3), full gene sequence

COX6B1 (cytochrome c oxidase subunit VIb polypeptide 1) (eg, mitochondrial respiratory chain complex IV deficiency), full gene sequence

CPT2 (carnitine palmitoyltransferase 2) (eg, carnitine palmitoyltransferase II deficiency), full gene sequence

CRX (cone-rod homeobox) (eg, cone-rod dystrophy 2, Leber congenital amaurosis), full gene sequence

CYP1B1 (cytochrome P450, family 1, subfamily B, polypeptide 1) (eg, primary congenital glaucoma), full gene sequence

EGR2 (early growth response 2) (eg, Charcot-Marie-Tooth), full gene sequence

EMD (emerin) (eg, Emery-Dreifuss muscular dystrophy), duplication/deletion analysis

EPM2A (epilepsy, progressive myoclonus type 2A, Lafora disease [laforin]) (eg, progressive myoclonus epilepsy), full gene sequence

FGF23 (fibroblast growth factor 23) (eg, hypophosphatemic rickets), full gene sequence

FGFR2 (fibroblast growth factor receptor 2) (eg, craniosynostosis, Apert syndrome, Crouzon syndrome), targeted sequence analysis (eg, exons 8, 10)

FGFR3 (fibroblast growth factor receptor 3) (eg, achondroplasia, hypochondroplasia), targeted sequence analysis (eg, exons 8, 11, 12, 13)

FHL1 (four and a half LIM domains 1) (eg, Emery-Dreifuss muscular dystrophy), full gene sequence

FKRP (fukutin related protein) (eg, congenital muscular dystrophy type 1C [MDC1C], limb-girdle muscular dystrophy [LGMD] type 2I), full gene sequence

FOXG1 (forkhead box G1) (eg, Rett syndrome), full gene sequence

FSHMD1A (facioscapulohumeral muscular dystrophy 1A) (eg, facioscapulohumeral muscular dystrophy), evaluation to detect abnormal (eg, deleted) alleles

FSHMD1A (facioscapulohumeral muscular dystrophy 1A) (eg, facioscapulohumeral muscular dystrophy), characterization of haplotype(s) (ie, chromosome 4A and 4B haplotypes)

GH1 (growth hormone 1) (eg, growth hormone deficiency), full gene sequence

GP1BB (glycoprotein Ib [platelet], beta polypeptide) (eg, Bernard-Soulier syndrome type B), full gene sequence

(For common deletion variants of alpha globin 1 and alpha globin 2 genes, use 81257)

HNF1B (HNF1 homeobox B) (eg, maturity-onset diabetes of the young [MODY]), duplication/deletion analysis

HRAS (v-Ha-ras Harvey rat sarcoma viral oncogene homolog) (eg, Costello syndrome), full gene sequence

HSD3B2 (hydroxy-delta-5-steroid dehydrogenase, 3 beta- and steroid delta-isomerase 2) (eg, 3-beta-hydroxysteroid dehydrogenase type II deficiency), full gene sequence

HSD11B2 (hydroxysteroid [11-beta] dehydrogenase 2) (eg, mineralocorticoid excess syndrome), full gene sequence

HSPB1 (heat shock 27kDa protein 1) (eg, Charcot-Marie-Tooth disease), full gene sequence

INS (insulin) (eg, diabetes mellitus), full gene sequence

KCNJ1 (potassium inwardly-rectifying channel, subfamily J, member 1) (eg, Bartter syndrome), full gene sequence

KCNJ10 (potassium inwardly-rectifying channel, subfamily J, member 10) (eg, SeSAME syndrome, EAST syndrome, sensorineural hearing loss), full gene sequence

LITAF (lipopolysaccharide-induced TNF factor) (eg, Charcot-Marie-Tooth), full gene sequence

MEFV (Mediterranean fever) (eg, familial Mediterranean fever), full gene sequence

MEN1 (multiple endocrine neoplasia I) (eg, multiple endocrine neoplasia type 1, Wermer syndrome), duplication/deletion analysis

MMACHC (methylmalonic aciduria [cobalamin deficiency] cblC type, with homocystinuria) (eg, methylmalonic acidemia and homocystinuria), full gene sequence

MPV17 (MpV17 mitochondrial inner membrane protein) (eg, mitochondrial DNA depletion syndrome), duplication/ deletion analysis

NDP (Norrie disease [pseudoglioma]) (eg, Norrie disease), full gene sequence

NDUFA1 (NADH dehydrogenase [ubiquinone] 1 alpha subcomplex, 1, 7.5kDa) (eg, Leigh syndrome, mitochondrial complex I deficiency), full gene sequence

NDUFAF2 (NADH dehydrogenase [ubiquinone] 1 alpha subcomplex, assembly factor 2) (eg, Leigh syndrome, mitochondrial complex I deficiency), full gene sequence

NDUFS4 (NADH dehydrogenase [ubiquinone] Fe-S protein 4, 18kDa [NADH-coenzyme Q reductase]) (eg, Leigh syndrome, mitochondrial complex I deficiency), full gene sequence

NIPA1 (non-imprinted in Prader-Willi/Angelman syndrome 1) (eg, spastic paraplegia), full gene sequence

NLGN4X (neuroligin 4, X-linked) (eg, autism spectrum disorders), duplication/deletion analysis

NPC2 (Niemann-Pick disease, type C2 [epididymal secretory protein E1]) (eg, Niemann-Pick disease type C2), full gene sequence

NR0B1 (nuclear receptor subfamily 0, group B, member 1) (eg, congenital adrenal hypoplasia), full gene sequence

PDX1 (pancreatic and duodenal homeobox 1) (eg, maturity-onset diabetes of the young [MODY]), full gene sequence

PHOX2B (paired-like homeobox 2b) (eg, congenital central hypoventilation syndrome), full gene sequence

PIK3CA (phosphatidylinositol-4,5-bisphosphate 3-kinase, catalytic subunit alpha) (eg, colorectal cancer), targeted sequence analysis (eg, exons 9 and 20)

PLP1 (proteolipid protein 1) (eg, Pelizaeus-Merzbacher disease, spastic paraplegia), duplication/deletion analysis

PQBP1 (polyglutamine binding protein 1) (eg, Renpenning syndrome), duplication/deletion analysis

PRNP (prion protein) (eg, genetic prion disease), full gene sequence

PROP1 (PROP paired-like homeobox 1) (eg, combined pituitary hormone deficiency), full gene sequence

PRPH2 (peripherin 2 [retinal degeneration, slow]) (eg, retinitis pigmentosa), full gene sequence

PRSS1 (protease, serine, 1 [trypsin 1]) (eg, hereditary pancreatitis), full gene sequence

RAF1 (v-raf-1 murine leukemia viral oncogene homolog 1) (eg, LEOPARD syndrome), targeted sequence analysis (eg, exons 7, 12, 14, 17)

RET (ret proto-oncogene) (eg, multiple endocrine neoplasia, type 2B and familial medullary thyroid carcinoma), common variants (eg, M918T, 2647_2648delinsTT, A883F)

RHO (rhodopsin) (eg, retinitis pigmentosa), full gene sequence

RP1 (retinitis pigmentosa 1) (eg, retinitis pigmentosa), full gene sequence

SCN1B (sodium channel, voltage-gated, type I, beta) (eg, Brugada syndrome), full gene sequence

SCO2 (SCO cytochrome oxidase deficient homolog 2 [SCO1L]) (eg, mitochondrial respiratory chain complex IV deficiency), full gene sequence

SDHC (succinate dehydrogenase complex, subunit C, integral membrane protein, 15kDa) (eg, hereditary paraganglioma-pheochromocytoma syndrome), duplication/deletion analysis

SDHD (succinate dehydrogenase complex, subunit D, integral membrane protein) (eg, hereditary paraganglioma), full gene sequence

SGCG (sarcoglycan, gamma [35kDa dystrophin-associated glycoprotein]) (eg, limb-girdle muscular dystrophy), duplication/deletion analysis

SH2D1A (SH2 domain containing 1A) (eg, X-linked lymphoproliferative syndrome), full gene sequence

SLC16A2 (solute carrier family 16, member 2 [thyroid hormone transporter]) (eg, specific thyroid hormone cell transporter deficiency, Allan-Herndon-Dudley syndrome), duplication/deletion analysis

SLC25A20 (solute carrier family 25 [carnitine/ acylcarnitine translocase], member 20) (eg, carnitine-acylcarnitine translocase deficiency), duplication/deletion analysis

SLC25A4 (solute carrier family 25 [mitochondrial carrier; adenine nucleotide translocator], member 4) (eg, progressive external ophthalmoplegia), full gene sequence

SOD1 (superoxide dismutase 1, soluble) (eg, amyotrophic lateral sclerosis), full gene sequence

SPINK1 (serine peptidase inhibitor, Kazal type 1) (eg, hereditary pancreatitis), full gene sequence

STK11 (serine/threonine kinase 11) (eg, Peutz-Jeghers syndrome), duplication/deletion analysis

TACO1 (translational activator of mitochondrial encoded cytochrome c oxidase I) (eg, mitochondrial respiratory chain complex IV deficiency), full gene sequence

THAP1 (THAP domain containing, apoptosis associated protein 1) (eg, torsion dystonia), full gene sequence

TOR1A (torsin family 1, member A [torsin A]) (eg, torsion dystonia), full gene sequence

TP53 (tumor protein 53) (eg, tumor samples), targeted sequence analysis of 2-5 exons

TTPA (tocopherol [alpha] transfer protein) (eg, ataxia), full gene sequence

TTR (transthyretin) (eg, familial transthyretin amyloidosis), full gene sequence

TWIST1 (twist homolog 1 [Drosophila]) (eg, Saethre-Chotzen syndrome), full gene sequence

TYR (tyrosinase [oculocutaneous albinism IA]) (eg, oculocutaneous albinism IA), full gene sequence

USH1G (Usher syndrome 1G [autosomal recessive]) (eg, Usher syndrome, type 1), full gene sequence

VHL (von Hippel-Lindau tumor suppressor) (eg, von Hippel-Lindau familial cancer syndrome), full gene sequence

VWF (von Willebrand factor) (eg, von Willebrand disease type 1C), targeted sequence analysis (eg, exons 26, 27, 37)

ZEB2 (zinc finger E-box binding homeobox 2) (eg, Mowat-Wilson syndrome), duplication/deletion analysis

ZNF41 (zinc finger protein 41) (eg, X-linked mental retardation 89), full gene sequence

▲ **81405** Molecular pathology procedure, Level 6 (eg, analysis of 6-10 exons by DNA sequence analysis, mutation scanning or duplication/deletion variants of 11-25 exons, regionally targeted cytogenomic array analysis)

ABCD1 (ATP-binding cassette, sub-family D [ALD], member 1) (eg, adrenoleukodystrophy), full gene sequence

ACADS (acyl-CoA dehydrogenase, C-2 to C-3 short chain) (eg, short chain acyl-CoA dehydrogenase deficiency), full gene sequence

ACTA2 (actin, alpha 2, smooth muscle, aorta) (eg, thoracic aortic aneurysms and aortic dissections), full gene sequence

ACTC1 (actin, alpha, cardiac muscle 1) (eg, familial hypertrophic cardiomyopathy), full gene sequence

ANKRD1 (ankyrin repeat domain 1) (eg, dilated cardiomyopathy), full gene sequence

APTX (aprataxin) (eg, ataxia with oculomotor apraxia 1), full gene sequence

ARSA (arylsulfatase A) (eg, arylsulfatase A deficiency), full gene sequence

BCKDHA (branched chain keto acid dehydrogenase E1, alpha polypeptide) (eg, maple syrup urine disease, type 1A), full gene sequence

BCS1L (BCS1-like [S. cerevisiae]) (eg, Leigh syndrome, mitochondrial complex III deficiency, GRACILE syndrome), full gene sequence

BMPR2 (bone morphogenetic protein receptor, type II [serine/threonine kinase]) (eg, heritable pulmonary arterial hypertension), duplication/deletion analysis

CASQ2 (calsequestrin 2 [cardiac muscle]) (eg, catecholaminergic polymorphic ventricular tachycardia), full gene sequence

CASR (calcium-sensing receptor) (eg, hypocalcemia), full gene sequence

CDKL5 (cyclin-dependent kinase-like 5) (eg, early infantile epileptic encephalopathy), duplication/deletion analysis

CHRNA4 (cholinergic receptor, nicotinic, alpha 4) (eg, nocturnal frontal lobe epilepsy), full gene sequence

CHRNB2 (cholinergic receptor, nicotinic, beta 2 [neuronal]) (eg, nocturnal frontal lobe epilepsy), full gene sequence

COX10 (COX10 homolog, cytochrome c oxidase assembly protein) (eg, mitochondrial respiratory chain complex IV deficiency), full gene sequence

COX15 (COX15 homolog, cytochrome c oxidase assembly protein) (eg, mitochondrial respiratory chain complex IV deficiency), full gene sequence

CPOX (coproporphyrinogen oxidase) (eg, hereditary coproporphyria), full gene sequence

CTRC (chymotrypsin C) (eg, hereditary pancreatitis), full gene sequence

CYP11B1 (cytochrome P450, family 11, subfamily B, polypeptide 1) (eg, congenital adrenal hyperplasia), full gene sequence

CYP17A1 (cytochrome P450, family 17, subfamily A, polypeptide 1) (eg, congenital adrenal hyperplasia), full gene sequence

CYP21A2 (cytochrome P450, family 21, subfamily A, polypeptide2) (eg, steroid 21-hydroxylase isoform, congenital adrenal hyperplasia), full gene sequence

Cytogenomic constitutional targeted microarray analysis of chromosome 22q13 by interrogation of genomic regions for copy number and single nucleotide polymorphism (SNP) variants for chromosomal abnormalities

(When performing genome-wide cytogenomic constitutional microarray analysis, see 81228, 81229)

(Do not report analyte-specific molecular pathology procedures separately when the specific analytes are included as part of the microarray analysis of chromosome 22q13)

(Do not report 88271 when performing cytogenomic microarray analysis)

DBT (dihydrolipoamide branched chain transacylase E2) (eg, maple syrup urine disease, type 2), duplication/deletion analysis

DCX (doublecortin) (eg, X-linked lissencephaly), full gene sequence

DES (desmin) (eg, myofibrillar myopathy), full gene sequence

DFNB59 (deafness, autosomal recessive 59) (eg, autosomal recessive nonsyndromic hearing impairment), full gene sequence

DGUOK (deoxyguanosine kinase) (eg, hepatocerebral mitochondrial DNA depletion syndrome), full gene sequence

DHCR7 (7-dehydrocholesterol reductase) (eg, Smith-Lemli-Opitz syndrome), full gene sequence

EIF2B2 (eukaryotic translation initiation factor 2B, subunit 2 beta, 39kDa) (eg, leukoencephalopathy with vanishing white matter), full gene sequence

EMD (emerin) (eg, Emery-Dreifuss muscular dystrophy), full gene sequence

ENG (endoglin) (eg, hereditary hemorrhagic telangiectasia, type 1), duplication/deletion analysis

EYA1 (eyes absent homolog 1 [Drosophila]) (eg, branchio-oto-renal [BOR] spectrum disorders), duplication/deletion analysis

FGFR1 (fibroblast growth factor receptor 1) (eg, Kallmann syndrome 2), full gene sequence

FH (fumarate hydratase) (eg, fumarate hydratase deficiency, hereditary leiomyomatosis with renal cell cancer), full gene sequence

FKTN (fukutin) (eg, limb-girdle muscular dystrophy [LGMD] type 2M or 2L), full gene sequence

FTSJ1 (FtsJ RNA methyltransferase homolog 1 [E. coli]) (eg, X-linked mental retardation 9), duplication/deletion analysis

GABRG2 (gamma-aminobutyric acid [GABA] A receptor, gamma 2) (eg, generalized epilepsy with febrile seizures), full gene sequence

GCH1 (GTP cyclohydrolase 1) (eg, autosomal dominant dopa-responsive dystonia), full gene sequence

GDAP1 (ganglioside-induced differentiation-associated protein 1) (eg, Charcot-Marie-Tooth disease), full gene sequence

GFAP (glial fibrillary acidic protein) (eg, Alexander disease), full gene sequence

GHR (growth hormone receptor) (eg, Laron syndrome), full gene sequence

GHRHR (growth hormone releasing hormone receptor) (eg, growth hormone deficiency), full gene sequence

GLA (galactosidase, alpha) (eg, Fabry disease), full gene sequence

HNF1A (HNF1 homeobox A) (eg, maturity-onset diabetes of the young [MODY]), full gene sequence

HNF1B (HNF1 homeobox B) (eg, maturity-onset diabetes of the young [MODY]), full gene sequence

HTRA1 (HtrA serine peptidase 1) (eg, macular degeneration), full gene sequence

IDS (iduronate 2-sulfatase) (eg, mucopolysacchridosis, type II), full gene sequence

IL2RG (interleukin 2 receptor, gamma) (eg, X-linked severe combined immunodeficiency), full gene sequence

ISPD (isoprenoid synthase domain containing) (eg, muscle-eye-brain disease, Walker-Warburg syndrome), full gene sequence

KRAS (Kirsten rat sarcoma viral oncogene homolog) (eg, Noonan syndrome), full gene sequence

LAMP2 (lysosomal-associated membrane protein 2) (eg, Danon disease), full gene sequence

LDLR (low density lipoprotein receptor) (eg, familial hypercholesterolemia), duplication/deletion analysis

MEN1 (multiple endocrine neoplasia I) (eg, multiple endocrine neoplasia type 1, Wermer syndrome), full gene sequence

MMAA (methylmalonic aciduria [cobalamine deficiency] type A) (eg, MMAA-related methylmalonic acidemia), full gene sequence

MMAB (methylmalonic aciduria [cobalamine deficiency] type B) (eg, MMAA-related methylmalonic acidemia), full gene sequence

MPI (mannose phosphate isomerase) (eg, congenital disorder of glycosylation 1b), full gene sequence

MPV17 (MpV17 mitochondrial inner membrane protein) (eg, mitochondrial DNA depletion syndrome), full gene sequence

MPZ (myelin protein zero) (eg, Charcot-Marie-Tooth), full gene sequence

MTM1 (myotubularin 1) (eg, X-linked centronuclear myopathy), duplication/deletion analysis

MYL2 (myosin, light chain 2, regulatory, cardiac, slow) (eg, familial hypertrophic cardiomyopathy), full gene sequence

MYL3 (myosin, light chain 3, alkali, ventricular, skeletal, slow) (eg, familial hypertrophic cardiomyopathy), full gene sequence

MYOT (myotilin) (eg, limb-girdle muscular dystrophy), full gene sequence

NDUFS7 (NADH dehydrogenase [ubiquinone] Fe-S protein 7, 20kDa [NADH-coenzyme Q reductase]) (eg, Leigh syndrome, mitochondrial complex I deficiency), full gene sequence

NDUFS8 (NADH dehydrogenase [ubiquinone] Fe-S protein 8, 23kDa [NADH-coenzyme Q reductase]) (eg, Leigh syndrome, mitochondrial complex I deficiency), full gene sequence

NDUFV1 (NADH dehydrogenase [ubiquinone] flavoprotein 1, 51kDa) (eg, Leigh syndrome, mitochondrial complex I deficiency), full gene sequence

NEFL (neurofilament, light polypeptide) (eg, Charcot-Marie-Tooth), full gene sequence

NF2 (neurofibromin 2 [merlin]) (eg, neurofibromatosis, type 2), duplication/deletion analysis

NLGN3 (neuroligin 3) (eg, autism spectrum disorders), full gene sequence

NLGN4X (neuroligin 4, X-linked) (eg, autism spectrum disorders), full gene sequence

NPHP1 (nephronophthisis 1 [juvenile]) (eg, Joubert syndrome), deletion analysis, and duplication analysis, if performed

NPHS2 (nephrosis 2, idiopathic, steroid-resistant [podocin]) (eg, steroid-resistant nephrotic syndrome), full gene sequence

NSD1 (nuclear receptor binding SET domain protein 1) (eg, Sotos syndrome), duplication/deletion analysis

OTC (ornithine carbamoyltransferase) (eg, ornithine transcarbamylase deficiency), full gene sequence

PAFAH1B1 (platelet-activating factor acetylhydrolase 1b, regulatory subunit 1 [45kDa]) (eg, lissencephaly, Miller-Dieker syndrome), duplication/deletion analysis

PARK2 (Parkinson protein 2, E3 ubiquitin protein ligase [parkin]) (eg, Parkinson disease), duplication/deletion analysis

PCCA (propionyl CoA carboxylase, alpha polypeptide) (eg, propionic acidemia, type 1), duplication/deletion analysis

PCDH19 (protocadherin 19) (eg, epileptic encephalopathy), full gene sequence

PDHA1 (pyruvate dehydrogenase [lipoamide] alpha 1) (eg, lactic acidosis), duplication/deletion analysis

PDHB (pyruvate dehydrogenase [lipoamide] beta) (eg, lactic acidosis), full gene sequence

PINK1 (PTEN induced putative kinase 1) (eg, Parkinson disease), full gene sequence

PKLR (pyruvate kinase, liver and RBC) (eg, pyruvate kinase deficiency), full gene sequence

PLP1 (proteolipid protein 1) (eg, Pelizaeus-Merzbacher disease, spastic paraplegia), full gene sequence

POU1F1 (POU class 1 homeobox 1) (eg, combined pituitary hormone deficiency), full gene sequence

PRX (periaxin) (eg, Charcot-Marie-Tooth disease), full gene sequence

PQBP1 (polyglutamine binding protein 1) (eg, Renpenning syndrome), full gene sequence

PSEN1 (presenilin 1) (eg, Alzheimer disease), full gene sequence

RAB7A (RAB7A, member RAS oncogene family) (eg, Charcot-Marie-Tooth disease), full gene sequence

RAI1 (retinoic acid induced 1) (eg, Smith-Magenis syndrome), full gene sequence

REEP1 (receptor accessory protein 1) (eg, spastic paraplegia), full gene sequence

RET (ret proto-oncogene) (eg, multiple endocrine neoplasia, type 2A and familial medullary thyroid carcinoma), targeted sequence analysis (eg, exons 10, 11, 13-16)

RPS19 (ribosomal protein S19) (eg, Diamond-Blackfan anemia), full gene sequence

RRM2B (ribonucleotide reductase M2 B [TP53 inducible]) (eg, mitochondrial DNA depletion), full gene sequence

SCO1 (SCO cytochrome oxidase deficient homolog 1) (eg, mitochondrial respiratory chain complex IV deficiency), full gene sequence

SDHB (succinate dehydrogenase complex, subunit B, iron sulfur) (eg, hereditary paraganglioma), full gene sequence

SDHC (succinate dehydrogenase complex, subunit C, integral membrane protein, 15kDa) (eg, hereditary paraganglioma-pheochromocytoma syndrome), full gene sequence

SGCA (sarcoglycan, alpha [50kDa dystrophin-associated glycoprotein]) (eg, limb-girdle muscular dystrophy), full gene sequence

SGCB (sarcoglycan, beta [43kDa dystrophin-associated glycoprotein]) (eg, limb-girdle muscular dystrophy), full gene sequence

SGCD (sarcoglycan, delta [35kDa dystrophin-associated glycoprotein]) (eg, limb-girdle muscular dystrophy), full gene sequence

SGCE (sarcoglycan, epsilon) (eg, myoclonic dystonia), duplication/deletion analysis

SGCG (sarcoglycan, gamma [35kDa dystrophin-associated glycoprotein]) (eg, limb-girdle muscular dystrophy), full gene sequence

SHOC2 (soc-2 suppressor of clear homolog) (eg, Noonan-like syndrome with loose anagen hair), full gene sequence

SHOX (short stature homeobox) (eg, Langer mesomelic dysplasia), full gene sequence

SIL1 (SIL1 homolog, endoplasmic reticulum chaperone [S. cerevisiae]) (eg, ataxia), full gene sequence

SLC2A1 (solute carrier family 2 [facilitated glucose transporter], member 1) (eg, glucose transporter type 1 [GLUT 1] deficiency syndrome), full gene sequence

SLC16A2 (solute carrier family 16, member 2 [thyroid hormone transporter]) (eg, specific thyroid hormone cell transporter deficiency, Allan-Herndon-Dudley syndrome), full gene sequence

SLC22A5 (solute carrier family 22 [organic cation/carnitine transporter], member 5) (eg, systemic primary carnitine deficiency), full gene sequence

SLC25A20 (solute carrier family 25 [carnitine/acylcarnitine translocase], member 20) (eg, carnitine-acylcarnitine translocase deficiency), full gene sequence

SMAD4 (SMAD family member 4) (eg, hemorrhagic telangiectasia syndrome, juvenile polyposis), duplication/deletion analysis

SPAST (spastin) (eg, spastic paraplegia), duplication/deletion analysis

SPG7 (spastic paraplegia 7 [pure and complicated autosomal recessive]) (eg, spastic paraplegia), duplication/deletion analysis

SPRED1 (sprouty-related, EVH1 domain containing 1) (eg, Legius syndrome), full gene sequence

STAT3 (signal transducer and activator of transcription 3 [acute-phase response factor]) (eg, autosomal dominant hyper-IgE syndrome), targeted sequence analysis (eg, exons 12, 13, 14, 16, 17, 20, 21)

STK11 (serine/threonine kinase 11) (eg, Peutz-Jeghers syndrome), full gene sequence

SURF1 (surfeit 1) (eg, mitochondrial respiratory chain complex IV deficiency), full gene sequence

TARDBP (TAR DNA binding protein) (eg, amyotrophic lateral sclerosis), full gene sequence

TBX5 (T-box 5) (eg, Holt-Oram syndrome), full gene sequence

TCF4 (transcription factor 4) (eg, Pitt-Hopkins syndrome), duplication/deletion analysis

TGFBR1 (transforming growth factor, beta receptor 1) (eg, Marfan syndrome), full gene sequence

TGFBR2 (transforming growth factor, beta receptor 2) (eg, Marfan syndrome), full gene sequence

THRB (thyroid hormone receptor, beta) (eg, thyroid hormone resistance, thyroid hormone beta receptor deficiency), full gene sequence or targeted sequence analysis of >5 exons

TK2 (thymidine kinase 2, mitochondrial) (eg, mitochondrial DNA depletion syndrome), full gene sequence

TNNC1 (troponin C type 1 [slow]) (eg, hypertrophic cardiomyopathy or dilated cardiomyopathy), full gene sequence

TNNI3 (troponin I, type 3 [cardiac]) (eg, familial hypertrophic cardiomyopathy), full gene sequence

TP53 (tumor protein 53) (eg, Li-Fraumeni syndrome, tumor samples), full gene sequence or targeted sequence analysis of >5 exons

TPM1 (tropomyosin 1 [alpha]) (eg, familial hypertrophic cardiomyopathy), full gene sequence

TSC1 (tuberous sclerosis 1) (eg, tuberous sclerosis), duplication/deletion analysis

TYMP (thymidine phosphorylase) (eg, mitochondrial DNA depletion syndrome), full gene sequence

VWF (von Willebrand factor) (eg, von Willebrand disease type 2N), targeted sequence analysis (eg, exons 18-20, 23-25)

WT1 (Wilms tumor 1) (eg, Denys-Drash syndrome, familial Wilms tumor), full gene sequence

ZEB2 (zinc finger E-box binding homeobox 2) (eg, Mowat-Wilson syndrome), full gene sequence

▲ **81407**   Molecular pathology procedure, Level 8 (eg, analysis of 26-50 exons by DNA sequence analysis, mutation scanning or duplication/deletion variants of >50 exons, sequence analysis of multiple genes on one platform)

ABCC8 (ATP-binding cassette, sub-family C [CFTR/MRP], member 8) (eg, familial hyperinsulinism), full gene sequence

AGL (amylo-alpha-1, 6-glucosidase, 4-alpha-glucanotransferase) (eg, glycogen storage disease type III), full gene sequence

AHI1 (Abelson helper integration site 1) (eg, Joubert syndrome), full gene sequence

ASPM (asp [abnormal spindle] homolog, microcephaly associated [Drosophila]) (eg, primary microcephaly), full gene sequence

CHD7 (chromodomain helicase DNA binding protein 7) (eg, CHARGE syndrome), full gene sequence

COL4A4 (collagen, type IV, alpha 4) (eg, Alport syndrome), full gene sequence

COL4A5 (collagen, type IV, alpha 5) (eg, Alport syndrome), duplication/deletion analysis

COL6A1 (collagen, type VI, alpha 1) (eg, collagen type VI-related disorders), full gene sequence

COL6A2 (collagen, type VI, alpha 2) (eg, collagen type VI-related disorders), full gene sequence

COL6A3 (collagen, type VI, alpha 3) (eg, collagen type VI-related disorders), full gene sequence

CREBBP (CREB binding protein) (eg, Rubinstein-Taybi syndrome), full gene sequence

F8 (coagulation factor VIII) (eg, hemophilia A), full gene sequence

JAG1 (jagged 1) (eg, Alagille syndrome), full gene sequence

KDM5C (lysine [K]-specific demethylase 5C) (eg, X-linked mental retardation), full gene sequence

KIAA0196 (KIAA0196) (eg, spastic paraplegia), full gene sequence

L1CAM (L1 cell adhesion molecule) (eg, MASA syndrome, X-linked hydrocephaly), full gene sequence

LAMB2 (laminin, beta 2 [laminin S]) (eg, Pierson syndrome), full gene sequence

MYBPC3 (myosin binding protein C, cardiac) (eg, familial hypertrophic cardiomyopathy), full gene sequence

MYH6 (myosin, heavy chain 6, cardiac muscle, alpha) (eg, familial dilated cardiomyopathy), full gene sequence

MYH7 (myosin, heavy chain 7, cardiac muscle, beta) (eg, familial hypertrophic cardiomyopathy, Liang distal myopathy), full gene sequence

MYO7A (myosin VIIA) (eg, Usher syndrome, type 1), full gene sequence

NOTCH1 (notch 1) (eg, aortic valve disease), full gene sequence

NPHS1 (nephrosis 1, congenital, Finnish type [nephrin]) (eg, congenital Finnish nephrosis), full gene sequence

OPA1 (optic atrophy 1) (eg, optic atrophy), full gene sequence

PCDH15 (protocadherin-related 15) (eg, Usher syndrome, type 1), full gene sequence

PKD1 (polycystic kidney disease 1 [autosomal dominant]) (eg, polycystic kidney disease), full gene sequence

PLCE1 (phospholipase C, epsilon 1) (eg, nephrotic syndrome type 3), full gene sequence

SCN1A (sodium channel, voltage-gated, type 1, alpha subunit) (eg, generalized epilepsy with febrile seizures), full gene sequence

SCN5A (sodium channel, voltage-gated, type V, alpha subunit) (eg, familial dilated cardiomyopathy), full gene sequence

SLC12A1 (solute carrier family 12 [sodium/potassium/chloride transporters], member 1) (eg, Bartter syndrome), full gene sequence

SLC12A3 (solute carrier family 12 [sodium/chloride transporters], member 3) (eg, Gitelman syndrome), full gene sequence

SPG11 (spastic paraplegia 11 [autosomal recessive]) (eg, spastic paraplegia), full gene sequence

SPTBN2 (spectrin, beta, non-erythrocytic 2) (eg, spinocerebellar ataxia), full gene sequence

Pathology and Laboratory 80047-89398, 0001U-0061U

TMEM67 (transmembrane protein 67) (eg, Joubert syndrome), full gene sequence

TSC2 (tuberous sclerosis 2) (eg, tuberous sclerosis), full gene sequence

USH1C (Usher syndrome 1C [autosomal recessive, severe]) (eg, Usher syndrome, type 1), full gene sequence

VPS13B (vacuolar protein sorting 13 homolog B [yeast]) (eg, Cohen syndrome), duplication/deletion analysis

WDR62 (WD repeat domain 62) (eg, primary autosomal recessive microcephaly), full gene sequence

Rationale

Five Tier 2 codes (81401, 81403, 81404, 81405, 81407) have been revised because 27 gene tests have been moved to new Tier 1 codes for 2019: 19 tests from code 81401; one test from code 81403; four tests from code 81404; two tests from code 81405; and one test from code 81407.

Refer to the codebook and the Rationale for codes 81171-81289 and 81329-81344 for a full discussion of these changes. In addition, code 81400 has been revised with the deletion of the SMN1 (survival of motor neuron 1, telomeric) (eg, spinal muscular atrophy), exon 7 deletion gene test.

Genomic Sequencing Procedures and Other Molecular Multianalyte Assays

81442   Noonan spectrum disorders (eg, Noonan syndrome, cardio-facio-cutaneous syndrome, Costello syndrome, LEOPARD syndrome, Noonan-like syndrome), genomic sequence analysis panel, must include sequencing of at least 12 genes, including *BRAF, CBL, HRAS, KRAS, MAP2K1, MAP2K2, NRAS, PTPN11, RAF1, RIT1, SHOC2,* and *SOS1*

● **81443**   Genetic testing for severe inherited conditions (eg, cystic fibrosis, Ashkenazi Jewish-associated disorders [eg, Bloom syndrome, Canavan disease, Fanconi anemia type C, mucolipidosis type VI, Gaucher disease, Tay-Sachs disease], beta hemoglobinopathies, phenylketonuria, galactosemia), genomic sequence analysis panel, must include sequencing of at least 15 genes (eg, *ACADM, ARSA, ASPA, ATP7B, BCKDHA, BCKDHB, BLM, CFTR, DHCR7, FANCC, G6PC, GAA, GALT, GBA, GBE1, HBB, HEXA, IKBKAP, MCOLN1, PAH)*

▶(If spinal muscular atrophy testing is performed separately, use 81401)◀

▶(If testing is performed only for Ashkenazi Jewish-associated disorders, use 81412)◀

▶(If *FMR1* [expanded allele] testing is performed separately, use 81243)◀

▶(If hemoglobin A testing is performed separately, use 81257)◀

▶(Do not report 81443 in conjunction with 81412)◀

Rationale

Code 81443 has been added to the Genomic Sequencing Procedures (GSP) and Other Molecular Multianalyte Assays section to report genetic testing for severe inherited conditions. Four parenthetical notes have been added to provide instruction on the appropriate reporting of this code.

The GSP section includes analyses of genes that are relevant to specific clinical conditions (eg, aortic dysfunction or dilation, hereditary breast cancer-related disorders). The GSP codes include, but are not limited to, specific genes or types of genes in the analysis. Code 81443 describes a genomic sequencing analysis panel. It is distinct from other GSP codes because it is not limited to analysis of specific genes or types of genes. In addition, code 81443 tests for multiple conditions (eg, Bloom syndrome, cystic fibrosis).

At least 15 genes must be sequenced in order to report code 81443. Examples of genes are included in the code descriptor. Ashkenazi Jewish testing is *included* in code 81443. However, if testing is *only* performed for Ashkenazi Jewish disorders, then code 81412 should be reported because the test is not performed for multiple disorders as indicated in code 81443. At times, testing for FMR1, spinal muscular atrophy, or hemoglobin A may be performed in addition to the panel included in code 81443. Therefore, testing for these conditions may be reported separately. Parenthetical notes have been added following code 81443 directing users to the appropriate codes for these tests.

Clinical Example (81443)

A 30-year-old pregnant female presents at initial obstetrics visit. Following ACOG 2017 guidance, she is counseled on carrier screening options and chooses to pursue an expanded carrier screening panel. A whole blood sample is submitted to the laboratory for testing.

Description of Procedure (81443)

High-quality DNA is isolated from the patient's blood sample. DNA targets are enriched by hybrid capture and the products undergo massively parallel DNA sequencing of the coding regions and intron/exon boundaries. The pathologist or other qualified healthcare professional evaluates the reads to identify nucleotide sequence variants. The pathologist or other qualified healthcare professional composes a report, which specifies the patient's mutation status. The report is edited, signed, and the results are communicated to appropriate caregivers.

Multianalyte Assays with Algorithmic Analyses

● **81518**   Oncology (breast), mRNA, gene expression profiling by real-time RT-PCR of 11 genes (7 content and 4 housekeeping), utilizing formalin-fixed paraffin-embedded tissue, algorithms reported as percentage risk for metastatic recurrence and likelihood of benefit from extended endocrine therapy

81519   Oncology (breast), mRNA, gene expression profiling by real-time RT-PCR of 21 genes, utilizing formalin-fixed paraffin-embedded tissue, algorithm reported as recurrence score

Rationale

A new Category I Multianalyte Assay with Algorithmic Analysis (MAAA) code 81518 has been established to report the prognostic ability of breast-cancer index for assessing the risk of distant (metastatic) recurrence. Unlisted code 81479 was previously used, however, it does not adequately address the reporting of the prognostic ability of breast cancer index for assessing risk of distant (metastatic) recurrence In addition, the usage volume and clinical importance of this test warrant its own code. A separate listing of this code that includes the proprietary test name has been added to Appendix O.

Clinical Example (81518)

A 50-year-old female presents with early-stage, hormone receptor-positive (HR+) invasive breast cancer, stage T1cN0M0. The tumor is Nottingham Grade 2. The patient is prescribed adjuvant endocrine therapy with tamoxifen. The physician orders a test for gene expression profiling to inform on the risk of metastasis and the likely benefit of extended endocrine therapy.

Description of Procedure (81518)

Extract and convert RNA from tumor-enriched, formalin-fixed paraffin-embedded tissue to cDNA by reverse transcription, and perform real-time polymerase chain reaction (RT-PCR) to measure the expression of 11 genes: 7 genes for content and 4 housekeeping genes for normalization. The assay then uses algorithms that report an individualized risk of metastatic recurrence up to 10 years post-diagnosis and the likelihood of benefit from extended endocrine therapy.

81595   Cardiology (heart transplant), mRNA, gene expression profiling by real-time quantitative PCR of 20 genes (11 content and 9 housekeeping), utilizing subfraction of peripheral blood, algorithm reported as a rejection risk score

● **81596**   Infectious disease, chronic hepatitis C virus (HCV) infection, six biochemical assays (ALT, A2-macroglobulin, apolipoprotein A-1, total bilirubin, GGT, and haptoglobin) utilizing serum, prognostic algorithm reported as scores for fibrosis and necroinflammatory activity in liver

Rationale

MAAA code 81596 has been added to report MAAA for measuring fibrosis and necroinflammatory activity in the liver, which was previously reported with administrative MAAA code 0001M. For 2019, administrative MAAA code 0001M has been deleted and the test described therein has been assigned to the Category I MAAA code 81596. Code 81596 has been added to Appendix O.

Clinical Example (81596)

A 64-year-old male with confirmed chronic hepatitis C virus (HCV) infection presents to his primary care physician. A serum sample is submitted to the laboratory for a quantitative biochemical assay of six liver markers with algorithm to estimate extent of liver fibrosis and inform whether liver biopsy and/or HCV direct acting antiviral therapy is indicated.

Description of Procedure (81596)

Measure the patient's serum sample for alanine aminotransferase (ALT), A2-macroglobulin, apolipoprotein A-1, total bilirubin, gamma–glutamyl transferase (GGT), and haptoglobin. Analyze the quantitative results of the six-biochemical tests using a proprietary algorithm to provide a numerical score for liver fibrosis and a numerical score for necroinflammatory activity.

★ = Telemedicine   ✛ = Add-on code   ✗ = FDA approval pending   # = Resequenced code   ⊘ = Modifier 51 exempt

Chemistry

82638   Dibucaine number

(Dichloroethane, use 82441)

(Dichloromethane, use 82441)

(Diethylether, use 84600)

● **82642**   Dihydrotestosterone (DHT)

▶(For dihydrotestosterone analysis for anabolic drug testing, see 80327, 80328)◀

Rationale

A distinct code to describe dihydrotestosterone testing for medical purposes has been re-established with the development of code 82642 for the 2019 code set. Instructional parenthetical notes have been included within the Drug Assay and Chemistry subsections to direct users to the correct code to report anabolic steroid testing.

Code 82642 is intended to identify the testing processes utilized to identify dihydrotestosterone (DHT) testing for medical purposes as opposed to testing for drugs of abuse or other circumstances. In 2015, a code specific to DHT was deleted in support of the establishment of the new Drug Assay subsection. Re-establishment of a code for this test alleviates a lack of specificity in the currently available codes (80327, 80328), which identifies drugs of abuse testing only. Drugs of abuse codes may be used to identify testosterone testing to specify levels of testosterone use/overuse, such as in drug abuse. Code 84403 may be used to identify total testosterone within the patient. However, none of these codes is appropriate to identify analysis of DHT for medical purposes (genetic and hormonal diagnostics). Instructional cross-references have been added to direct users to the appropriate codes for the specific type of testosterone testing being provided.

Clinical Example (82642)

A 17-year-old patient with female external genitalia was referred to an endocrine clinic with primary amenorrhea, virilization, and lack of secondary sex characteristics. The physician ordered hormonal assays that included dihydrotestosterone.

Description of Procedure (82642)

Submit serum sample to the laboratory for dihydrotestosterone testing. Measure dihydrotestosterone using high-pressure liquid chromatography with tandem mass spectrometry detection after liquid-liquid extraction. Report the quantitative dihydrotestosterone result to the patient's physician.

83718   Lipoprotein, direct measurement; high density cholesterol (HDL cholesterol)

83719   VLDL cholesterol

83721   LDL cholesterol

● **83722**   small dense LDL cholesterol

(For fractionation by high resolution electrophoresis or ultracentrifugation, use 83701)

(For lipoprotein particle numbers and subclasses analysis by nuclear magnetic resonance spectroscopy, use 83704)

Rationale

Code 83722 has been added to report direct small dense low-density lipoprotein (LDL) cholesterol measurement. Currently, there are codes for direct measurement of high-density lipoprotein (HDL) cholesterol (83718); very low-density lipoprotein (VLDL) cholesterol (83719); and LDL cholesterol (83721). Small dense LDL cholesterol, as described in code 83722, is LDL cholesterol that is smaller and denser than common LDL cholesterol. Small dense LDL cholesterol may be a factor in atherosclerosis risk.

Clinical Example (83722)

A 59-year-old male presents with a family history of heart disease, coronary stents, hypertension, abnormal lipids, and chest pain. Medications include statins and antihypertensives. His fasting lipids reveal normal total cholesterol, increased triglycerides, normal direct LDL cholesterol, and normal calculated LDL cholesterol, with decreased HDL cholesterol. A blood specimen is submitted to the laboratory for a direct small dense LDL cholesterol measurement.

Description of Procedure (83722)

The laboratory performs a direct small dense LDL cholesterol measurement on an automated chemistry analyzer. The assay consists of two steps, including well-characterized surfactants and enzymes that selectively react with certain groups of lipoproteins. Measure small dense LDL cholesterol using automated enzymatic analysis. Send the test results to the ordering physician.

Cytopathology

88164   Cytopathology, slides, cervical or vaginal (the Bethesda System); manual screening under physician supervision

88165 with manual screening and rescreening under physician supervision

88166 with manual screening and computer-assisted rescreening under physician supervision

88167 with manual screening and computer-assisted rescreening using cell selection and review under physician supervision

▶(For collection of specimen via fine needle aspiration biopsy, see 10004, 10005, 10006, 10007, 10008, 10009, 10010, 10011, 10012, 10021)◀

88172 Cytopathology, evaluation of fine needle aspirate; immediate cytohistologic study to determine adequacy for diagnosis, first evaluation episode, each site

(The evaluation episode represents a complete set of cytologic material submitted for evaluation and is independent of the number of needle passes or slides prepared. A separate evaluation episode occurs if the proceduralist provider obtains additional material from the same site, based on the prior immediate adequacy assessment, or a separate lesion is aspirated)

88173 interpretation and report

(Report one unit of 88173 for the interpretation and report from each anatomic site, regardless of the number of passes or evaluation episodes performed during the aspiration procedure)

▶(For fine needle aspirate biopsy, see 10004, 10005, 10006, 10007, 10008, 10009, 10010, 10011, 10012, 10021)◀

(Do not report 88172, 88173 in conjunction with 88333 and 88334 for the same specimen)

Rationale

Parenthetical notes within the Cytopathology subsection for Pathology and Laboratory procedures following codes 88167 and 88173 have been revised to direct users to the correct codes to report fine-needle aspiration-biopsy procedures (10004-10012, 10021).

Refer to the codebook and the Rationale for codes 10004-10012 and 10021 for a full discussion of these changes.

Surgical Pathology

88309 **Level VI** - Surgical pathology, gross and microscopic examination

Bone resection

Breast, mastectomy - with regional lymph nodes

Colon, segmental resection for tumor

Colon, total resection

Esophagus, partial/total resection

Extremity, disarticulation

Fetus, with dissection

Larynx, partial/total resection - with regional lymph nodes

Lung - total/lobe/segment resection

Pancreas, total/subtotal resection

Prostate, radical resection

Small intestine, resection for tumor

Soft tissue tumor, extensive resection

Stomach - subtotal/total resection for tumor

Testis, tumor

Tongue/tonsil -resection for tumor

Urinary bladder, partial/total resection

Uterus, with or without tubes and ovaries, neoplastic

Vulva, total/subtotal resection

▶(For fine needle aspiration biopsy, see 10004, 10005, 10006, 10007, 10008, 10009, 10010, 10011, 10012, 10021)◀

(For evaluation of fine needle aspirate, see 88172-88173)

(Do not report 88302-88309 on the same specimen as part of Mohs surgery)

Rationale

A parenthetical note within the Surgical Pathology subsection for Pathology and Laboratory procedures following code 88309 has been revised to direct users to the correct codes to report fine-needle aspiration-biopsy procedures (10004-10012, 10021).

Refer to the codebook and the Rationale for codes 10004-10012 and 10021 for a full discussion of the changes.

Proprietary Laboratory Analyses

▶(0004U has been deleted)◀

0005U Oncology (prostate) gene expression profile by real-time RT-PCR of 3 genes *(ERG, PCA3,* and *SPDEF)*, urine, algorithm reported as risk score

★ = Telemedicine + = Add-on code ✔ = FDA approval pending # = Resequenced code ⊘ = Modifier 51 exempt

▲ **0006U**   Detection of interacting medications, substances, supplements and foods, 120 or more analytes, definitive chromatography with mass spectrometry, urine, description and severity of each interaction identified, per date of service

✕**0007U**   Drug test(s), presumptive, with definitive confirmation of positive results, any number of drug classes, urine, includes specimen verification including DNA authentication in comparison to buccal DNA, per date of service

▶(For additional PLA code with identical clinical descriptor, see 0020U. See Appendix O to determine appropriate code assignment)◀

▶(0015U has been deleted)◀

● **0018U**   Oncology (thyroid), microRNA profiling by RT-PCR of 10 microRNA sequences, utilizing fine needle aspirate, algorithm reported as a positive or negative result for moderate to high risk of malignancy

● **0019U**   Oncology, RNA, gene expression by whole transcriptome sequencing, formalin-fixed paraffin-embedded tissue or fresh frozen tissue, predictive algorithm reported as potential targets for therapeutic agents

✕● **0020U**   Drug test(s), presumptive, with definitive confirmation of positive results, any number of drug classes, urine, with specimen verification including DNA authentication in comparison to buccal DNA, per date of service

▶(For additional PLA code with identical clinical descriptor, see 0007U. See Appendix O to determine appropriate code assignment)◀

● **0021U**   Oncology (prostate), detection of 8 autoantibodies (ARF 6, NKX3-1, 5'-UTR-BMI1, CEP 164, 3'-UTR-Ropporin, Desmocollin, AURKAIP-1, CSNK2A2), multiplexed immunoassay and flow cytometry serum, algorithm reported as risk score

● **0022U**   Targeted genomic sequence analysis panel, non-small cell lung neoplasia, DNA and RNA analysis, 23 genes, interrogation for sequence variants and rearrangements, reported as presence/absence of variants and associated therapy(ies) to consider

● **0023U**   Oncology (acute myelogenous leukemia), DNA, genotyping of internal tandem duplication, p.D835, p.I836, using mononuclear cells, reported as detection or non-detection of *FLT3* mutation and indication for or against the use of midostaurin

● **0024U**   Glycosylated acute phase proteins (GlycA), nuclear magnetic resonance spectroscopy, quantitative

● **0025U**   Tenofovir, by liquid chromatography with tandem mass spectrometry (LC-MS/MS), urine, quantitative

● **0026U**   Oncology (thyroid), DNA and mRNA of 112 genes, next-generation sequencing, fine needle aspirate of thyroid nodule, algorithmic analysis reported as a categorical result ("Positive, high probability of malignancy" or "Negative, low probability of malignancy")

● **0027U**   *JAK2 (Janus kinase 2)* (eg, myeloproliferative disorder) gene analysis, targeted sequence analysis exons 12-15

● **0028U**   *CYP2D6 (cytochrome P450, family 2, subfamily D, polypeptide 6)* (eg, drug metabolism) gene analysis, copy number variants, common variants with reflex to targeted sequence analysis

● **0029U**   Drug metabolism (adverse drug reactions and drug response), targeted sequence analysis (ie, *CYP1A2, CYP2C19, CYP2C9, CYP2D6, CYP3A4, CYP3A5, CYP4F2, SLCO1B1, VKORC1* and rs12777823)

● **0030U**   Drug metabolism (warfarin drug response), targeted sequence analysis (ie, *CYP2C9, CYP4F2, VKORC1,* rs12777823)

● **0031U**   *CYP1A2 (cytochrome P450 family 1, subfamily A, member 2)* (eg, drug metabolism) gene analysis, common variants (ie, *1F, *1K, *6, *7)

● **0032U**   *COMT (catechol-O-methyltransferase)* (eg, drug metabolism) gene analysis, c.472G>A (rs4680) variant

● **0033U**   *HTR2A (5-hydroxytryptamine receptor 2A), HTR2C (5-hydroxytryptamine receptor 2C)* (eg, citalopram metabolism) gene analysis, common variants (ie, *HTR2A* rs7997012 [c.614-2211T>C], *HTR2C* rs3813929 [c.-759C>T] and rs1414334 [c.551-3008C>G])

● **0034U**   *TPMT (thiopurine S-methyltransferase), NUDT15 (nudix hydroxylase 15)* (eg, thiopurine metabolism) gene analysis, common variants (ie, *TPMT *2, *3A, *3B, *3C, *4, *5, *6, *8, *12; NUDT15 *3, *4, *5)

● **0035U**   Neurology (prion disease), cerebrospinal fluid, detection of prion protein by quaking-induced conformational conversion, qualitative

● **0036U**   Exome (ie, somatic mutations), paired formalin-fixed paraffin-embedded tumor tissue and normal specimen, sequence analyses

● **0037U**   Targeted genomic sequence analysis, solid organ neoplasm, DNA analysis of 324 genes, interrogation for sequence variants, gene copy number amplifications, gene rearrangements, microsatellite instability and tumor mutational burden

● **0038U**   Vitamin D, 25 hydroxy D2 and D3, by LC-MS/MS, serum microsample, quantitative

● **0039U**   Deoxyribonucleic acid (DNA) antibody, double stranded, high avidity

● **0040U**   *BCR/ABL1 (t(9;22))* (eg, chronic myelogenous leukemia) translocation analysis, major breakpoint, quantitative

● **0041U**   Borrelia burgdorferi, antibody detection of 5 recombinant protein groups, by immunoblot, IgM

● **0042U**   Borrelia burgdorferi, antibody detection of 12 recombinant protein groups, by immunoblot, IgG

● **0043U**   Tick-borne relapsing fever Borrelia group, antibody detection to 4 recombinant protein groups, by immunoblot, IgM

● **0044U** Tick-borne relapsing fever Borrelia group, antibody detection to 4 recombinant protein groups, by immunoblot, IgG

● **0045U** Oncology (breast ductal carcinoma in situ), mRNA, gene expression profiling by real-time RT-PCR of 12 genes (7 content and 5 housekeeping), utilizing formalin-fixed paraffin-embedded tissue, algorithm reported as recurrence score

● **0046U** *FLT3 (fms-related tyrosine kinase 3)* (eg, acute myeloid leukemia) internal tandem duplication (ITD) variants, quantitative

● **0047U** Oncology (prostate), mRNA, gene expression profiling by real-time RT-PCR of 17 genes (12 content and 5 housekeeping), utilizing formalin-fixed paraffin-embedded tissue, algorithm reported as a risk score

● **0048U** Oncology (solid organ neoplasia), DNA, targeted sequencing of protein-coding exons of 468 cancer-associated genes, including interrogation for somatic mutations and microsatellite instability, matched with normal specimens, utilizing formalin-fixed paraffin-embedded tumor tissue, report of clinically significant mutation(s)

● **0049U** *NPM1 (nucleophosmin)* (eg, acute myeloid leukemia) gene analysis, quantitative

● **0050U** Targeted genomic sequence analysis panel, acute myelogenous leukemia, DNA analysis, 194 genes, interrogation for sequence variants, copy number variants or rearrangements

● **0051U** Prescription drug monitoring, evaluation of drugs present by LC-MS/MS, urine, 31 drug panel, reported as quantitative results, detected or not detected, per date of service

● **0052U** Lipoprotein, blood, high resolution fractionation and quantitation of lipoproteins, including all five major lipoprotein classes and subclasses of HDL, LDL, and VLDL by vertical auto profile ultracentrifugation

● **0053U** Oncology (prostate cancer), FISH analysis of 4 genes (*ASAP1, HDAC9, CHD1,* and *PTEN*), needle biopsy specimen, algorithm reported as probability of higher tumor grade

● **0054U** Prescription drug monitoring, 14 or more classes of drugs and substances, definitive tandem mass spectrometry with chromatography, capillary blood, quantitative report with therapeutic and toxic ranges, including steady-state range for the prescribed dose when detected, per date of service

● **0055U** Cardiology (heart transplant), cell-free DNA, PCR assay of 96 DNA target sequences (94 single nucleotide polymorphism targets and two control targets), plasma

● **0056U** Hematology (acute myelogenous leukemia), DNA, whole genome next-generation sequencing to detect gene rearrangement(s), blood or bone marrow, report of specific gene rearrangement(s)

● **0057U** Oncology (solid organ neoplasia), mRNA, gene expression profiling by massively parallel sequencing for analysis of 51 genes, utilizing formalin-fixed paraffin-embedded tissue, algorithm reported as a normalized percentile rank

● **0058U** Oncology (Merkel cell carcinoma), detection of antibodies to the Merkel cell polyoma virus oncoprotein (small T antigen), serum, quantitative

● **0059U** Oncology (Merkel cell carcinoma), detection of antibodies to the Merkel cell polyoma virus capsid protein (VP1), serum, reported as positive or negative

● **0060U** Twin zygosity, genomic-targeted sequence analysis of chromosome 2, using circulating cell-free fetal DNA in maternal blood

● **0061U** Transcutaneous measurement of five biomarkers (tissue oxygenation [StO_2], oxyhemoglobin [$ctHbO_2$], deoxyhemoglobin [ctHbR], papillary and reticular dermal hemoglobin concentrations [ctHb1 and ctHb2]), using spatial frequency domain imaging (SFDI) and multi-spectral analysis

Rationale

A total of 44 new proprietary laboratory analyses (PLA) codes have been established for the 2019 CPT code set. PLA test codes will be released and posted online on a quarterly basis (fall, winter, spring, and summer) in data files, which are available online at https://www.ama-assn.org/practice-management/cpt-pla-codes. New codes are effective the quarter following their publication.

Other changes include the deletion of codes 0004U and 0015U, and the revision of code 0006U to report detection of interacting medications, substances, supplements, and food.

A new symbol has also been added to the code set to identify duplicate PLA codes. In the instance when more than one PLA code has an identical descriptor, the codes will be denoted by the symbol ✣. To determine the appropriate code to report, reference Appendix O as the code may only be differentiated by the listed proprietary name in Appendix O.

Medicine

In the Medicine section, a total of 29 codes have been added and 17 codes have been revised.

The Vaccine, Toxoids subsection includes a new vaccine code (90689) to report quadrivalent influenza virus vaccine.

Throughout the Psychiatry subsections, exclusionary parenthetical notes to preclude reporting the new adaptive behavior services codes in conjunction with other codes in this subsection have been added.

In the Ophthalmology section, a new guideline to identify how electroretinography (ERG) is used to evaluate function of the retina and optic nerve of the eye has been added. In addition, two new codes have been added: code 92273 to identify full field, and code 92274 to identify multifocal ERG services.

Numerous changes have been made to the Cardiovascular section. The "Implantable and Wearable Cardiac Device Evaluation" subsection has been revised to "Implantable, Insertable, and Wearable Cardiac Device Evaluation." In addition, the introductory guidelines and definitions have been revised to address the differences between the leadless pacemaker and implantable monitors. A new code (93264) to report remote monitoring of a wireless pulmonary artery pressure sensor has also been added. In addition, several codes have been revised to allow for more appropriate and consistent reporting.

Throughout the Neurology and Neuromuscular Procedures subsection, introductory and exclusionary parenthetical notes to preclude reporting the new electronic analysis of implanted neurostimulator pulse codes in conjunction with other codes in this subsection have been added. In addition, a new chart to provide additional instructions on the appropriate reporting of face-to-face time for brain neurostimulator analysis with programming services has been added.

In the Adaptive Behavior Services subsection, introductory guidelines and definitions have been revised to address the differences between behavior assessments and instruments and procedures. Several new codes to report behavior identification assessments and protocol modification services have been added too. In addition, two new charts to guide the appropriate selection of codes have also been added.

In the Central Nervous System Assessments/Tests subsection, introductory guidelines and definitions have been revised to address the differences between neurological testing and examination services. Several new codes to report developmental, neurobehavioral, psychological, and neuropsychological testing evaluations have been added too. In addition, a new chart to guide the appropriate selection of codes and performance testing by a physician or other qualified health care professional, clinical staff, or technician has been added.

Other subsections with changes include Health and Behavior Assessment, Physical Medicine and Rehabilitation, and Special Services, Procedures and Reports.

Summary of Additions, Deletions, and Revisions

The summary of changes shows the actual changes that have been made to the code descriptors.

New codes appear with a bullet (●) and are indicated as "Code added." Revised codes are preceded with a triangle (▲). Within revised codes, or if a code symbol has been deleted, the deleted language and code symbol appears with a ~~strikethrough~~ (⊖), while new text appears underlined.

The ⊮ symbol is used to identify codes for vaccines that are pending FDA approval. The # symbol is used to identify codes that have been resequenced. CPT add-on codes are annotated by the + symbol.

The ⊘ symbol is used to identify codes that are exempt from the use of modifier 51. The ★ symbol is used to identify codes that may be used for reporting telemedicine services. The Ж is used to identify proprietary laboratory analyses (PLA) test that has an identical descriptor as another PLA test.

Code	Description
✴●90689	Code added
●92273	Code added
●92274	Code added
92275	~~Electroretinography with interpretation and report~~
#●93264	Code added
▲93279	Programming device evaluation (in person) with iterative adjustment of the implantable device to test the function of the device and select optimal permanent programmed values with analysis, review and report by a physician or other qualified health care professional; single lead <u>pacemaker system or leadless</u> pacemaker system <u>in one cardiac chamber</u>
▲93285	~~implantable loop recorder system~~<u>subcutaneous cardiac rhythm monitor system</u>
▲93286	Peri-procedural device evaluation (in person) and programming of device system parameters before or after a surgery, procedure, or test with analysis, review and report by a physician or other qualified health care professional; single, dual, or multiple lead <u>pacemaker system, or leadless</u> pacemaker system
▲93288	Interrogation device evaluation (in person) with analysis, review and report by a physician or other qualified health care professional, includes connection, recording and disconnection per patient encounter; single, dual, or multiple lead <u>pacemaker system, or leadless</u> pacemaker system
▲93290	implantable cardiovascular <u>physiologic</u> monitor system, including analysis of 1 or more recorded physiologic cardiovascular data elements from all internal and external sensors
▲93291	~~implantable loop recorder system~~<u>subcutaneous cardiac rhythm monitor system</u>, including heart rhythm derived data analysis
▲93294	Interrogation device evaluation(s) (remote), up to 90 days; single, dual, or multiple lead <u>pacemaker system, or leadless</u> pacemaker system with interim analysis, review(s) and report(s) by a physician or other qualified health care professional
▲93296	single, dual, or multiple lead <u>pacemaker system, leadless</u> pacemaker system, or implantable defibrillator system, remote data acquisition(s), receipt of transmissions and technician review, technical support and distribution of results
▲93297	Interrogation device evaluation(s), (remote) up to 30 days; implantable cardiovascular <u>physiologic</u> monitor system, including analysis of 1 or more recorded physiologic cardiovascular data elements from all internal and external sensors, analysis, review(s) and report(s) by a physician or other qualified health care professional
★▲93298	~~implantable loop recorder system~~<u>subcutaneous cardiac rhythm monitor system</u>, including analysis of recorded heart rhythm data, analysis, review(s) and report(s) by a physician or other qualified health care professional
★▲93299	implantable cardiovascular <u>physiologic</u> monitor system or ~~implantable loop recorder system~~<u>subcutaneous cardiac rhythm monitor system</u>, remote data acquisition(s), receipt of transmissions and technician review, technical support and distribution of results

Code	Description
▲94780	Car seat/bed testing for airway integrity, ~~neonate~~<u>for infants through 12 months of age</u>, with continual ~~nursing~~<u>clinical staff</u> observation and continuous recording of pulse oximetry, heart rate and respiratory rate, with interpretation and report; 60 minutes
+▲94781	each additional full 30 minutes (List separately in addition to code for primary procedure)
#●95836	Code added
▲95970	Electronic analysis of implanted neurostimulator pulse generator ~~system~~/transmitter (eg, ~~rate~~<u>contact group[s]</u>, ~~pulse~~<u>interleaving,</u> amplitude, pulse ~~duration~~<u>width</u>, frequency [Hz], ~~configuration of wave form~~<u>on/off cycling, burst,</u> magnet mode, ~~battery status~~<u>dose lockout</u>, ~~electrode selectability~~<u>patient selectable parameters</u>, ~~output modulation~~<u>responsive neurostimulation</u>, ~~cycling~~<u>detection algorithms</u>, ~~impedance~~<u>closed loop parameters,</u> and ~~patient compliance measurements)~~<u>passive parameters) with brain, cranial nerve</u>, spinal cord, ~~or~~peripheral ~~(ie, cranial~~nerve, ~~peripheral nerve,~~<u>or</u> sacral nerve, ~~neuromuscular)~~neurostimulator pulse generator/transmitter, without ~~reprogramming~~<u>programming</u>
▲95971	<u>with</u> simple spinal cord~~, or peripheral (ie,~~ peripheral nerve <u>(eg,</u> sacral nerve~~, neuromuscular)~~ neurostimulator pulse generator/transmitter~~, with intraoperative~~ programming by physician or ~~subsequent programming~~<u>other qualified health care professional</u>
▲95972	<u>with</u> complex spinal cord~~, or peripheral (ie,~~ peripheral ~~nerve, sacral~~nerve~~, neuromuscular) (except cranial~~<u>eg, sacral</u> nerve) neurostimulator pulse generator/transmitter~~, with intraoperative~~ programming by physician or ~~subsequent programming~~<u>other qualified health care professional</u>
95974	~~complex cranial nerve neurostimulator pulse generator/transmitter, with intraoperative or subsequent programming, with or without nerve interface testing, first hour~~
95975	~~complex cranial nerve neurostimulator pulse generator/transmitter, with intraoperative or subsequent programming, each additional 30 minutes after first hour (List separately in addition to code for primary procedure)~~
●95976	Code added
●95977	Code added
#●95983	Code added
#+●95984	Code added
95978	~~Electronic analysis of implanted neurostimulator pulse generator system (eg, rate, pulse amplitude and duration, battery status, electrode selectability and polarity, impedance and patient compliance measurements), complex deep brain neurostimulator pulse generator/transmitter, with initial or subsequent programming; first hour~~
95979	~~each additional 30 minutes after first hour (List separately in addition to code for primary procedure)~~
#●97151	Code added
#●97152	Code added
#●97153	Code added
#●97154	Code added
#●97155	Code added
#●97156	Code added
#●97157	Code added
#●97158	Code added

Code	Description
96101	~~Psychological testing (includes psychodiagnostic assessment of emotionality, intellectual abilities, personality and psychopathology, eg, MMPI, Rorschach, WAIS), per hour of the psychologist's or physician's time, both face-to-face time administering tests to the patient and time interpreting these test results and preparing the report~~
96102	~~Psychological testing (includes psychodiagnostic assessment of emotionality, intellectual abilities, personality and psychopathology, eg, MMPI and WAIS), with qualified health care professional interpretation and report, administered by technician, per hour of technician time, face-to-face~~
96103	~~Psychological testing (includes psychodiagnostic assessment of emotionality, intellectual abilities, personality and psychopathology, eg, MMPI), administered by a computer, with qualified health care professional interpretation and report~~
96111	Developmental testing, (includes assessment of motor, language, social, adaptive, and/or cognitive functioning by standardized developmental instruments) with interpretation and report
●96112	Code added
+●96113	Code added
★▲96116	Neurobehavioral status exam (clinical assessment of thinking, reasoning and judgment, [eg, acquired knowledge, attention, language, memory, planning and problem solving, and visual spatial abilities]), ~~per hour of the psychologist's or physician's time~~by physician or other qualified health care professional, both face-to-face time with the patient and time interpreting test results and preparing the report; first hour
96118	~~Neuropsychological testing (eg, Halstead-Reitan Neuropsychological Battery, Wechsler Memory Scales and Wisconsin Card Sorting Test), per hour of the psychologist's or physician's time, both face-to-face time administering tests to the patient and time interpreting these test results and preparing the report~~
96119	~~Neuropsychological testing (eg, Halstead-Reitan Neuropsychological Battery, Wechsler Memory Scales and Wisconsin Card Sorting Test), with qualified health care professional interpretation and report, administered by technician, per hour of technician time, face-to-face~~
96120	~~Neuropsychological testing (eg, Wisconsin Card Sorting Test), administered by a computer, with qualified health care professional interpretation and report~~
+●96121	Code added
●96130	Code added
+●96131	Code added
●96132	Code added
+●96133	Code added
●96136	Code added
+●96137	Code added
●96138	Code added
+●96139	Code added
●96146	Code added
99090	~~Analysis of clinical data stored in computers (eg, ECGs, blood pressures, hematologic data)~~

★=Telemedicine   +=Add-on code   ✗=FDA approval pending   #=Resequenced code   ⊘=Modifier 51 exempt

Medicine Guidelines

Imaging Guidance

▶When imaging guidance or imaging supervision and interpretation is included in a procedure, guidelines for image documentation and report, included in the guidelines for Radiology (including Nuclear Medicine and Diagnostic Ultrasound) will apply. Imaging guidance should not be reported for use of a non-imaging guided tracking or localizing system (eg, radar signals, electromagnetic signals). Imaging guidance should only be reported when an imaging modality (eg, radiography, fluoroscopy, ultrasonography, magnetic resonance imaging, computed tomography, or nuclear medicine) is used and is appropriately documented.◀

Rationale

The guidelines in the Imaging Guidance subsection of the Medicine Guidelines section have been revised to clarify reporting for nonimaging guidance. Imaging guidance should not be reported when a nonimaging-guided modality (eg, radar signals, electromagnetic signals) is used. Instead, it should only be reported when an imaging modality (eg, radiography, fluoroscopy, ultrasonography, magnetic resonance imaging, computed tomography, or nuclear medicine) is used and is appropriately documented.

Medicine

Vaccines, Toxoids

✎● **90689** Influenza virus vaccine, quadrivalent (IIV4), inactivated, adjuvanted, preservative free, 0.25 mL dosage, for intramuscular use

Rationale

New vaccine product code 90689 has been established in the Vaccines, Toxoids subsection to report pediatric quadrivalent influenza vaccine. Code 90689 describes an adjuvanted (ie, addition of enhancer that improves protection), inactivated (ie, previously killed virus using heat or formaldehyde), preservative-free, quadrivalent flu vaccine for pediatric population usage. Administration of the vaccine is reported separately using codes 90460-90472 (immunization administration for vaccines/toxoids). Code 90689 carries the US Food and Drug Administration (FDA) approval-pending symbol (✎); therefore, interim updates on the FDA status of this code will be reflected on the AMA CPT website at www.ama-assn.org/go/cpt-vaccine, under the CPT Category I Vaccine Codes on a semiannual basis (July 1 and January 1).

The Centers for Disease Control and Prevention Advisory Committee on Immunization Practices (ACIP) has not assigned a US vaccine abbreviation for this vaccine. Visit the AMA CPT website for updates on the US vaccine abbreviation status for this vaccine.

Clinical Example (90689)

A 6-month-old male infant presents for an influenza immunization.

Description of Procedure (90689)

Evaluate the injection site; apply antisepsis, and administer the injection intramuscularly.

Psychiatry

Psychiatry services include diagnostic services, psychotherapy, and other services to an individual, family, or group. Patient condition, characteristics, or situational factors may require services described as being with interactive complexity. Services may be provided to a patient in crisis. Services are provided in all settings of care and psychiatry services codes are reported without regard to setting. Services may be provided by a physician or other qualified health care professional. Some psychiatry services may be reported with **Evaluation and Management Services** (99201-99255, 99281-99285, 99304-99337, 99341-99350) or other services when performed. **Evaluation and Management Services** (99201-99285, 99304-99337, 99341-99350) may be reported for treatment of psychiatric conditions, rather than using **Psychiatry Services** codes, when appropriate.

Hospital care in treating a psychiatric inpatient or partial hospitalization may be initial or subsequent in nature (see 99221-99233).

Some patients receive hospital evaluation and management services only and others receive hospital evaluation and management services and other procedures. If other procedures such as electroconvulsive therapy or psychotherapy are rendered in addition to hospital evaluation and management services, these may be listed separately (eg, hospital care services [99221-99223, 99231-99233] plus electroconvulsive therapy [90870]), or when psychotherapy is done, with appropriate code(s) defining psychotherapy services.

Consultation for psychiatric evaluation of a patient includes examination of a patient and exchange of information with the primary physician and other informants such as nurses or family members, and preparation of a report. These services may be reported using consultation codes (see **Consultations**).

▶(Do not report 90785-90899 in conjunction with 90839, 90840, 97151, 97152, 97153, 97154, 97155, 97156, 97157, 97158, 0362T, 0373T)◀

Rationale

In support of the establishment of codes 97151-97158 (adaptive behavior services) and deletion of codes 0359T-0361T, 0363T-0372T, and 0374T, the exclusionary parenthetical note following the psychiatry guidelines has been revised to reflect these changes.

Refer to the codebook and the Rationale for codes 97151-97158, 0362T, and 0373T for a full discussion of these changes.

Interactive Complexity

✚ **90785** Interactive complexity (List separately in addition to the code for primary procedure)

★ = Telemedicine   ✚ = Add-on code   ✎ = FDA approval pending   # = Resequenced code   ⊘ = Modifier 51 exempt

(Use 90785 in conjunction with codes for diagnostic psychiatric evaluation [90791, 90792], psychotherapy [90832, 90834, 90837], psychotherapy when performed with an evaluation and management service [90833, 90836, 90838, 99201-99255, 99304-99337, 99341-99350], and group psychotherapy [90853])

(Do not report 90785 in conjunction with 90839, 90840, or in conjunction with E/M services when no psychotherapy service is also reported)

▶(Do not report 90785 in conjunction with 90839, 90840, 97151, 97152, 97153, 97154, 97155, 97156, 97157, 97158, 0362T, 0373T)◀

Rationale

In support of the establishment of codes 97151-97158 (adaptive behavior services) and deletion of codes 0359T-0361T, 0363T-0372T, and 0374T, the exclusionary parenthetical note following code 90785 (interactive complexity) has been revised to reflect these changes.

Refer to the codebook and the Rationale for codes 97151-97158, 0362T, and 0373T for a full discussion of these changes.

Psychiatric Diagnostic Procedures

Psychiatric diagnostic evaluation is an integrated biopsychosocial assessment, including history, mental status, and recommendations. The evaluation may include communication with family or other sources and review and ordering of diagnostic studies.

Psychiatric diagnostic evaluation with medical services is an integrated biopsychosocial and medical assessment, including history, mental status, other physical examination elements as indicated, and recommendations. The evaluation may include communication with family or other sources, prescription of medications, and review and ordering of laboratory or other diagnostic studies.

In certain circumstances one or more other informants (family members, guardians, or significant others) may be seen in lieu of the patient. Codes 90791, 90792 may be reported more than once for the patient when separate diagnostic evaluations are conducted with the patient and other informants. Report services as being provided to the patient and not the informant or other party in such circumstances. Codes 90791, 90792 may be reported once per day and not on the same day as an evaluation and management service performed by the same individual for the same patient.

The psychiatric diagnostic evaluation may include interactive complexity services when factors exist that

complicate the delivery of the psychiatric procedure. These services should be reported with add-on code 90785 used in conjunction with the diagnostic psychiatric evaluation codes 90791, 90792.

Codes 90791, 90792 are used for the diagnostic assessment(s) or reassessment(s), if required, and do not include psychotherapeutic services. Psychotherapy services, including for crisis, may not be reported on the same day.

▶(Do not report 90791-90899 in conjunction with 90839, 90840, 97151, 97152, 97153, 97154, 97155, 97156, 97157, 97158, 0362T, 0373T)◀

★ **90791**   Psychiatric diagnostic evaluation

★ **90792**   Psychiatric diagnostic evaluation with medical services

▶(Do not report 90791 or 90792 in conjunction with 99201-99337, 99341-99350, 99366-99368, 99401-99444, 97151, 97152, 97153, 97154, 97155, 97156, 97157, 97158, 0362T, 0373T)◀

(Use 90785 in conjunction with 90791, 90792 when the diagnostic evaluation includes interactive complexity services)

Rationale

In support of the establishment of codes 97151-97158 (adaptive behavior services) and deletion of codes 0359T-0361T, 0363T-0372T, and 0374T, the exclusionary parenthetical notes following the psychiatric diagnostic procedures guidelines and code 90792 have been revised to reflect these changes.

Refer to the codebook and the Rationale for codes 97151-97158, 0362T, and 0373T for a full discussion of these changes.

Other Psychotherapy

★ **90847**   Family psychotherapy (conjoint psychotherapy) (with patient present), 50 minutes

(Do not report 90846, 90847 for family psychotherapy services less than 26 minutes)

▶(Do not report 90846, 90847 in conjunction with 97151, 97152, 97153, 97154, 97155, 97156, 97157, 97158, 0362T, 0373T)◀

90849   Multiple-family group psychotherapy

90853   Group psychotherapy (other than of a multiple-family group)

(Use 90853 in conjunction with 90785 for the specified patient when group psychotherapy includes interactive complexity)

▶(Do not report 90853 in conjunction with 97151, 97152, 97153, 97154, 97155, 97156, 97157, 97158, 0362T, 0373T)◀

Rationale

In support of the establishment of codes 97151-97158 (adaptive behavior services) and deletion of codes 0359T-0361T, 0363T-0372T, and 0374T, the exclusionary parenthetical notes following codes 90847 (family psychotherapy) and 90853 (group psychotherapy) have been revised to reflect these changes.

Refer to the codebook and the Rationale for codes 97151-97158, 0362T, and 0373T for a full discussion of these changes.

Other Psychiatric Services or Procedures

▶(For electronic analysis with programming, when performed, of vagal nerve neurostimulators, see 95970, 95976, 95977)◀

★✚ **90863** Pharmacologic management, including prescription and review of medication, when performed with psychotherapy services (List separately in addition to the code for primary procedure)

(Use 90863 in conjunction with 90832, 90834, 90837)

(For pharmacologic management with psychotherapy services performed by a physician or other qualified health care professional who may report evaluation and management codes, use the appropriate evaluation and management codes 99201-99255, 99281-99285, 99304-99337, 99341-99350 and the appropriate psychotherapy with evaluation and management service 90833, 90836, 90838)

(Do not count time spent on providing pharmacologic management services in the time used for selection of the psychotherapy service)

Rationale

The parenthetical note listed within the Other Psychiatric Services or Procedures subsection of the Psychiatry (Psychiatric Diagnostic Procedures) listing has been revised in conjunction with changes made to reporting neurostimulator services. These changes include the addition of language that standardizes the parenthetical note by adding the term "electronic" and "with programming when performed" to match instructions in other sections regarding neurostimulation. It also adds codes 95976 and 95977 because these codes include language regarding cranial nerve stimulator programming (vagus nerve is a cranial nerve) and by removing deleted codes 95974 and 95975.

Refer to the codebook and the Rationale for codes 95970-95972, 95976-95984 for a full discussion of these changes.

90865 Narcosynthesis for psychiatric diagnostic and therapeutic purposes (eg, sodium amobarbital (Amytal) interview)

90887 Interpretation or explanation of results of psychiatric, other medical examinations and procedures, or other accumulated data to family or other responsible persons, or advising them how to assist patient

▶(Do not report 90887 in conjunction with 97151, 97152, 97153, 97154, 97155, 97156, 97157, 97158, 0362T, 0373T)◀

Rationale

In support of the establishment of codes 97151-97158 (adaptive behavior services) and deletion of codes 0359T-0361T, 0363T-0372T, and 0374T, the exclusionary parenthetical note following code 90887 has been revised to reflect these changes.

Refer to the codebook and the Rationale for codes 97151-97158, 0362T, and 0373T for a full discussion of these changes.

★ = Telemedicine   ✚ = Add-on code   ✗ = FDA approval pending   # = Resequenced code   ⊘ = Modifier 51 exempt

Gastroenterology

Other Procedures

91200   Liver elastography, mechanically induced shear wave (eg, vibration), without imaging, with interpretation and report

▶(Do not report 91200 in conjunction with 76981, 76982, 76983)◀

Rationale

In support of the establishment of codes 76981, 76982, and 76983, a new parenthetical note has been added following code 91200 in the Gastroenterology section.

Refer to the codebook and the Rationale for codes 76981, 76982, and 76983 for a full discussion of these changes.

Ophthalmology

Special Ophthalmological Services

Other Specialized Services

For prescription, fitting, and/or medical supervision of ocular prosthetic (artificial eye) adaptation by a physician, see evaluation and management services including office or other outpatient services (99201-99215), office or other outpatient consultations (99241-99245) or general ophthalmological service codes 92002-92014.

▶Electroretinography (ERG) is used to evaluate function of the retina and optic nerve of the eye, including photoreceptors and ganglion cells. A number of techniques are used which target different areas of the eye, including full field (flash and flicker) (92273) for a global response of photoreceptors of the retina, multifocal (92274) for photoreceptors in multiple separate locations in the retina including the macula, and pattern (0509T) for retinal ganglion cells. Multiple additional terms and techniques are used to describe various types of ERG. If the technique used is not specifically named in the code descriptors for 92273, 92274, or 0509T, use the unlisted procedure code 92499.◀

92265   Needle oculoelectromyography, 1 or more extraocular muscles, 1 or both eyes, with interpretation and report

92270   Electro-oculography with interpretation and report

(For vestibular function tests with recording, see 92537, 92538, 92540, 92541, 92542, 92544, 92545, 92546, 92547, 92548)

(Do not report 92270 in conjunction with 92537, 92538, 92540, 92541, 92542, 92544, 92545, 92546, 92547, 92548)

(To report saccadic eye movement testing with recording, use 92700)

● **92273**   Electroretinography (ERG), with interpretation and report; full field (ie, ffERG, flash ERG, Ganzfeld ERG)

● **92274**   multifocal (mfERG)

▶(For pattern ERG, use 0509T)◀

▶(92275 has been deleted. To report electroretinography, see 92273, 92274, 0509T)◀

(For electronystagmography for vestibular function studies, see 92541 et seq)

(For ophthalmic echography (diagnostic ultrasound), see 76511-76529)

Rationale

Code 92275, *Electroretinography with interpretation and report,* has been deleted and two new codes (92273, 92274 [electroretinography {ERG}]) have been added to the Ophthalmology/Special Ophthalmological Services/Other Specialized Services section. New guidelines and parenthetical notes have also been added to provide instruction on the appropriate use of these two new codes.

Two methods of ERG testing (full field ERG [ffERG] and multifocal ERG [mfERG]) were in clinical use when code 92275 was added to the CPT code set. The work involved in each of these methods was similar and there was no need to distinguish them with different CPT codes. However, in 2015, a Centers for Medicare & Medicaid Services (CMS) analysis identified code 92275 as potentially misvalued due to a sharp increase in utilization. This increase in clinical use was due to the use of code 92275 to report a different ERG test called pattern ERG (PERG). Code 92275 was never intended to report PERG. Therefore, in order to accommodate appropriate coding and tracking of the different types of ERG testing, it was determined that separate codes should be established to properly distinguish mfERG, ffERG, and PERG testing.

Code 92273 describes ffERG, which measures overall retinal function. Code 92274 describes mfERG, which provides tracings of multiple locations in the retina.

Medicine 90281-99607

Interpretation and report are included in both codes 92273 and 92274 and, therefore, it must be performed in order to report both codes. The new guidelines explain ffERG and mfERG testing and provide additional instruction on the reporting of these procedures.

Category III code 0509T has been added to report PERG testing. Refer to the codebook and the Rationale for code 0509T for a full discussion of these changes.

Clinical Example (92273)

A 17-year-old male presents with a history of declining near vision with evidence of a peripheral pigmentary retinopathy.

Description of Procedure (92273)

Examine multiple images for waveform, latency, and amplitude. Compare with patterns associated with known retinal dystrophies and formulate a diagnosis, potential genotypes, prognosis, and potential therapeutic options.

Clinical Example (92274)

A 50-year-old female presents with loss of vision in the inferonasal field with corresponding narrowing of the retinal vessels in the superotemporal retina with clinical diagnosis of outer retinal damage in this zone.

Description of Procedure (92274)

Examine multiple images for waveform, latency, and amplitude. Compare with patterns associated with known retinal dystrophies and toxicities and formulate a diagnosis, potential genotypes, prognosis, and potential therapeutic options.

92285   External ocular photography with interpretation and report for documentation of medical progress (eg, close-up photography, slit lamp photography, goniophotography, stereo-photography)

(For tear film imaging, use 0330T)

▶(For meibomian gland imaging, use 0507T)◀

Rationale

A parenthetical note has been added in the Medicine section following code 92285 to direct users to use new code 0507T for meibomian gland imaging.

Refer to the codebook and the Rationale for code 0505T for a full discussion of these changes.

Special Otorhinolaryngologic Services

92507   Treatment of speech, language, voice, communication, and/or auditory processing disorder; individual

▶(Do not report 92507 in conjunction with 97153, 97155)◀

92508   group, 2 or more individuals

▶(Do not report 92508 in conjunction with 97154, 97158)◀

(For auditory rehabilitation, prelingual hearing loss, use 92630)

(For auditory rehabilitation, postlingual hearing loss, use 92633)

(For cochlear implant programming, see 92601-92604)

Rationale

In support of the establishment of codes 97151-97158 (adaptive behavior services) and deletion of codes 0359T-0361T, 0363T-0372T, and 0374T, the exclusionary parenthetical notes following codes 92507 and 92508 (otorhinolaryngologic) have been revised to reflect these changes.

Refer to the codebook and the Rationale for codes 97151-97158, 0362T, and 0373T for a full discussion of these changes.

Cardiovascular

Cardiography

(For echocardiography, see 93303-93350)

(For acoustic cardiography services, use 93799)

93000   Electrocardiogram, routine ECG with at least 12 leads; with interpretation and report

93005   tracing only, without interpretation and report

93010   interpretation and report only

(For ECG monitoring, see 99354-99360)

▶(Do not report 93000, 93005, 93010 in conjunction with, 0525T, 0526T, 0527T, 0528T, 0529T, 0530T, 0531T, 0532T)◀

★ = Telemedicine   ✚ = Add-on code   ✗ = FDA approval pending   # = Resequenced code   ⊘ = Modifier 51 exempt

Cardiovascular Monitoring Services

Cardiovascular monitoring services are diagnostic medical procedures using in-person and remote technology to assess cardiovascular rhythm (ECG) data. Holter monitors (93224-93227) include up to 48 hours of continuous recording. Mobile cardiac telemetry monitors (93228, 93229) have the capability of transmitting a tracing at any time, always have internal ECG analysis algorithms designed to detect major arrhythmias, and transmit to an attended surveillance center. Event monitors (93268-93272) record segments of ECGs with recording initiation triggered either by patient activation or by an internal automatic, pre-programmed detection algorithm (or both) and transmit the recorded electrocardiographic data when requested (but cannot transmit immediately based upon the patient or algorithmic activation rhythm) and require attended surveillance.

Attended surveillance: is the immediate availability of a remote technician to respond to rhythm or device alert transmissions from a patient, either from an implanted or wearable monitoring or therapy device, as they are generated and transmitted to the remote surveillance location or center.

Electrocardiographic rhythm derived elements: elements derived from recordings of the electrical activation of the heart including, but not limited to heart rhythm, rate, ST analysis, heart rate variability, T-wave alternans.

Mobile cardiovascular telemetry (MCT): continuously records the electrocardiographic rhythm from external electrodes placed on the patient's body. Segments of the ECG data are automatically (without patient intervention) transmitted to a remote surveillance location by cellular or landline telephone signal. The segments of the rhythm, selected for transmission, are triggered automatically (MCT device algorithm) by rapid and slow heart rates or by the patient during a symptomatic episode. There is continuous real time data analysis by preprogrammed algorithms in the device and

attended surveillance of the transmitted rhythm segments by a surveillance center technician to evaluate any arrhythmias and to determine signal quality. The surveillance center technician reviews the data and notifies the physician or other qualified health care professional depending on the prescribed criteria.

►ECG rhythm derived elements are distinct from physiologic data, even when the same device is capable of producing both. Implantable cardiovascular physiologic monitor device services are always separately reported from implantable cardioverter-defibrillator (ICD) service.◄

93224	External electrocardiographic recording up to 48 hours by continuous rhythm recording and storage; includes recording, scanning analysis with report, review and interpretation by a physician or other qualified health care professional
93264	Code is out of numerical sequence. See 93272-93280
★ **93268**	External patient and, when performed, auto activated electrocardiographic rhythm derived event recording with symptom-related memory loop with remote download capability up to 30 days, 24-hour attended monitoring; includes transmission, review and interpretation by a physician or other qualified health care professional
★ **93270**	recording (includes connection, recording, and disconnection)
★ **93271**	transmission and analysis
★ **93272**	review and interpretation by a physician or other qualified health care professional

►(For subcutaneous cardiac rhythm monitoring, see 33285, 93285, 93291, 93298, 93299)◄

▶Implantable, Insertable, and Wearable Cardiac Device Evaluations◀

▶Cardiac device evaluation services are diagnostic medical procedures using in-person and remote technology to assess device therapy and cardiovascular physiologic data. Codes 93260, 93261, 93279-93299 describe this technology and technical/professional and service center practice. Codes 93260, 93261, 93279-93292 are reported per procedure. Codes 93293, 93294, 93295, 93296 are reported no more than **once** every 90 days. Do not report 93293, 93294, 93295, 93296, if the monitoring period is less than 30 days. Codes 93297, 93298 are reported no more than **once** up to every 30 days, per patient. Do not report 93297-93299, if the monitoring period is less than 10 days. Do not report 93264 if the monitoring period is less than 30 days. Code 93264 is reported no more than once up to every 30 days, per patient.

A service center may report 93296 or 93299 during a period in which a physician or other qualified health care professional performs an in-person interrogation device evaluation. The same individual may not report an in-person and remote interrogation of the same device during the same period. Report only remote services when an in-person interrogation device evaluation is performed during a period of remote interrogation device evaluation. A period is established by the initiation of the remote monitoring or the 91st day of a pacemaker or implantable defibrillator monitoring or the 31st day of monitoring a subcutaneous cardiac rhythm monitor or implantable cardiovascular physiologic monitor, and extends for the subsequent 90 or 30 days respectively, for which remote monitoring is occurring. Programming device evaluations and in-person interrogation device evaluations may not be reported on the same date by the same individual. Programming device evaluations and remote interrogation device evaluations may both be reported during the remote interrogation device evaluation period.◀

For monitoring by wearable devices, see 93224-93272.

▶ECG rhythm derived elements are distinct from physiologic data, even when the same device is capable of producing both. Implantable cardiovascular physiologic monitor services are always separately reported from implantable defibrillator services. When cardiac rhythm data are derived from an implantable defibrillator or pacemaker, do not report subcutaneous cardiac rhythm monitor services with pacemaker or implantable defibrillator services.◀

Do not report 93268-93272 when performing 93260, 93261, 93279-93289, 93291-93296, or 93298-93299. Do not report 93040, 93041, 93042 when performing 93260, 93261, 93279-93289, 93291-93296, or 93298-93299.

The pacemaker and implantable defibrillator interrogation device evaluations, peri-procedural device evaluations and programming, and programming device evaluations may not be reported in conjunction with pacemaker or implantable defibrillator device and/or lead insertion or revision services by the same individual.

The following definitions and instructions apply to codes 93260, 93261, 93279-93299.

▶*Attended surveillance:* the immediate availability of a remote technician to respond to rhythm or device alert transmissions from a patient, either from an implanted, inserted, or wearable monitoring or therapy device, as they are generated and transmitted to the remote surveillance location or center.

Device, leadless: a leadless cardiac pacemaker system that includes a pulse generator with built-in battery and electrode for implantation into the cardiac chamber via a transcatheter approach.◀

Device, single lead: a pacemaker or implantable defibrillator with pacing and sensing function in only one chamber of the heart or a subcutaneous electrode.

Device, dual lead: a pacemaker or implantable defibrillator with pacing and sensing function in only two chambers of the heart.

Device, multiple lead: a pacemaker or implantable defibrillator with pacing and sensing function in three or more chambers of the heart.

Electrocardiographic rhythm derived elements: elements derived from recordings of the electrical activation of the heart including, but not limited to heart rhythm, rate, ST analysis, heart rate variability, T-wave alternans.

▶*Implantable cardiovascular physiologic monitor:* an implantable cardiovascular device used to assist the physician or other qualified health care professional in the management of non-rhythm related cardiac conditions such as heart failure. The device collects longitudinal physiologic cardiovascular data elements from one or more internal sensors (such as right ventricular pressure, pulmonary artery pressure, left atrial pressure, or an index of lung water) and/or external sensors (such as blood pressure or body weight) for patient assessment and management. The data are stored and transmitted by either local telemetry or remotely to an Internet-based file server or surveillance technician. The function of the implantable cardiovascular physiologic monitor may be an additional function of an implantable cardiac device (eg, implantable defibrillator) or a function of a stand-alone device. When implantable cardiovascular physiologic monitor functionality is

Medicine 90281-99607

included in an implantable defibrillator device or pacemaker, the implantable cardiovascular physiologic monitor data and the implantable defibrillator or pacemaker, heart rhythm data such as sensing, pacing, and tachycardia detection therapy are distinct and, therefore, the monitoring processes are distinct.

Implantable defibrillator: two general categories of implantable defibrillators exist: transvenous implantable pacing cardioverter-defibrillator (ICD) and subcutaneous implantable defibrillator (SICD). An implantable pacing cardioverter-defibrillator device provides high-energy and low-energy stimulation to one or more chambers of the heart to terminate rapid heart rhythms called tachycardia or fibrillation. Implantable pacing cardioverter-defibrillators also have pacemaker functions to treat slow heart rhythms called bradycardia. In addition to the tachycardia and bradycardia functions, the implantable pacing cardioverter-defibrillator may or may not include the functionality of an implantable cardiovascular physiologic monitor or a subcutaneous cardiac rhythm monitor. The subcutaneous implantable defibrillator uses a single subcutaneous electrode to treat ventricular tachyarrhythmias. Subcutaneous implantable defibrillators differ from transvenous implantable pacing cardioverter-defibrillators in that subcutaneous implantable defibrillators do not provide antitachycardia pacing or chronic pacing. For subcutaneous implantable defibrillator device evaluation, see 93260, 93261.

Interrogation device evaluation: an evaluation of an implantable device such as a cardiac pacemaker, implantable defibrillator, implantable cardiovascular physiologic monitor, or subcutaneous cardiac rhythm monitor. Using an office, hospital, or emergency room instrument or via a remote interrogation system, stored and measured information about the lead(s) when present, sensor(s) when present, battery and the implanted device function, as well as data collected about the patient's heart rhythm and heart rate is retrieved. The retrieved information is evaluated to determine the current programming of the device and to evaluate certain aspects of the device function such as battery voltage, lead impedance, tachycardia detection settings, and rhythm treatment settings.

The components that must be evaluated for the various types of implantable or insertable cardiac devices are listed below. (The required components for both remote and in-person interrogations are the same.)

  Pacemaker: programmed parameters, with or without lead(s), battery, capture and sensing function and heart rhythm.◄

  Implantable defibrillator: programmed parameters, lead(s), battery, capture and sensing function, presence or absence of therapy for ventricular tachyarrhythmias and underlying heart rhythm.

▶*Implantable cardiovascular physiologic monitor:* programmed parameters and analysis of at least one recorded physiologic cardiovascular data element from either internal or external sensors.

Subcutaneous cardiac rhythm monitor: programmed parameters and the heart rate and rhythm during recorded episodes from both patient initiated and device algorithm detected events, when present.

Interrogation device evaluation (remote): a procedure performed for patients with pacemakers, implantable defibrillators, or subcutaneous cardiac rhythm monitors using data obtained remotely. All device functions, including the programmed parameters, lead(s), battery, capture and sensing function, presence or absence of therapy for ventricular tachyarrhythmias (for implantable defibrillators) and underlying heart rhythm are evaluated.

The components that must be evaluated for the various types of implantable or insertable cardiac devices are listed below. (The required components for both remote and in person interrogations are the same.)

  Pacemaker: programmed parameters, with or without lead(s), battery, capture and sensing function, and heart rhythm.◄

  Implantable defibrillator: programmed parameters, lead(s), battery, capture and sensing function, presence or absence of therapy for ventricular tachyarrhythmias, and underlying heart rhythm.

▶*Implantable cardiovascular physiologic monitor:* programmed parameters and analysis of at least one recorded physiologic cardiovascular data element from either internal or external sensors.

Subcutaneous cardiac rhythm monitor: programmed parameters and the heart rate and rhythm during recorded episodes from both patient-initiated and device algorithm detected events, when present.

Pacemaker: an implantable device that provides low energy localized stimulation to one or more chambers of the heart to initiate contraction in that chamber. Two general categories of pacemakers exist: (1) pacemakers with a subcutaneous generator plus transvenous/ epicardial lead(s); and (2) leadless pacemakers. A leadless pacemaker does not require a subcutaneous pocket for the generator. It combines a miniaturized generator with an integrated electrode for implantation in a heart chamber via a transcatheter approach.

Peri-procedural device evaluation and programming: an evaluation of an implantable device system (either a pacemaker or implantable defibrillator) to adjust the device to settings appropriate for the patient prior to a surgery, procedure, or test. The device system data are interrogated to evaluate the lead(s) when present, sensor(s), and battery in addition to review of stored information, including patient and system measurements. The device is programmed to settings appropriate for the surgery, procedure, or test, as required. A second evaluation and programming are performed after the surgery, procedure, or test to provide settings appropriate to the post procedural situation, as required. If one performs both the pre- and post-evaluation and programming service, the appropriate code, either 93286 or 93287, would be reported two times. If one performs the pre-surgical service and a separate individual performs the post-surgical service, each reports either 93286 or 93287 only one time.◄

Physiologic cardiovascular data elements: data elements from one or more internal sensors (such as right ventricular pressure, left atrial pressure or an index of lung water) and/or external sensors (such as blood pressure or body weight) for patient assessment and management. It does not include ECG rhythm derived data elements.

►*Programming device evaluation (in person):* a procedure performed for patients with a pacemaker, implantable defibrillator, or subcutaneous cardiac rhythm monitor. All device functions, including the battery, programmable settings and lead(s), when present, are evaluated. To assess capture thresholds, iterative adjustments (eg, progressive changes in pacing output of a pacing lead) of the programmable parameters are conducted. The iterative adjustments provide information that permits the operator to assess and select the most appropriate final program parameters to provide for consistent delivery of the appropriate therapy and to verify the function of the device. The final program parameters may or may not change after evaluation.◄

The programming device evaluation includes all of the components of the interrogation device evaluation (remote) or the interrogation device evaluation (in person), and it includes the selection of patient specific programmed parameters depending on the type of device.

The components that must be evaluated for the various types of programming device evaluations are listed below. (See also required interrogation device evaluation [remote and in person] components above.)

►*Pacemaker:* programmed parameters, lead(s) when present, battery, capture and sensing function, and heart rhythm. Often, but not always, the sensor rate response, lower and upper heart rates, AV intervals, pacing voltage and pulse duration, sensing value, and diagnostics will be adjusted during a programming evaluation.◄

Implantable defibrillator: programmed parameters, lead(s), battery, capture and sensing function,

presence or absence of therapy for ventricular tachyarrhythmias and underlying heart rhythm. Often, but not always, the sensor rate response, lower and upper heart rates, AV intervals, pacing voltage and pulse duration, sensing value, and diagnostics will be adjusted during a programming evaluation. In addition, ventricular tachycardia detection and therapies are sometimes altered depending on the interrogated data, patient's rhythm, symptoms, and condition.

►*Subcutaneous cardiac rhythm monitor:* programmed parameters and the heart rhythm during recorded episodes from both patient initiated and device algorithm detected events. Often, but not always, the tachycardia and bradycardia detection criteria will be adjusted during a programming evaluation.

Subcutaneous cardiac rhythm monitor: an implantable or insertable device that continuously records the electrocardiographic rhythm triggered automatically by rapid, irregular, and/or slow heart rates or by the patient during a symptomatic episode. The cardiac rhythm monitor function may be the only function of the device or it may be part of a pacemaker or implantable defibrillator device. The data are stored and transmitted by either local telemetry or remotely to an Internet-based file server or surveillance technician. Extraction of data and compilation or report for physician or qualified health care professional interpretation is usually performed in the office setting.

Transtelephonic rhythm strip pacemaker evaluation: service of transmission of an electrocardiographic rhythm strip over the telephone by the patient using a transmitter and recorded by a receiving location using a receiver/recorder (also commonly known as transtelephonic pacemaker monitoring). The electrocardiographic rhythm strip is recorded both with and without a magnet applied over the pacemaker. The rhythm strip is evaluated for heart rate and rhythm, atrial and ventricular capture (if observed) and atrial and ventricular sensing (if observed). In addition, the battery status of the pacemaker is determined by measurement of the paced rate on the electrocardiographic rhythm strip recorded with the magnet applied. For remote monitoring of an implantable wireless pulmonary artery pressure sensor, use 93264.

Implantable wireless pulmonary artery sensor: an implantable cardiovascular device used to assist the physician or other qualified health care professional in monitoring heart failure. The device collects longitudinal physiologic cardiovascular data elements from an internal sensor located in the pulmonary artery. The data are transmitted and stored remotely to an Internet-based file server.◄

#● 93264 Remote monitoring of a wireless pulmonary artery pressure sensor for up to 30 days, including at least weekly downloads of pulmonary artery pressure recordings, interpretation(s), trend analysis, and report(s) by a physician or other qualified health care professional

▶(Report 93264 only once per 30 days)◀

▶(Do not report 93264 if download[s], interpretation[s], trend analysis, and report[s] do not occur at least weekly during the 30-day time period)◀

▶(Do not report 93264 if review does not occur at least weekly during the 30-day time period)◀

▶(Do not report 93264 if monitoring period is less than 30 days)◀

▲ 93279 Programming device evaluation (in person) with iterative adjustment of the implantable device to test the function of the device and select optimal permanent programmed values with analysis, review and report by a physician or other qualified health care professional; single lead pacemaker system or leadless pacemaker system in one cardiac chamber

(Do not report 93279 in conjunction with 93286, 93288)

93280   dual lead pacemaker system

(Do not report 93280 in conjunction with 93286, 93288)

93281   multiple lead pacemaker system

(Do not report 93281 in conjunction with 93286, 93288)

93282   single lead transvenous implantable defibrillator system

(Do not report 93282 in conjunction with 93260, 93287, 93289, 93745)

93283   dual lead transvenous implantable defibrillator system

(Do not report 93283 in conjunction with 93287, 93289)

93284   multiple lead transvenous implantable defibrillator system

(Do not report 93284 in conjunction with 93287, 93289)

 # 93260   implantable subcutaneous lead defibrillator system

(Do not report 93260 in conjunction with 93261, 93282, 93287)

(Do not report 93260 in conjunction with pulse generator and lead insertion or repositioning codes 33240, 33241, 33262, 33270, 33271, 33272, 33273)

▲ 93285   subcutaneous cardiac rhythm monitor system

▶(Do not report 93285 in conjunction with 33285, 93279-93284, 93291)◀

▲ 93286 Peri-procedural device evaluation (in person) and programming of device system parameters before or after a surgery, procedure, or test with analysis, review and report by a physician or other qualified health care professional; single, dual, or multiple lead pacemaker system, or leadless pacemaker system

(Report 93286 once before and once after surgery, procedure, or test, when device evaluation and programming is performed before and after surgery, procedure, or test)

(Do not report 93286 in conjunction with 93279-93281, 93288, 0408T, 0409T, 0410T, 0411T, 0414T, 0415T)

93287   single, dual, or multiple lead implantable defibriliator system

(Report 93287 once before and once after surgery, procedure, or test, when device evaluation and programming is performed before and after surgery, procedure, or test)

(Do not report 93287 in conjunction with 93260, 93261, 93282, 93283, 93284, 93289, 0408T, 0409T, 0410T, 0411T, 0414T, 0415T)

▲ 93288 Interrogation device evaluation (in person) with analysis, review and report by a physician or other qualified health care professional, includes connection, recording and disconnection per patient encounter; single, dual, or multiple lead pacemaker system, or leadless pacemaker system

(Do not report 93288 in conjunction with 93279-93281, 93286, 93294, 93296)

93289   single, dual, or multiple lead transvenous implantable defibrillator system, including analysis of heart rhythm derived data elements

(For monitoring physiologic cardiovascular data elements derived from an implantable defibrillator, use 93290)

(Do not report 93289 in conjunction with 93261, 93282, 93283, 93284, 93287, 93295, 93296)

 # 93261   implantable subcutaneous lead defibrillator system

(Do not report 93261 in conjunction with 93260, 93287, 93289)

(Do not report 93261 in conjunction with pulse generator and lead insertion or repositioning codes 33240, 33241, 33262, 33270, 33271, 33272, 33273)

▲ 93290   implantable cardiovascular physiologic monitor system, including analysis of 1 or more recorded physiologic cardiovascular data elements from all internal and external sensors

(For heart rhythm derived data elements, use 93289)

(Do not report 93290 in conjunction with 93297, 93299)

▲ 93291   subcutaneous cardiac rhythm monitor system, including heart rhythm derived data analysis

▶(Do not report 93291 in conjunction with 33285, 93288-93290, 93298, 93299)◀

93292   wearable defibrillator system

(Do not report 93292 in conjunction with 93745)

—— *Coding Tip* ——

Instructions for Reporting Pacemaker and Interrogation Device Evaluations

Codes 93293-93296 are reported no more than once every 90 days. Do not report 93293-93296 if the monitoring period is less than 30 days.

CPT Coding Guidelines, Cardiovascular, Cardiography Implantable and Wearable Cardiac Device Evaluations

93293   Transtelephonic rhythm strip pacemaker evaluation(s) single, dual, or multiple lead pacemaker system, includes recording with and without magnet application with analysis, review and report(s) by a physician or other qualified health care professional, up to 90 days

(Do not report 93293 in conjunction with 93294)

(For in person evaluation, see 93040, 93041, 93042)

(Report 93293 only once per 90 days)

▲ 93294   Interrogation device evaluation(s) (remote), up to 90 days; single, dual, or multiple lead pacemaker system, or leadless pacemaker system with interim analysis, review(s) and report(s) by a physician or other qualified health care professional

(Do not report 93294 in conjunction with 93288, 93293)

(Report 93294 only once per 90 days)

93295   single, dual, or multiple lead implantable defibrillator system with interim analysis, review(s) and report(s) by a physician or other qualified health care professional

(For remote monitoring of physiologic cardiovascular data elements derived from an ICD, use 93297)

(Do not report 93295 in conjunction with 93289)

(Report 93295 only once per 90 days)

▲ 93296   single, dual, or multiple lead pacemaker system, leadless pacemaker system, or implantable defibrillator system, remote data acquisition(s), receipt of transmissions and technician review, technical support and distribution of results

(Do not report 93296 in conjunction with 93288, 93289, 93299)

(Report 93296 only once per 90 days)

▲ 93297   Interrogation device evaluation(s), (remote) up to 30 days; implantable cardiovascular physiologic monitor system, including analysis of 1 or more recorded physiologic cardiovascular data elements from all internal and external sensors, analysis, review(s) and report(s) by a physician or other qualified health care professional

(For heart rhythm derived data elements, use 93295)

▶(Do not report 93297 in conjunction with 93264, 93290, 93298)◀

(Report 93297 only once per 30 days)

★▲ 93298   subcutaneous cardiac rhythm monitor system, including analysis of recorded heart rhythm data, analysis, review(s) and report(s) by a physician or other qualified health care professional

▶(Do not report 93298 in conjunction with 33285, 93291, 93297)◀

(Report 93298 only once per 30 days)

★▲ 93299   implantable cardiovascular physiologic monitor system or subcutaneous cardiac rhythm monitor system, remote data acquisition(s), receipt of transmissions and technician review, technical support and distribution of results

▶(For remote monitoring of an implantable wireless pulmonary artery pressure sensor, use 93264)◀

▶(Do not report 93299 in conjunction with 93264, 93290, 93291, 93296)◀

(Report 93299 only once per 30 days)

Rationale

A large number of revisions have been made to the guidelines and codes in the Implantable and Wearable Cardiac Device Evaluations subsection, including a revision to the subsection title to include the word "Insertable" (Implantable, Insertable, and Wearable Cardiac Device Evaluations).

Code 93264 has been established for remote monitoring of a wireless pulmonary artery pressure sensor for up to 30 days. In addition, the implantable and wearable cardiac device evaluations guidelines have been revised to further define an implantable wireless pulmonary artery sensor.

The procedure described by code 93264 specifically involves pulmonary artery pressure measurements performed and transmitted by the patient and the population receiving this service requires intense follow-up in both the optimization and continuation phase. Recurrences of congestive heart failure and recurrent hospitalization rates for this group of patients are very high. For this reason, at least weekly provider-to-patient contact with review of pulmonary artery measurements is required within a 30-day period. Code 93264 should not be reported if the monitoring is less than 30 days. For the implantation of wireless pulmonary artery pressure sensor, see code 33289. Refer to the codebook and the Rationale for code 33289 for a full discussion of these changes.

In support of the conversion of Category III codes 0387T-0391T (leadless pacemaker services) to Category I codes 33274 and 33275, changes have been made to the Implantable and Wearable Cardiac Device Evaluations subsection. Codes 93279, 93286, 93288, 93294, and 93296 (device evaluation) have been revised to include evaluation of leadless pacemakers. "Insertable" has been added to the subsection title (Implantable, Insertable, and Wearable Cardiac Device Evaluations) because leadless pacemakers are inserted via catheter through the femoral vein, rather than worn by the patient or implanted. A definition for leadless device has been added to the implantable, insertable, and wearable cardiac device evaluations guidelines. Refer to the codebook and the Rationales for codes 33274 and 33275 and the deletion of codes 0387T-0391T for a full discussion of these changes.

In support of the device terminology used in new codes 33285 and 33286 (subcutaneous cardiac rhythm monitor), the device terminology has also been revised in the Medicine/Cardiovascular Monitoring Services subsection. Specifically, the descriptors of codes 93285, 93291, 93298, and 93299, device definitions in the guidelines, and relevant parenthetical notes in this subsection have been revised to "subcutaneous cardiac rhythm monitor" in place of the former "implantable loop recorder." Terminology changes have also been made to codes 93290, 93297, and 93299 and associated guidelines by adding the qualifier "physiologic" to "implantable cardiovascular monitor." This revision clarifies the function of the device and draws a clearer distinction between this device and subcutaneous cardiac rhythm monitor. Refer to the codebook and the Rationale for codes 93285 and 93286 for a full discussion of these changes.

Clinical Example (93264)

A 69-year-old male with heart failure, preserved left ventricular ejection fraction, and mild renal insufficiency with an implanted pulmonary artery (PA) pressure monitoring system is undergoing continued hemodynamic monitoring.

Description of Procedure (93264)

Interpret data and analyze trends from the 18-second waveforms and corresponding systolic, diastolic, and mean PA pressures from patient-transmitted data weekly during the 30-day period. Evaluate appropriateness of the current programmed parameters and alerts.

Cardiac Catheterization

⊘ **93451**   Right heart catheterization including measurement(s) of oxygen saturation and cardiac output, when performed

▶(Do not report 93451 in conjunction with 33289, 93453, 93456, 93457, 93460, 93461)◀

(Do not report 93451 in conjunction with 0345T for diagnostic left and right heart catheterization procedures intrinsic to the valve repair procedure)

Rationale

In accordance with the addition of code 33289, the parenthetical note following code 93451 has been revised to preclude the use of code 33289 with code 93451.

Refer to the codebook and the Rationale for code 33289 for a full discussion of these changes.

Injection Procedures

+ **93563**   Injection procedure during cardiac catheterization including imaging supervision, interpretation, and report; for selective coronary angiography during congenital heart catheterization (List separately in addition to code for primary procedure)

+ **93564**   for selective opacification of aortocoronary venous or arterial bypass graft(s) (eg, aortocoronary saphenous vein, free radial artery, or free mammary artery graft) to one or more coronary arteries and in situ arterial conduits (eg, internal mammary), whether native or used for bypass to one or more coronary arteries during congenital heart catheterization, when performed (List separately in addition to code for primary procedure)

(Do not report 93563, 93564 in conjunction with 0345T for coronary angiography intrinsic to the valve repair procedure)

+ **93565**   for selective left ventricular or left atrial angiography (List separately in addition to code for primary procedure)

(Do not report 93563-93565 in conjunction with 93452-93461)

(Use 93563-93565 in conjunction with 93530-93533)

+ **93566**   for selective right ventricular or right atrial angiography (List separately in addition to code for primary procedure)

(Use 93566 in conjunction with 93451, 93453, 93456, 93457, 93460, 93461, 93530-93533)

Medicine 90281-99607

▶(Do not report 93566 in conjunction with 33274 for right ventriculography performed during leadless pacemaker insertion)◀

Rationale

In support of the deletion of code 0387T and the establishment of code 33274, the exclusionary parenthetical note following code 93566 has been revised with the removal of code 0387T and the inclusion of code 33274.

Refer to the codebook and the Rationale for codes 33274 and 0387T for a full discussion of these changes.

+ **93567** for supravalvular aortography (List separately in addition to code for primary procedure)

(Use 93567 in conjunction with 93451-93461, 93530-93533)

(For non-supravalvular thoracic aortography or abdominal aortography performed at the time of cardiac catheterization, use the appropriate radiological supervision and interpretation codes [36221, 75600-75630])

+ **93568** for pulmonary angiography (List separately in addition to code for primary procedure)

(Use 93568 in conjunction with 93451, 93453, 93456, 93457, 93460, 93461, 93530-93533, 93582, 93583)

+ **93571** Intravascular Doppler velocity and/or pressure derived coronary flow reserve measurement (coronary vessel or graft) during coronary angiography including pharmacologically induced stress; initial vessel (List separately in addition to code for primary procedure)

(Use 93571 in conjunction with 92920, 92924, 92928, 92933, 92937, 92941, 92943, 92975, 93454-93461, 93563, 93564)

▶(Do not report 93571 in conjunction with 0523T)◀

+ **93572** each additional vessel (List separately in addition to code for primary procedure)

(Use 93572 in conjunction with 93571)

(Intravascular distal coronary blood flow velocity measurements include all Doppler transducer manipulations and repositioning within the specific vessel being examined, during coronary angiography or therapeutic intervention [eg, angioplasty])

(For unlisted cardiac catheterization procedure, use 93799)

▶(Do not report 93572 in conjunction with 0523T)◀

Rationale

In accordance with the addition of code 0523T, a new parenthetical note has been added following code 93571 to preclude the use of codes 93571 and 93572 with code 0523T.

Refer to the codebook and the Rationale for code 0523T for a full discussion of these changes.

Pulmonary

Pulmonary Diagnostic Testing and Therapies

▲ **94780** Car seat/bed testing for airway integrity, for infants through 12 months of age, with continual clinical staff observation and continuous recording of pulse oximetry, heart rate and respiratory rate, with interpretation and report; 60 minutes

(Do not report 94780 for less than 60 minutes)

(Do not report 94780 in conjunction with 93040-93042, 94760, 94761, 99468-99472, 99477-99480)

+▲ **94781** each additional full 30 minutes (List separately in addition to code for primary procedure)

(Use 94781 in conjunction with 94780)

Rationale

An editorial revision has been made to codes 94780 and 94781 to replace the term "neonate" (ie, 28 days of age or younger) with the phrase "for infants through 12 months of age." These codes have also been revised by replacing "nursing" with "clinical staff." These changes were made to specify that medical necessity of the test is related to gestational and respiratory maturity rather than chronological age. It is for this reason that "neonate" has been deleted from the code descriptor and replaced with "for infants through 12 months of age" to allow this code to be used for the population that most needs it.

This service is typically performed by clinical staff, such as respiratory therapists or nurses. Accordingly, "nursing" has been deleted and replaced with "clinical staff" to more specifically identify the individuals providing the service.

★ = Telemedicine   ✚ = Add-on code   ✗ = FDA approval pending   # = Resequenced code   ⊘ = Modifier 51 exempt

Medicine 90281-99607

Neurology and Neuromuscular Procedures

Routine Electroencephalography (EEG)

95829   Code is out of numerical sequence. See 95827-95832

95830   Insertion by physician or other qualified health care professional of sphenoidal electrodes for electroencephalographic (EEG) recording

►Electrocorticography◄

►Electrocorticography (ECoG) is the recording of EEG from electrodes directly on or in the brain.

Code 95829 describes intraoperative recordings of ECoG from electrode arrays implanted in or placed directly on the brain exposed during surgery. Code 95829 includes review and interpretation during surgery.

Code 95836 describes recording of ECoG from electrodes chronically implanted on or in the brain. Chronically implanted electrodes allow for intracranial recordings to continue after the patient has been discharged from the hospital. Code 95836 includes unattended ECoG recording with storage for later review and interpretation during a single 30-day period. Code 95836 may be reported only once for each 30-day period. The dates encompassed by the 30-day period must be documented in the report.

For report of programming for a brain neurostimulator pulse generator/transmitter during the ECoG (95836) 30-day period, see 95983, 95984.◄

 # 95829   Electrocorticogram at surgery (separate procedure)

#● 95836   Electrocorticogram from an implanted brain neurostimulator pulse generator/transmitter, including recording, with interpretation and written report, up to 30 days

   ►(Report 95836 only once per 30 days)◄

   ►(Do not report 95836 in conjunction with 95957)◄

   ►(For programming a brain neurostimulator pulse generator/transmitter when performed in conjunction with ECoG [95836], see 95983, 95984)◄

Rationale

New code 95836 has been established, code 95829 relocated, and new Electrocorticography subsection with guidelines added to identify electrocorticography (ECoG) performed over a 30-day period. In addition, parenthetical notes have been added to direct users regarding the intended use of the new code, as well as to direct users to codes for programming for chronic electrocorticography procedures.

Code 95836 is intended to identify ECoG performed over a 30-day period, ie, it identifies reporting for ongoing outpatient recording and interpretation of ECoG data after the patient has been discharged from the hospital. Note that this includes recording that uses electrodes that are placed in or on the brain with the intent of capturing electrocorticographic events/data over the course of a period of time that does not exceed 30 days. Review and interpretation of ECoG data usually occurs multiple times during the cycle in order to obtain a number of readings that may then be evaluated as parts of a total service. Therefore, this code should be reported only once during the 30-day period (as noted in the parenthetical note following code 95836).

This differs from the intended use of code 95829, which identifies ECoG recording that is performed intraoperatively. Code 95829 was relocated from the Routine Electroencephalography (EEG) section to the Electrocorticography subsection so that it is grouped together with other codes that describe similar services.

Additional parenthetical notes restrict reporting of ECoG (95836) in conjunction with digital analysis of EEG (95957) and direct users to the correct codes to report for programming for brain neurostimulators.

Clinical Example (95836)

A 30-year-old female with medically refractory partial onset seizures occurring several times per month has been treated with a surgically implanted intracranial responsive neurostimulator. Stored electrocorticograms (ECoG) are interpreted.

Description of Procedure (95836)

Perform ECoG review by navigating to the ECoG section of the Web-based application. Physician reviews each of the 100 to 140 seizure files, approximately nine pages each, identifying which are true seizure detections, where each real seizure started, whether electroshocks stopped the seizure, and if so, how many shocks were necessary to stop the seizure. When false detections are identified, review them to determine which detection parameters triggered the detection so they can be considered for adjustments. Review the brain location of detections to determine if seizures are arising from more than one site because if all seizures arise from one site in the long term then the site can be considered for surgical resection. Compare the intensity of electroshock stimulations delivered to prior settings to determine if these intensities, electrodes used, and frequencies improved stopping seizures. Based on the intracranial ECoG recordings that have been collected over the prior month, physician determines whether the most recent settings improved stopping seizures compared to prior settings. If improvements occurred, physician must decide if continuing further changes of these parameters are warranted. If there are false detections or if no improvement occurred, then seizure data reviewed in this session are used to model new detection parameter settings in an attempt to better capture the patient's seizure activity. New detection parameters can be simulated in digital models and applied to the stored intracranial ECoGs to determine if the new proposed settings will detect seizures more accurately or earlier in the seizure. After new detection parameters have been developed, tested, and finalized, save the new detection parameters for later separate neurostimulator programming performed in a separate procedure.

Muscle and Range of Motion Testing

95831 Muscle testing, manual (separate procedure) with report; extremity (excluding hand) or trunk

95836 Code is out of numerical sequence. See 95827-95832

Intraoperative Neurophysiology

#+ 95941 Continuous intraoperative neurophysiology monitoring, from outside the operating room (remote or nearby) or for monitoring of more than one case while in the operating room, per hour (List separately in addition to code for primary procedure)

(Use 95941 in conjunction with the study performed, 92585, 95822, 95860-95870, 95907-95913, 95925, 95926, 95927, 95928, 95929, 95930-95937, 95938, 95939)

(For time spent waiting on standby before monitoring, use 99360)

(For electrocorticography, use 95829)

(For intraoperative EEG during nonintracranial surgery, use 95955)

(For intraoperative functional cortical or subcortical mapping, see 95961-95962)

▶(For intraoperative neurostimulator programming, see 95971, 95972, 95976, 95977, 95983, 95984)◀

Rationale

The parenthetical note following code 95941 has been revised in conjunction with changes made to neurostimulator services reporting. This includes removal of "and analysis," removal of codes 95970 and 95975, and addition of codes 95971, 95972, 95976, 95977, 95983, and 95984 to the guideline.

Refer to the codebook and the Rationale for codes 95970-95972 and 95976-95984 for a full discussion of these changes.

Neurostimulators, Analysis-Programming

▶Electronic analysis of an implanted neurostimulator pulse generator/transmitter involves documenting settings and electrode impedances of the system parameters prior to programming. Programming involves adjusting the system parameter(s) to address clinical signs and patient symptoms. Parameters available for programming can vary between systems and may need to be adjusted multiple times during a single programming session. The iterative adjustments to parameters provide information that is required for the physician or other qualified health care professional to assess and select the most appropriate final program parameters to provide for consistent delivery of appropriate therapy. The values of the final program parameters may differ from the starting values after the programming session.

Examples of parameters include: contact group(s), interleaving, amplitude, pulse width, frequency (Hz), on/off cycling, burst, magnet mode, dose lockout, patient-selectable parameters, responsive neurostimulation, detection algorithms, closed-loop parameters, and passive parameters. Not all parameters are available for programming in every neurostimulator pulse generator/transmitter.

For coding purposes, a neurostimulator system is considered implanted when the electrode array(s) is inserted into the target area for either permanent or trial placement.

There are several types of implantable neurostimulator pulse generator/transmitters and they are differentiated by the nervous system region that is stimulated. A brain neurostimulator may stimulate either brain surface regions (cortical stimulation) or deep brain structures (deep brain stimulation). A brain neurostimulation system consists of array(s) that targets one or more of these regions.

►Physician or Other Qualified Health Care Professional Face-to-Face Time for Brain Neurostimulator Analysis With Programming	Code(s)
Less than 8 minutes	Not reported
8-22 minutes	95983 X 1
23-37 minutes	95983 X 1 + 95984 X 1
38-52 minutes	95983 X 1 + 95984 X 2
53-67 minutes	95983 X 1 + 95984 X 3
68 minutes or longer	add units of 95984◄

A cranial nerve neurostimulator targets the fibers of the cranial nerves or their branches and divisions. There are 12 pairs of cranial nerves (see nerve anatomy figure on page 706 [of the codebook]). Each cranial nerve has its origin in the brain and passes through one or more foramina in the skull to innervate extracranial structures. A cranial nerve neurostimulator stimulates the nerve fibers of either the extracranial or intracranial portion(s) of one or more cranial nerve(s) (eg, vagus nerve, trigeminal nerve).

A spinal cord or peripheral nerve neurostimulator targets nerve(s) that originate in the spinal cord and exit the spine through neural foramina and gives rise to peripheral nerves. The peripheral nervous system consists of the nerves and ganglia outside of the brain and spinal cord. Peripheral nerves may give rise to independent branches or branches that combine with other peripheral nerves in neural plexuses (ie, brachial plexus, lumbosacral plexus). Under the lumbosacral plexus, the sacral nerves (specifically S2, S3, S4) are located in the lower back just above the tailbone. Neurostimulation of the sacral nerves affect pelvic floor muscles and urinary organs (eg, bladder, urinary sphincter).

Cranial nerve, spinal cord, peripheral nerve, and sacral nerve neurostimulator analysis with programming (95971, 95972, 95976, 95977) are reported based on the number of parameters adjusted during a programming session. Brain neurostimulator analysis with programming (95983, 95984) is reported based on physician or other qualified health care professional face-to-face time.

Code 95970 describes electronic analysis of the implanted brain, cranial nerve, spinal cord, peripheral nerve, or sacral nerve neurostimulator pulse generator/ transmitter without programming. Electronic analysis is inherent to implantation codes 43647, 43648, 43881, 43882, 61850, 61860, 61863, 61864, 61867, 61868, 61870, 61880, 61885, 61886, 61888, 63650, 63655, 63661, 63662, 63663, 63664, 63685, 63688, 64553, 64555, 64561, 64566, 64568, 64569, 64570, 64575, 64580, 64581, 64585, 64590, 64595, and is not separately reportable at the same operative session.

Codes 95971, 95972, 95976, 95977 describe electronic analysis with simple or complex programming of the implanted neurostimulator pulse generator/transmitter. Simple programming of a neurostimulator pulse generator/transmitter includes adjustment of one to three parameter(s). Complex programming includes adjustment of more than three parameters. For purposes of counting the number of parameters being programmed, a single parameter that is adjusted two or more times during a programming session counts as one parameter.

Code 95971 describes electronic analysis with simple programming of an implanted spinal cord or peripheral nerve (eg, sacral nerve) neurostimulator pulse generator/ transmitter.

Code 95972 describes electronic analysis with complex programming of an implanted spinal cord or peripheral nerve (eg, sacral nerve) neurostimulator pulse generator/ transmitter.

Code 95976 describes electronic analysis with simple programming of an implanted cranial nerve neurostimulator pulse generator/transmitter.

Code 95977 describes electronic analysis with complex programming of an implanted cranial nerve neurostimulator pulse generator/transmitter.

Codes 95983, 95984 describe electronic analysis with programming of an implanted brain neurostimulator pulse generator/transmitter. Code 95983 is reported for the first 15 minutes of physician or other qualified health care professional face-to-face time for analysis and programming. Code 95984 is reported for each additional 15 minutes. A unit of service is attained when the mid-point is passed. Physician or other qualified health care professional face-to-face time of less than eight minutes is not separately reportable.◄

Code 95980 describes intraoperative electronic analysis of an implanted gastric neurostimulator pulse generator system, with programming; code 95981 describes subsequent analysis of the device; code 95982 describes

Medicine 90281-99607

subsequent analysis and reprogramming. For electronic analysis and reprogramming of gastric neurostimulator, lesser curvature, see 95980-95982.

►Codes 95971, 95972, 95976, 95977, 95983, 95984 are reported when programming a neurostimulator is performed by a physician or other qualified health care professional. Programming may be performed in the operating room, postoperative care unit, inpatient, and/or outpatient setting. Programming a neurostimulator in the operating room is not inherent in the service represented by the implantation code and may be reported by either the implanting surgeon or other qualified health care professional, when performed.

Test stimulations are typically performed during an implantation procedure (43647, 43648, 43881, 43882, 61850, 61860, 61863, 61864, 61867, 61868, 61870, 61880, 61885, 61886, 61888, 63650, 63655, 63661, 63662, 63663, 63664, 63685, 63688, 64553, 64555, 64561, 64566, 64568, 64569, 64570, 64575, 64580, 64581, 64585, 64590, 64595) to confirm correct target site placement of the electrode array(s) and/or to confirm the functional status of the system. Test stimulation is not considered electronic analysis or programming of the neurostimulator system (test stimulation is included in the service described by the implantation code) and should not be reported with 95970, 95971, 95972, 95980, 95981, 95982, 95983, 95984. Electronic analysis of a device (95970) is not reported separately at the time of implantation.◄

►(For insertion of neurostimulator pulse generator, see 61885, 61886, 63685, 64568, 64590)◄

►(For revision or removal of neurostimulator pulse generator or receiver, see 61888, 63688, 64569, 64570, 64595)◄

►(For implantation of neurostimulator electrodes, see 43647, 43881, 61850-61870, 63650, 63655, 64553-64581. For revision or removal of neurostimulator electrodes, see 43648, 43882, 61880, 63661, 63662, 63663, 63664, 64569, 64570, 64585)◄

▲ 95970   Electronic analysis of implanted neurostimulator pulse generator/transmitter (eg, contact group[s], interleaving, amplitude, pulse width, frequency [Hz], on/off cycling, burst, magnet mode, dose lockout, patient selectable parameters, responsive neurostimulation, detection algorithms, closed loop parameters, and passive parameters) by physician or other qualified health care professional; with brain, cranial nerve, spinal cord, peripheral nerve, or sacral nerve, neurostimulator pulse generator/transmitter, without programming

►(Do not report 95970 in conjunction with 43647, 43648, 43881, 43882, 61850, 61860, 61863, 61864, 61867, 61868, 61870, 61880, 61885, 61886, 61888, 63650, 63655, 63661, 63662, 63663, 63664, 63685, 63688, 64553, 64555, 64561, 64566, 64568, 64569, 64570, 64575, 64580, 64581, 64585, 64590, 64595, during the same operative session)◄

►(Do not report 95970 in conjunction with 95971, 95972, 95976, 95977, 95983, 95984)◄

▲ 95971   with simple spinal cord or peripheral nerve (eg, sacral nerve) neurostimulator pulse generator/transmitter programming by physician or other qualified health care professional

►(Do not report 95971 in conjunction with 95972)◄

▲ 95972   with complex spinal cord or peripheral nerve (eg, sacral nerve) neurostimulator pulse generator/transmitter programming by physician or other qualified health care professional

►(95974, 95975 have been deleted. To report, see 95976, 95977)◄

● 95976   with simple cranial nerve neurostimulator pulse generator/transmitter programming by physician or other qualified health care professional

►(Do not report 95976 in conjunction with 95977)◄

● 95977   with complex cranial nerve neurostimulator pulse generator/transmitter programming by physician or other qualified health care professional

#● 95983   with brain neurostimulator pulse generator/transmitter programming, first 15 minutes face-to-face time with physician or other qualified health care professional

#+● 95984   with brain neurostimulator pulse generator/transmitter programming, each additional 15 minutes face-to-face time with physician or other qualified health care professional (List separately in addition to code for primary procedure)

►(Use 95984 in conjunction with 95983)◄

►(95978, 95979 have been deleted. To report, see 95983, 95984)◄

95980   Electronic analysis of implanted neurostimulator pulse generator system (eg, rate, pulse amplitude and duration, configuration of wave form, battery status, electrode selectability, output modulation, cycling, impedance and patient measurements) gastric neurostimulator pulse generator/transmitter; intraoperative, with programming

95981   subsequent, without reprogramming

95982   subsequent, with reprogramming

(For intraoperative or subsequent analysis, with programming, when performed, of vagus nerve trunk stimulator used for blocking therapy [morbid obesity], see 0312T, 0317T)

95983   Code is out of numerical sequence. See 95976-95981

95984   Code is out of numerical sequence. See 95976-95981

Rationale

New codes have been added, existing codes revised, four codes deleted, and two new tables included in multiple sections of the CPT code set to clarify reporting cranial, cranial nerve, spinal, peripheral nerve, and sacral nerve neurostimulator services. In addition, a number of guideline revisions have been made to define existing neurostimulator programming and analysis services.

The AMA/Specialty Society Relative Value Scale (RVS) Update Committee (RUC) had recommended a review of codes 95971 and 95972 for high-volume growth. Survey results indicated that although the service identified by code 95972 was valued at one hour, the service was typically performed in 30 minutes or less. As a result of concerns regarding incorrect reporting and misvaluation of these services, changes have been made to the neurostimulator programming services codes to better represent the efforts necessary to perform each type of neurostimulator service.

The guidelines within the neurostimulator services subsection have been revised to better differentiate electronic analysis services from true programming of a neurostimulator device by including definitions for electronic analysis services and programming. Typically, electronic analysis of the neurostimulator device involves documenting system parameters and ascertaining the functionality of the device. This allows the physician or other qualified health care professional (QHP) the ability to ensure that the device is working correctly, including checking all parameters that the device is designed to affect. This also ensures that the device has been appropriately placed to affect the targeted body area for treatment of the condition. Programming involves iterative manipulation of the parameters to identify the correct settings to treat the condition. The guidelines deliberately focus on the efforts provided during programming that may result in necessary revision(s) of the final parameters in order to provide the appropriate therapy. In addition, the guidelines acknowledge that multiple adjustments may be needed during a single programming session to accurately assess the settings that are needed to provide the treatment.

The guidelines also focus on specifically identifying the different types of parameters that may be available in the neurostimulator device and on providing information about what is considered as "implanted." This provides better insight regarding the complexity of the parameters and how implanted neurostimulator devices are used.

Differences between the nervous system components that are treated are also identified in the guidelines. The definitions and anatomical explanations within the guidelines provide additional insight regarding the efforts necessary to treat these areas. This helps in understanding the differences represented in the coding structure for these different nervous system components, which includes identifying and defining the differences between brain (may involve surface [cortical] stimulation versus deep brain structures), cranial nerve, spinal cord, and peripheral nerve stimulation. A new anatomical illustration of the cranial nerves highlighting the different cranial nerves has been added to provide further clarification regarding the specific cranial nerves that are included for reporting for cranial nerve neurostimulation.

The differentiation of each type of nervous system component allows better explanation regarding the granularity in reporting mechanisms for the different nervous system components. Cranial nerve, spinal cord, peripheral nerve, and sacral nerve neurostimulators services are reported based on the number of parameters, while brain neurostimulators (that have device components that directly contact the brain) are reported according to the face-to-face time provided by the physician/QHP.

Special instruction is provided regarding the intended use of code 95970. This is important because this code is used to report electronic analysis for any of the nervous system components. There is no programming involved in performing this service; therefore, it is inherently included as part of the placement procedure required to implant any of the neurostimulator devices. Guidelines throughout the code set within each anatomic location (including within the neurostimulator services section) provide consistent instruction that placement of the device inherently includes analyzing the device to ensure that it has been placed appropriately and is working according to the intended specifications of the device. The guidelines also include a listing of codes that inherently include the 95970 service.

The use of simple and complex electronic analysis and programming codes for neurostimulator devices that are not placed directly on the brain (ie, cranial nerve, spinal cord, peripheral nerve, and sacral nerve stimulators) are also explained. As noted, these codes are differentiated by identifying if the procedure is simple or complex, and by determining what nervous system anatomy is being analyzed and programmed. To provide a better explanation regarding the new method of reporting vs the former method, the guidelines include definitions that identify the number of parameters that are included for simple programming vs complex programming. Definitions also reiterate what each code is used to identify. This includes a description for cranial neurostimulator services and reminder that these specific services are reported based on time. Further clarification regarding time reporting for cranial neurostimulation services is also provided via the use of a table that provides the codes that may be used according to the time range spent providing the service. It is specifically noted that brain neurostimulation of less than eight minutes is not separately reportable.

The guidelines also specify who may report these services (ie, physicians/QHPs) and in what settings these services may be provided. They identify a caveat regarding programming of a neurostimulator in the operating room. Because different practitioners may place the device and test it as opposed to programming the device, the guideline provides instruction that the programming may be reported by either the implanting surgeon or other QHP, when performed.

The guidelines reiterate that test stimulations to confirm correct target-site placement of the electrode array and to confirm the functional status of the system is inherently included in the placement services. Electronic analysis (95970) of the device is inherently included as part of the placement service and, therefore, it is not separately reported at the time of implantation.

Additional parenthetical notes that follow the guidelines and direct users to codes for insertion of neurostimulator services, revision/removal of neurostimulators, and implantation of electrodes have been revised to include all codes that identify these services respectively.

Coinciding with the language revisions made to the guidelines are revisions to the codes themselves. These include: (1) addition of analysis parameters to the parent code 95970; (2) addition of physician/QHP as appropriate; (3) addition of language that specifies anatomy within the codes; (4) addition of new codes 95976-95977 and 95983-95984 to complement the existing codes by providing coding mechanisms for simple vs complex cranial nerve stimulation and time component reporting for brain neurostimulators; (5) deletion of codes 95974, 95975, 95978, and 95979 to accommodate the addition of the new codes; and (6) addition of exclusionary, add-on, and instructional parenthetical notes that restrict or direct reporting for these codes in congruity with the explanations provided within the guidelines for these services.

Clinical Example (95970)

A 56-year-old male with an implanted nerve stimulator returns to the clinic for device analysis without programming.

Description of Procedure (95970)

Verify populated patient-specific data in the programming equipment, including patient demographics and device history. Perform electronic analysis of the implanted neurostimulator pulse generator/transmitter (eg, contact group[s], interleaving, amplitude, pulse width, frequency [Hz], on/off cycling, burst, magnet mode, dose lockout, patient selectable parameters, responsive neurostimulation, detection algorithms, closed loop parameters, and passive parameters). Document the diagnostic analysis, including battery state, current program settings, and impedance of electrodes, as well as any event logs from the programming equipment and patient device interrogation in the patient's medical record. No program settings are changed.

Clinical Example (95971)

A 56-year-old patient with a condition that requires nerve stimulation returns for simple programming of the implanted neurostimulator pulse generator system in which three or fewer of the parameters are adjusted.

Description of Procedure (95971)

Link programmer with patient programmer (handheld device). Interrogate patient's neurostimulator device. Review preset program settings by switching with handheld programmer between programs and record patient sensation. Change the lead configuration. Change amplitude until stimulation is felt if appropriate then maintain that configuration. If inappropriate, repeat process until appropriate response is obtained. Assess three parameters and change as necessary. Re-sync new program with patient's handheld programmer.

Clinical Example (95972)

A 56-year-old patient with a condition that requires nerve stimulation returns for complex programming of the implanted neurostimulator pulse generator system in which four or more parameters are adjusted.

Description of Procedure (95972)

Link programmer with patient programmer (handheld device). Interrogate patient's neurostimulator device. Review preset program settings by switching with handheld programmer between programs and record patient sensation. Change the lead configuration. Change amplitude until stimulation is felt if appropriate then maintain that configuration. If inappropriate, then repeat process until appropriate response is obtained. Assess four or more parameters and change as necessary. Re-sync new program with patient's handheld programmer.

Clinical Example (95976)

A 35-year-old female with intractable epilepsy had a vagus nerve stimulator (VNS) surgically implanted for better seizure control. The patient returns to clinic for VNS electronic analysis and programming in which three or fewer of the parameters are adjusted.

Description of Procedure (95976)

Verify populated patient-specific data in the programming equipment, including patient demographics and device history. Perform electronic analysis of the implanted neurostimulator pulse generator/transmitter (eg, contact group[s], interleaving, amplitude, pulse width, frequency [Hz], on/off cycling, burst, magnet mode, dose lockout, patient selectable parameters, responsive neurostimulation, detection algorithms, closed loop parameters, and passive parameters). Document the diagnostic analysis, including battery state, current program settings, and impedance of electrodes, as well as any event logs from the programming equipment and patient device interrogation, in the patient's medical record. Turn attention to the stimulation parameters to achieve optimal therapeutic stimulation of the vagus nerve. Adjust three or fewer parameters (eg, current, frequency, pulse width, and train duration, magnet mode, or sensing), as limited by pain, respiratory, and/or swallowing problems. The physician or other qualified health care professional conducts multiple stimulation trials, adjusting the three or fewer parameters until optimal therapeutic stimulation is achieved.

Clinical Example (95977)

A 35-year-old female with intractable epilepsy had a VNS surgically implanted for better seizure control. The patient returns to clinic for VNS electronic analysis and programming in which four or more of the parameters are adjusted.

Description of Procedure (95977)

Verify populated patient-specific data in the programming equipment, including patient demographics and device history. Perform electronic analysis of the implanted neurostimulator pulse generator/transmitter (eg, contact group[s], interleaving, amplitude, pulse width, frequency [Hz], on/off cycling, burst, magnet mode, dose lockout, patient selectable parameters, responsive neurostimulation, detection algorithms, closed loop parameters, and passive parameters). Document the diagnostic analysis, including battery state, current program settings, and impedance of electrodes, as well as any event logs from the programming equipment and patient device interrogation, in the patient's medical record. Turn

attention to the stimulation parameters to achieve optimal therapeutic stimulation of the vagus nerve. Adjust four or more parameters (eg, current, frequency, pulse width, and train duration, magnet mode, or sensing), as limited by pain, respiratory, and/or swallowing problems. The physician or other qualified health care professional conducts multiple stimulation trials, adjusting the four or more parameters until optimal therapeutic stimulation is achieved.

Clinical Example (95983)

A 67-year-old male with Parkinson's disease had a brain neurostimulator surgically implanted and now returns to clinic for electronic analysis and programming by the physician or other qualified health care professional. (**Note:** Code 95983 is reported for the initial 15 minutes of face-to-face time with physician or other qualified health care professional for analysis and programming.]

Description of Procedure (95983)

Verify populated patient-specific data in the programming equipment, including patient demographics and device history. Perform electronic analysis of the implanted neurostimulator pulse generator/transmitter (eg, contact group[s], interleaving, amplitude, pulse width, frequency [Hz], on/off cycling, burst, magnet mode, dose lockout, patient selectable parameters, responsive neurostimulation, detection algorithms, closed loop parameters, and passive parameters). Document the diagnostic analysis, including battery state, current program settings, and impedance of electrodes, as well as any event logs from the programming equipment and patient device interrogation, in the patient's medical record. Turn attention to the stimulation parameters and electrode mapping. Each electrode contact on the array is systematically activated one at a time in monopolar mode as a cathode. The parameters are adjusted (eg, amplitude, frequency, pulse width, contact combinations, patient controllable parameters) while neurologic effects on symptoms and signs (eg, bradykinesia, rigidity) are noted as well as side effects (eg, twitching, pulling of face/contralateral limb). After electrode mapping, the physician or other qualified health care professional then determines which combination of parameters results in an optimal effect while minimizing adverse side effects and the final exit parameters are selected to balance benefits to bradykinesia and rigidity with least side effects.

Clinical Example (95984)

A 67-year-old male with Parkinson's disease had a brain neurostimulator surgically implanted and now returns to clinic for electronic analysis and programming that requires more than 15 minutes by the physician or other qualified health care professional. (**Note:** Code 95984 is reported for each additional 15 minutes of face-to-face time with physician or other qualified health care professional for the following analysis/programming work.)

Description of Procedure (95984)

Verify populated patient-specific data in the programming equipment, including patient demographics and device history. Perform electronic analysis of the implanted neurostimulator pulse generator/transmitter (eg, contact group[s], interleaving, amplitude, pulse width, frequency [Hz], on/off cycling, burst, magnet mode, dose lockout, patient selectable parameters, responsive neurostimulation, detection algorithms, closed loop parameters, and passive parameters). Document the diagnostic analysis, including battery state, current program settings, and impedance of electrodes, as well as any event logs from the programming equipment and patient device interrogation, in the patient's medical record. Turn attention to the stimulation parameters and electrode mapping. Each electrode contact on the array is systematically activated one at a time in monopolar mode as a cathode. The parameters are adjusted (eg, amplitude, frequency, pulse width, contact combinations, patient controllable parameters) while neurologic effects on symptoms and signs (eg, bradykinesia, rigidity) are noted as well as side effects (eg, twitching, pulling of face/contralateral limb). After electrode mapping, the physician or other qualified health care professional then determines which combination of parameters results in an optimal effect while minimizing adverse side effects and the final exit parameters are selected to balance benefits to bradykinesia and rigidity with least side effects. Document any additional final program measurements and any other relevant clinical information obtained from the additional programming in the patient's medical record.

Functional Brain Mapping

96020   Neurofunctional testing selection and administration during noninvasive imaging functional brain mapping, with test administered entirely by a physician or other qualified health care professional (ie, psychologist), with review of test results and report

(For functional magnetic resonance imaging [fMRI], brain, use 70555)

▶(Do not report 96020 in conjunction with 96112, 96113, 96116, 96121, 96130, 96131, 96132, 96133)◀

(Do not report 96020 in conjunction with 70554)

(Evaluation and Management services codes should not be reported on the same day as 96020)

Rationale

In accordance with the deletion of codes 96101, 96102, 96103, and 96120 and the addition of codes 96121, 96130, 96131, 96132, and 96133, the parenthetical note following code 96020 has been revised.

Refer to the codebook and the Rationale for codes 96101, 96102, 96103, 96120, 96121, 96130, 96131, 96132, and 96133 for a full discussion of these changes.

▶Adaptive Behavior Services◀

▶Adaptive behavior services address deficient adaptive behaviors (eg, impaired social, communication, or self-care skills), maladaptive behaviors (eg, repetitive and stereotypic behaviors, behaviors that risk physical harm to the patient, others, and/or property), or other impaired functioning secondary to deficient adaptive or maladaptive behaviors, including, but not limited to, instruction-following, verbal and nonverbal communication, imitation, play and leisure, social interactions, self-care, daily living, and personal safety.

Definitions

Functional behavior assessment: comprises descriptive assessment procedures designed to identify environmental events that occur just before and just after occurrences of potential target behaviors and that may influence those behaviors. That information may be gathered by interviewing the patient's caregivers; having caregivers complete checklists, rating scales, or questionnaires; and/or observing and recording occurrences of target behaviors and environmental events in everyday situations.

Functional analysis: an assessment procedure for evaluating the separate effects of each of several environmental events on a potential target behavior by systematically presenting and withdrawing each event to a patient multiple times and observing and measuring occurrences of the behavior in response to those events. Graphed data are analyzed visually to determine which events produced relatively high and low occurrences of the behavior.

Standardized instruments and procedures: include, but not limited to, behavior checklists, rating scales, and adaptive skill assessment instruments that comprise a fixed set of items and are administered and scored in a uniform way with all patients (eg, Pervasive Developmental Disabilities Behavior Inventory, Brigance Inventory of Early Development, Vineland Adaptive Behavior Scales).

▶*Nonstandardized instruments and procedures:* include, but not limited to, curriculum-referenced assessments, stimulus preference assessment procedures, and other procedures for assessing behaviors and associated environmental events that are specific to the individual patient and behaviors.◀

▶Adaptive Behavior Assessments◀

▶**Behavior identification assessment** (97151) is conducted by the physician or other qualified health care professional and may include analysis of pertinent past data (including medical diagnosis), a detailed behavioral history, patient observation, administration of standardized and/or non-standardized instruments and procedures, functional behavior assessment, functional analysis, and/or guardian/caregiver interview to identify and describe deficient adaptive behaviors, maladaptive behaviors, and other impaired functioning secondary to deficient adaptive or maladaptive behaviors. Code 97151 includes the physician's or other qualified health care professional's scoring of assessments, interpretation of results, discussion of findings and recommendations with the primary guardian(s)/caregiver(s), preparation of report, and development of plan of care, which may include behavior identification supporting assessment (97152) or behavior identification–supporting assessment with four required components (0362T).

Behavior identification supporting assessment (97152) is administered by a technician under the direction of a physician or other qualified health care professional. The physician or other qualified health care professional may or may not be on site during the face-to-face assessment process. Code 97152 includes the physician's or other qualified health care professional's interpretation of results and may include functional behavior assessment, functional analysis, and other structured observations and/or standardized and/or nonstandardized instruments and procedures to determine levels of adaptive and maladaptive behavior.

Codes 97152, 0362T may be reported separately with 97151 based on the time that the patient is face-to-face with one or more technician(s). Only count the time of one technician when two or more are present.

For behavior identification–supporting assessment with four required components, use 0362T.◀

―― *Coding Tip* ――――――――――

If the physician or other qualified health care professional personally performs the technician activities, his or her time engaged in these activities should be included as part of the required technician time to meet the components of the code.

――――――――――――――――

▶Guide to Selection of Codes 97152 and 0362T

	97152	0362T
Physician or other qualified health care professional required to be on site		✓
Physician or other qualified health care professional not required to be on site	✓	
Number of technicians	1	2 or more
Deficient adaptive behavior(s), maladaptive behavior(s), or other impaired functioning secondary to deficient adaptive or maladaptive behaviors	✓	
Destructive behavior(s)		✓
May include functional behavior assessment	✓	✓
May include functional analysis	✓	✓
Environment customized to patient and behavior		✓◀

#● 97151   **Behavior identification assessment,** administered by a physician or other qualified health care professional, each 15 minutes of the physician's or other qualified health care professional's time face-to-face with patient and/or guardian(s)/caregiver(s) administering assessments and discussing findings and recommendations, and non-face-to-face analyzing past data, scoring/interpreting the assessment, and preparing the report/treatment plan

#● 97152   **Behavior identification-supporting assessment,** administered by one technician under the direction of a physician or other qualified health care professional, face-to-face with the patient, each 15 minutes

▶(97151, 97152, 0362T may be repeated on the same or different days until the behavior identification assessment [97151] and, if necessary, supporting assessment[s] [97152, 0362T], is complete)◀

▶(For psychiatric diagnostic evaluation, see 90791, 90792)◀

▶(For speech evaluations, see 92521, 92522, 92523, 92524)◀

▶(For occupational therapy evaluation, see 97165, 97166, 97167, 97168)◀

▶(For medical team conference, see 99366, 99367, 99368)◀

▶(For health and behavior assessment/intervention, see 96150, 96151, 96152, 96153, 96154, 96155)◀

▶(For neurobehavioral status exam, see 96116, 96121)◀

▶(For neuropsychological testing, see 96132, 96133, 96136, 96137, 96138, 96139, 96146)◀

Medicine 90281-99607

Medicine 90281-99607

Clinical Example (97151)

A 3-year-old male is brought in by his parents for an assessment. The patient has nonfunctional speech, poor eye contact, repetitive motor movements, tantrums with unexpected changes in routines, and ritualistic play. He does not respond to gestures or his name and has almost no imitative behavior.

Description of Procedure (97151)

Before the appointment, the qualified health care professional reviews the child's medical records, previous assessments, and records of any previous or current treatments. During the initial visit, the qualified health care professional conducts a structured interview with the parents to solicit their observations about the child's deficient adaptive behaviors (eg, impaired social, communication, or self-care skills), maladaptive behaviors, and other concerns. The qualified health care professional then conducts a series of indirect and direct assessments to identify potential skills to be strengthened and maladaptive behaviors to be reduced by treatment. Indirect assessments include standardized and nonstandardized scales and checklists completed by the parents and other caregivers to evaluate the patient's adaptive skills in several domains (eg, social, communication, play, self-help, community participation), as well as maladaptive behaviors. Direct assessments include a functional behavior assessment comprising an interview with the parents about environmental events that may precede and follow occurrences of maladaptive behaviors, and observations of the patient in several everyday settings to record occurrences of tantrums, repetitive movements, and other maladaptive behaviors, as well as environmental events that precede and follow those occurrences. Use the information from the functional behavior assessment to design functional analyses of tantrums and ritualistic behaviors. Use the data from all assessments to develop a treatment plan with potential goals and objectives, including social, communication, play and leisure, self-care, and other skills to be developed and maladaptive behaviors to be reduced, all defined in observable, measurable terms. For each treatment, the plan also specifies the current (baseline) level target; procedures for direct observation and measurement; conditions under which the behavior is to occur; a written protocol with instructions for implementing procedures to change the behavior and promote generalization of behavior changes; and criteria for mastery or attainment. The qualified health care professional and parents then meet to review the assessment results and proposed treatment plan and to select and prioritize goals and objectives. The qualified health care professional revises the treatment plan, as needed.

Clinical Example (97152)

A 10-year-old female requires an additional assessment for severe stereotypic behavior that interferes with acquisition of adaptive skills.

Description of Procedure (97152)

A behavior technician, under the direction of a qualified health care professional, observes and records occurrences of the patient's stereotypical behavior and environmental events that immediately precede and follow those occurrences. The technician then observes and records the patient's behavior and associated environmental events several times in a variety of situations (eg, structured intervention sessions, solitary play, play with others). The qualified health care professional reviews and analyzes the data from those observations.

▶Adaptive Behavior Treatment◀

▶**Adaptive behavior treatment** codes 97153, 97154, 97155, 97156, 97157, 97158, 0373T describe services that address specific treatment targets and goals based on results of previous assessments (see 97151, 97152, 0362T), and include ongoing assessment and adjustment of treatment protocols, targets, and goals.

Adaptive behavior treatment by protocol (97153) and **group adaptive behavior treatment by protocol** (97154) are administered by a technician under the direction of a physician or other qualified health care professional, utilizing a treatment protocol designed in advance by the physician or other qualified health care professional, who may or may not provide direction during the treatment. Code 97153 describes face-to-face services with one patient and code 97154 describes face-to-face services with two or more patients. Do not report 97154 if the group is larger than eight patients.

Adaptive behavior treatment with protocol modification (97155) is administered by a physician or other qualified health care professional face-to-face with a single patient. The physician or other qualified health care professional resolves one or more problems with the protocol and may simultaneously direct a technician in administering the modified protocol while the patient is present. Physician or other qualified health care professional direction to the technician without the patient present is not reported separately.

Family adaptive behavior treatment guidance and **multiple-family group adaptive behavior treatment guidance** (97156, 97157) are administered by a physician or other qualified health care professional face-to-face with guardian(s)/caregiver(s) and involve identifying potential treatment targets and training guardian(s)/caregiver(s) of one patient (97156) or

▶Guide to Selection of Codes 97153, 97155, and 0373T

	97153	97155	0373T
By protocol	✓		
With protocol modification		✓	✓
Physician or other qualified health care professional face-to-face with patient		✓	
Physician or other qualified health care professional required to be on site			✓
Physician or other qualified health care professional not required to be on site	✓		
Number of technicians	1	0-1	2 or more
Deficient adaptive behavior(s), maladaptive behavior(s), or other impaired functioning secondary to deficient adaptive or maladaptive behaviors	✓	✓	
Destructive behavior(s)		✓	✓
Environment customized to patient and behavior			✓◀

multiple patients (97157) to implement treatment protocols designed to address deficient adaptive or maladaptive behaviors. Services described by 97156 may be performed with or without the patient present. Services described by 97157 are performed without the patient present. Do not report 97157 if the group has more than eight patients' guardian(s)/caretaker(s).

Group adaptive behavior treatment with protocol modification (97158) is administered by a physician or other qualified health care professional face-to-face with multiple patients. The physician or other qualified health care professional monitors the needs of individual patients and adjusts the treatment techniques during the group sessions, as needed. In contrast to group adaptive behavior treatment by protocol (97154), protocol adjustments are made in real time rather than for a subsequent service. Do not report 97158 if the group has more than eight patients.

For adaptive behavior treatment with protocol modification with four required components, use 0373T.◀

—— Coding Tip ——

If the physician or other qualified health care professional personally performs the technician activities, his or her time engaged in these activities should be reported as technician time.

#● **97153**   **Adaptive behavior treatment by protocol,** administered by technician under the direction of a physician or other qualified health care professional, face-to-face with one patient, each 15 minutes

▶(Do not report 97153 in conjunction with 90785-90899, 92507, 96105-96155)◀

#● **97154**   **Group adaptive behavior treatment by protocol,** administered by technician under the direction of a physician or other qualified health care professional, face-to-face with two or more patients, each 15 minutes

▶(Do not report 97154 if the group has more than 8 patients)◀

▶(Do not report 97154 in conjunction with 90785-90899, 92508, 96105-96155, 97150)◀

#● **97155**   **Adaptive behavior treatment with protocol modification,** administered by physician or other qualified health care professional, which may include simultaneous direction of technician, face-to-face with one patient, each 15 minutes

▶(Do not report 97155 in conjunction with 90785-90899, 96105-96155, 92507)◀

#● **97156**   **Family adaptive behavior treatment guidance,** administered by physician or other qualified health care professional (with or without the patient present), face-to-face with guardian(s)/caregiver(s), each 15 minutes

▶(Do not report 97156 in conjunction with 90785-90899, 96105-96155)◀

#● **97157**   **Multiple-family group adaptive behavior treatment guidance,** administered by physician or other qualified health care professional (without the patient present), face-to-face with multiple sets of guardians/caregivers, each 15 minutes

▶(Do not report 97157 if the group has more than 8 families)◀

▶(Do not report 97156, 97157 in conjunction with 90785-90899, 96105-96155)◀

Medicine 90281-99607

#● **97158** **Group adaptive behavior treatment with protocol modification,** administered by physician or other qualified health care professional, face-to-face with multiple patients, each 15 minutes

▶(Do not report 97158 if the group has more than 8 patients)◀

▶(Do not report 97158 in conjunction with 90785-90899, 96105-96155, 92508, 97150)◀

Rationale

A new Adaptive Behavior Services subsection with new guidelines and eight new codes has been added. The new codes are categorized into two subsections within adaptive behavior services: (1) adaptive behavior assessments (97151, 97152); and (2) adaptive behavior treatments (97153-97158). These two subsections each have their own set of guidelines and definitions.

Prior to 2019, adaptive behavior services were reported with Category III codes 0359T-0363T (adaptive behavior assessments); 0364T-0372T (adaptive behavior treatment); and 0373T-0374T (exposure adaptive behavior treatment with protocol modification). Effective in 2019, codes 0359T, 0360T, 0361T, 0363T, 0364T-0372T, and 0374T have been converted to Category I codes. The code descriptors were evaluated to ensure they reflect current practice and have been modified accordingly when the services were converted to Category I codes. In addition, the remaining Category III codes 0362T and 0373T have been revised to reflect current practice. (See Table 1 to see the comparisons between reporting of adaptive behavior services **before** 2019 and **for** 2019.) Refer to the codebook and the Rationale for codes 0362T and 0373T for a full discussion of these changes.

Adaptive behavior identification assessment services are reported with codes 97151 and 97152. Code 97151 describes behavior identification assessment administered by a physician/QHP. Code 97152 describes behavior identification supporting assessment and is administered by a technician under a physician/QHP direction. Prior to 2019, adaptive behavior assessment services were described by five Category III codes that divided the services into behavior identification assessment (0359T); observational behavioral follow-up assessment (0360T, 0361T); and exposure behavioral follow-up assessment (0362T, 0363T). The "follow-up" terminology previously used has been removed for 2019 because the work involves structured observations of behavior rather than just a follow-up assessment. The term "exposure" in reference to exposure behavioral

assessment has been removed for 2019 because it was determined that providers are less familiar with this term than they are with the synonymous and more commonly used term "functional analysis." Code 97152 includes functional analysis when performed by the technician. This is stated in the adaptive behavior assessment guidelines, as well as the definition for functional analysis. Code 97151 is reported for 15 minutes of face-to-face time with the patient and/or guardian/caregiver and non-face-to-face time analyzing data, scoring/interpreting the assessment, and preparing the report/treatment plan. Code 97152 is reported for 15 minutes of face-to-face time with the patient and **does not** include non-face-to-face time.

Codes 97153-97158 describe adaptive behavior treatment services. They include treatment protocols designed by the physician/QHP. Adaptive behavior treatment services are reported for each 15 minutes of face-to-face time.

Prior to 2019, these services were reported with Category III codes 0364T-0369T. Adaptive behavior treatment services are divided into treatment of one patient (97153, 97155); treatment of a group of patients (ie, two to eight patients) (97154, 97158); family guidance with or without the patient present (97156); and multiple-family guidance without the patient present (97157). Codes 97154, 97157, and 97158 should not be reported for groups of more than eight individuals. Codes 97153 and 97154 are reported for treatment administered by a technician under a physician/other QHP direction. Codes 97155-97158 are reported for treatment administered by the physician/other QHP. However, code 97155 may include simultaneous physician/QHP direction of a technician. Codes 97155 and 97158 include modification of the treatment protocol.

Clinical Example (97153)

A 4-year-old female presents with deficits in language and social skills. She engages in perseverative speech on one or two preferred topics and displays strong emotional outbursts in response to small changes in routines or when preferred items are unavailable.

Description of Procedure (97153)

The qualified health care professional directs a technician in the implementation of treatment protocols and data-collection procedures. Treatment sessions comprising multiple planned opportunities for the child to practice each target skill are conducted by the technician daily in the family home and in community settings (eg, a playground, stores, church). The qualified health care professional reviews technician-recorded, graphed data frequently to assess the child's progress and determine if any treatment protocols need to be adjusted.

★ = Telemedicine   ✚ = Add-on code   ✗ = FDA approval pending   # = Resequenced code   ⊘ = Modifier 51 exempt

Table 1. Adaptive Behavior Services Comparison Table

Prior to 2019	Effective 2019
Category/Section/Subsection/Sub-Subsection	**Category/Section/Subsection/Sub-Subsection**
Category: III	**Category: I**
Section: **Category III Codes**	Section: **Medicine**
Subsection: **Adaptive Behavior Assessments**	Subsection: **Adaptive Behavior Services**

Adaptive Behavior Assessments	**Adaptive Behavior Assessments**
0359T Behavior identification assessment, by the physician or other qualified health care professional, face-to-face with patient and caregiver(s), includes administration of standardized and non-standardized tests, detailed behavioral history, patient observation and caregiver interview, interpretation of test results, discussion of findings and recommendations with the primary guardian(s)/caregiver(s), and preparation of report	#●**97151** Behavior identification assessment, administered by a physician or other qualified health care professional, each 15 minutes of the physician's or other qualified health care professional's time face-to-face with patient and/or guardian(s)/caregiver(s) administering assessments and discussing findings and recommendations, and non-face-to-face analyzing past data, scoring/interpreting the assessment, and preparing the report/treatment plan
0360T Observational behavioral follow-up assessment, includes physician or other qualified health care professional direction with interpretation and report, administered by one technician; first 30 minutes of technician time, face-to-face with the patient **+0361T** each additional 30 minutes of technician time, face-to-face with the patient (List separately in addition to code for primary service)	#●**97152** Behavior identification–supporting assessment, administered by one technician under the direction of a physician or other qualified health care professional, face-to-face with the patient, each 15 minutes
Adaptive Behavior Treatment	**Adaptive Behavior Treatment**
0364T Adaptive behavior treatment by protocol, administered by technician, face-to-face with one patient; first 30 minutes of technician time **+0365T** each additional 30 minutes of technician time (List separately in addition to code for primary procedure)	#●**97153** Adaptive behavior treatment by protocol, administered by technician under the direction of a physician or other qualified health care professional, face-to-face with one patient, each 15 minutes
0366T Group adaptive behavior treatment by protocol, administered by technician, face-to-face with two or more patients; first 30 minutes of technician time **+0367T** each additional 30 minutes of technician time (List separately in addition to code for primary procedure)	#●**97154** Group adaptive behavior treatment by protocol, administered by technician under the direction of a physician or other qualified health care professional, face-to-face with two or more patients, each 15 minutes
0368T Adaptive behavior treatment with protocol modification administered by physician or other qualified health care professional with one patient; first 30 minutes of patient face-to-face time **+0369T** each additional 30 minutes of patient face-to-face time (List separately in addition to code for primary procedure)	#●**97155** Adaptive behavior treatment with protocol modification administered by physician or other qualified health care professional, which may include simultaneous direction of technician, face-to-face with one patient, each 15 minutes
0370T Family adaptive behavior treatment guidance, administered by physician or other qualified health care professional (without the patient present)	#●**97156** Family adaptive behavior treatment guidance, administered by physician or other qualified health care professional (with or without the patient present), face-to-face with guardian(s)/caregiver(s), each 15 minutes
0371T Multiple-family group adaptive behavior treatment guidance, administered by physician or other qualified health care professional (without the patient present)	#●**97157** Multiple-family group adaptive behavior treatment guidance, administered by physician or other qualified health care professional (without the patient present), face-to-face with multiple sets of guardians/caregivers, each 15 minutes

Table 1. Adaptive Behavior Services Comparison Table

Prior to 2019	Effective 2019
Category/Section/Subsection/Sub-Subsection	Category/Section/Subsection/Sub-Subsection
Category: III	Category: I
Section: **Category III Codes**	Section: **Medicine**
Subsection: **Adaptive Behavior Assessments**	Subsection: **Adaptive Behavior Services**

Adaptive Behavior Assessments	Adaptive Behavior Treatment
0372T Adaptive behavior treatment social skills group, administered by physician or other qualified health care professional face-to-face with multiple patients	#●**97158** Group adaptive behavior treatment with protocol modification, administered by physician or other qualified health care professional, face-to-face with multiple patients, each 15 minutes
Section: Category III Codes	**Section: Category III Codes**
Adaptive Behavior Assessments	**Adaptive Behavior Assessments and Treatment**
0362T Exposure behavioral follow-up assessment, includes physician or other qualified health care professional direction with interpretation and report, administered by physician or other qualified health care professional with the assistance of one or more technicians; first 30 minutes of technician(s) time, face-to-face with the patient **+0363T** each additional 30 minutes of technician(s) time, face-to-face with the patient (List separately in addition to code for primary procedure)	▲**0362T** Behavior identification supporting assessment, each 15 minutes of technicians' time face-to-face with a patient, requiring the following components: ■ administration by the physician or other qualified health care professional who is on site; ■ with the assistance of two or more technicians; ■ for a patient who exhibits destructive behavior; ■ completion in an environment that is customized to the patient's behavior.
Exposure Adaptive Behavior Treatment With Protocol Modification	
0373T Exposure adaptive behavior treatment with protocol modification requiring two or more technicians for severe maladaptive behavior(s); first 60 minutes of technicians' time, face-to-face with patient **+0374T** each additional 30 minutes of technicians' time face-to-face with patient (List separately in addition to code for primary procedure)	▲**0373T** Adaptive behavior treatment with protocol modification, each 15 minutes of technicians' time face-to-face with a patient, requiring the following components: ■ administration by the physician or other qualified health care professional who is on site; ■ with the assistance of two or more technicians; ■ for a patient who exhibits destructive behavior; ■ completion in an environment that is customized, to the patient's behavior.

Clinical Example (97154)

A 7-year-old female exhibits deficits in social skills. Patient is verbal and has emerging social skills as a result of one-to-one therapy designed to teach basic communication and social interactions. Peer social skills training in a small group is recommended.

Description of Procedure (97154)

The qualified health care professional directs a technician in the implementation of treatment protocols and data-collection procedures during small-group activities. Group treatment sessions are conducted by the technician. The qualified health care professional reviews technician-recorded, graphed data frequently to

assess the child's progress and determine if any treatment protocols need to be adjusted.

Clinical Example (97155)

A 5-year-old male previously showed steady improvements in language and social skills at home as a result of one-to-one intensive applied behavior analysis intervention, but skill development seems to have reached a plateau recently.

Description of Procedure (97155)

To promote generalization of treatment gains across people and situations (outside the treatment context), the qualified health care professional modifies the written protocols previously used to incorporate procedures designed to build the child's language and social skills into daily home routines (eg, play, dressing, mealtimes) and directs the technician to implement the protocols with the child. The qualified health care professional demonstrates the procedures to the technician, and then has the technician implement the procedures with the child while the qualified health care professional observes and provides feedback.

Clinical Example (97156)

The parents of a 6-year-old male seek training on procedures for helping the child communicate using picture cards (skills he previously developed in adaptive behavior treatment sessions with technicians) during typical family routines.

Description of Procedure (97156)

The qualified health care professional trains the parents to use prompting and reinforcement to promote their child's use of picture cards and gestures to indicate his desire to stop an activity and to request help. The parents are trained to honor the "stop" and "help" requests when they occur. Training includes the qualified health care professional reviewing written treatment and data-collection protocols with the parents, demonstrating how to implement them in role-plays and with the child, and having the parents implement the protocols with the child while the qualified health care professional observes and provides feedback.

Clinical Example (97157)

The parents of a 3-year-old male, who has pervasive hyperactivity and no functional play, social, or communication skills, seek training on how to manage his hyperactive and disruptive behavior and help him develop appropriate play, social, and communication skills.

Description of Procedure (97157)

The qualified health care professional invites the parents to attend a training session with several sets of other parents. To start the session, the qualified health care professional asks each set of parents to identify one skill to be increased or one problem behavior to be decreased in their own child. The qualified health care professional describes how behavior analytic principles and procedures could be applied to the behavior identified by the parents of this 3-year-old patient. The qualified health care professional demonstrates a procedure (eg, prompting the child to speak instead of whining when he wants something, and not giving him preferred items when he whines). The parents then role-play using that

same procedure. Other group participants and the qualified health care professional provide feedback and make constructive suggestions. That process is repeated for skills/behaviors identified by other sets of parents. The qualified health care professional ends the group session by summarizing the main points, answering questions, and giving each set of parents a homework assignment to practice the skills they worked on during the session.

Clinical Example (97158)

A 13-year-old female is reported to be isolated from peers due to poor social skills and odd behavior. She has difficulty recognizing emotions in others and often annoys her peers because she tells the same joke over and over and talks incessantly about comic-book heroes.

Description of Procedure (97158)

The qualified health care professional includes sessions that focus on peer social skills in the patient's treatment plan in the group-participation treatment sessions. The qualified health care professional begins the group session by asking each patient to briefly describe two of their recent social encounters with peers, one that went well and one that did not. The qualified health care professional uses that information to develop a group activity in which each member has the opportunity to practice the skills he or she used in the encounters that went well and to problem solve the interactions that did not go well. The qualified health care professional helps each patient identify social cues that were interpreted correctly and incorrectly and what he or she could have done differently, and provides prompts and feedback individualized to each patient's skills. The qualified health care professional ends the session by summarizing the discussion and skills that were practiced, answering questions, and giving each patient an individualized homework assignment to practice a particular social skill, for which the patient is to determine what will constitute success and how they will measure it.

Central Nervous System Assessments/Tests (eg, Neuro-Cognitive, Mental Status, Speech Testing)

▶The following codes are used to report the services provided during testing of the central nervous system functions. The central nervous system assessments include, but are not limited to, memory, language, visual motor responses, and abstract reasoning/problem-solving abilities. It is accomplished by the combination of several types of testing procedures. Testing procedures include assessment of aphasia and cognitive performance testing, developmental screening and behavioral assessments and testing, and psychological/neuropsychological testing. The administration of these tests will generate material that will be formulated into a report or an automated result.◄

> (For development of cognitive skills, see 97127, 97533)

> (For dementia screens, [eg, Folstein Mini-Mental State Examination, by a physician or other qualified health care professional], see **Evaluation and Management** services codes)

> ►(Do not report assessment of aphasia and cognitive performance testing services [96105, 96125], developmental/behavioral screening and testing services [96110, 96112, 96113, 96127], and psychological/ neuropsychological testing services [96116, 96121, 96130, 96131, 96132, 96133, 96136, 96137, 96138, 96139, 96146] in conjunction with 97151, 97152, 97153, 97154, 97155, 97156, 97157, 97158, 0362T, 0373T)◄

►Definitions

Codes in this family (96105-96146) describe a number of services that are defined below:

Cognitive performance testing: assesses the patient's ability to complete specific functional tasks applicable to the patient's environment in order to identify or quantify specific cognitive deficits. The results are used to determine impairments and develop therapeutic goals and objectives.

Interactive feedback: used to convey the implications of psychological or neuropsychological test findings and diagnostic formulation. Based on patient-specific cognitive and emotional strengths and weaknesses, interactive feedback may include promoting adherence to medical and/or psychological treatment plans; educating and engaging the patient about his or her condition to maximize patient collaboration in their care; addressing safety issues; facilitating psychological coping; coordinating care; and engaging the patient in planning given the expected course of illness or condition, when performed.

Interpretation and report: performed by a physician or other qualified health care professional. In some circumstances, a result is generated through the use of a "computer", tablet(s), or other device(s).

Neurobehavioral status examination: a clinical assessment of cognitive functions and behavior, and may include an interview with the patient, other informant(s), and/or staff, as well as integration of prior history and other sources of clinical data with clinical decision making, further assessment and/or treatment planning and report. Evaluation domains may include acquired knowledge, attention, language, memory, planning and problem solving, and visual spatial abilities.

Neuropsychological testing evaluation services: typically include integration of patient data with other sources of clinical data, interpretation, clinical decision making, and treatment planning and report. It may include interactive feedback to the patient, family member(s) or caregiver(s), when performed. Evaluation domains for neuropsychological evaluation may include intellectual function, attention, executive function, language and communication, memory, visual-spatial function, sensorimotor function, emotional and personality features, and adaptive behavior.

Psychological testing evaluation services: typically include integration of patient data with other sources of clinical data, interpretation, clinical decision making, and treatment planning and report. It may include interactive feedback to the patient, family member(s) or caregiver(s) when performed. Evaluation domains for psychological evaluation may include emotional and interpersonal functioning, intellectual function, thought processes, personality, and psychopathology.

Standardized instruments: used in the performance of these services. Standardized instruments are validated tests that are administered and scored in a consistent or "standard" manner consistent with their validation.

Testing: administered by a physician, other qualified health care professional, and technician, or completed by the patient. The mode of completion can be manual (eg, paper and pencil) or via automated means.

Assessment of aphasia and cognitive performance testing, which includes interpretation and report, are described by 96105, 96125.

Developmental screening services are described by 96110. Developmental/behavioral testing services, which include interpretation and report, are described by 96112, 96113.

Neurobehavioral status examination, which includes interpretation and report, is described by 96116, 96121.

Psychological and neuropsychological test evaluation services, which include integration of patient data, interpretation of test results and clinical data, treatment planning and report, and interactive feedback, are described by 96130, 96131, 96132, 96133.

Testing and administration services (96136, 96137) are performed by a physician or other qualified health care professional. For 96136, 96137, do not include time for evaluation services (eg, integration of patient data or interpretation of test results). This time is included with psychological and neuropsychological test evaluation services (96130, 96131, 96132, 96133). Testing and administration services (96138, 96139) are performed by a technician. The tests selected, test administration and method of testing and scoring are the same, regardless whether the testing is performed by a physician, other qualified health care professional, or a technician, for 96136, 96137, 96138, 96139. Automated testing and result code 96146 describes testing performed by a single automated instrument with an automated result.

Some of these services are typically performed together. For example, psychological/neuropsychological testing evaluation services (96130, 96131, 96132, 96133) may be reported with psychological/neuropsychological test administration and scoring services (96136, 96137, 96138, 96139).

A requirement of testing services (96105, 96125, 96112, 96113, 96130, 96131, 96132, 96133, 96146) is that there is an interpretation and report when performed by a qualified health care professional, or a result when generated by automation. These services follow standard CPT time definitions (ie, a minimum of 16 minutes for 30 minutes codes and 31 minutes for 1-hour codes must be provided to report any per hour code). The time reported in 96116, 96121, 96130, 96131, 96132, 96133, 96125 is the face-to-face time with the patient and the time spent integrating and interpreting data.

Report the total time at the completion of the entire episode of evaluation.◄

▶(96101, 96102, 96103 have been deleted)◄

▶(To report psychological testing evaluation and administration and scoring services, see 96130, 96131, 96136, 96137, 96138, 96139, 96146)◄

▶(To report psychological test administration using a single automated instrument, use 96146)◄

▶Assessment of Aphasia and Cognitive Performance Testing◄

96105   Assessment of aphasia (includes assessment of expressive and receptive speech and language function, language comprehension, speech production ability, reading, spelling, writing, eg, by Boston Diagnostic Aphasia Examination) with interpretation and report, per hour

96125   Standardized cognitive performance testing (eg, Ross Information Processing Assessment) per hour of a qualified health care professional's time, both face-to-face time administering tests to the patient and time interpreting these test results and preparing the report

▶(To report neuropsychological testing evaluation and administration and scoring services, see 96132, 96133, 96136, 96137, 96138, 96139, 96146)◄

▶Developmental/Behavioral Screening and Testing◄

96110   Developmental screening (eg, developmental milestone survey, speech and language delay screen), with scoring and documentation, per standardized instrument

(For an emotional/behavioral assessment, use 96127)

▶(96111 has been deleted)◄

▶(To report developmental testing, see 96112, 96113)◄

● 96112   Developmental test administration (including assessment of fine and/or gross motor, language, cognitive level, social, memory and/or executive functions by standardized developmental instruments when performed), by physician or other qualified health care professional, with interpretation and report; first hour

+● 96113   each additional 30 minutes (List separately in addition to code for primary procedure)

96127   Brief emotional/behavioral assessment (eg, depression inventory, attention-deficit/hyperactivity disorder [ADHD] scale), with scoring and documentation, per standardized instrument

(For developmental screening, use 96110)

Clinical Example (96112)

A 5-year-old male previously diagnosed with autism, but not enrolled in early intervention due to family circumstances, presents for extended developmental testing after he could not be successfully assessed for kindergarten entry.

Description of Procedure (96112)

Multiple standardized tests of fine and gross motor, expressive and receptive language, visual/spatial problem solving, and social interactions were administered during which child-examiner interactions and perceived difficulty engaging the patient provided additional diagnostic information. The parent was present during the testing, and explanation of observed behaviors was briefly noted to the mother as the testing progressed. The test results were scored, and a report was developed integrating the standardized results, informal observations, medical, developmental, and behavioral history.

Clinical Example (96113)

A 5-year-old male previously diagnosed with autism, but not enrolled in early intervention due to family circumstances, presents for extended developmental testing after he could not be successfully assessed for kindergarten entry. Patient requires an additional 30 minutes of extended developmental testing beyond the first hour.

Medicine 90281-99607

Central Nervous System Assessments/Tests (eg, Neuro-Cognitive, Mental Status, Speech Testing) Tables

Assessment of Aphasia and Cognitive Performance Testing

Code	Unit	Cognitive Services		Test Administration/Scoring		Interpretation and Report or Automated Result	
		Evaluation	Interactive Feedback	Physician or Qualified Health Care Professional	Technician	Physician or Qualified Health Care Professional	Automated Result
96105	Per hour	X		X		X	
96125	Per hour	X		X		X	

Developmental/Behavioral Screening and Testing

Code	Unit	Cognitive Services		Test Administration/Scoring		Interpretation and Report or Automated Result	
		Evaluation	Interactive Feedback	Physician or Qualified Health Care Professional	Clinical Staff	Physician or Qualified Health Care Professional	Automated Result
96110	Per instrument				X		
96112	Per hour	X		X		X	
+96113	Per hour (add-on)	X		X		X	
96127	Per instrument				X		

Psychological/Neuropsychological Testing

Code	Unit	Cognitive Services		Test Administration/ Scoring		Interpretation and Report or Automated Result	
		Evaluation	Interactive Feedback	Physician or Qualified Health Care Professional	Technician	Physician or Qualified Health Care Professional	Automated Result
Neurobehavioral Status Examination							
96116	Per hour	X		X		X	
+96121	Per hour (add-on)	X		X		X	
Testing Evaluation Services							
96130	Per hour	X	X	Not included in Code	Not Included in Code	X	
+96131	Per hour (add-on)	X	X	Not included in Code	Not Included in Code	X	
96132	Per hour	X	X	Not included in Code	Not Included in Code	X	
+96133	Per hour (add-on)	X	X	Not included in Code	Not Included in Code	X	
Test Administration & Scoring							
96136	Per 30 min	Not included in Code	Not Included in Code	X		Not included in Code	Not Included in Code
+96137	Per 30 min (add-on)	Not included in Code	Not included in Code	X		Not included in Code	Not Included in Code
96138	Per 30 min	Not included in Code	Not included in Code		X	Not included in Code	Not Included in Code
+96139	Per 30 min (add-on)	Not included in Code	Not included in Code		X	Not included in Code	Not Included in Code
Automated Testing and Result							
96146	Automated report(s)	Not included in Code	Not Included in Code				X

★ =Telemedicine   ✛ =Add-on code   ✦ =FDA approval pending   # =Resequenced code   ⃠ =Modifier 51 exempt

Description of Procedure (96113)

Multiple standardized tests of fine and gross motor, expressive and receptive language, visual/spatial problem solving, and social interactions were administered during which child-examiner interactions and perceived difficulty engaging the patient provided additional diagnostic information. The parent was present during the testing, and explanation of observed behaviors was briefly noted to the mother as the testing progressed. The test results were scored.

▶Psychological/Neuropsychological Testing◀

▶Neurobehavioral Status Examination◀

★▲ **96116**   Neurobehavioral status exam (clinical assessment of thinking, reasoning and judgment, [eg, acquired knowledge, attention, language, memory, planning and problem solving, and visual spatial abilities]), by physician or other qualified health care professional, both face-to-face time with the patient and time interpreting test results and preparing the report; first hour

▶(96118, 96119, 96120 have been deleted)◀

▶(To report neuropsychological testing evaluation and administration and scoring services, see 96132, 96133, 96136, 96137, 96138, 96139, 96146)◀

▶(To report psychological test administration using a single automated instrument, use 96146)◀

+● **96121**   each additional hour (List separately in addition to code for primary procedure)

▶(Use 96121 in conjunction with 96116)◀

96125   Code is out of numerical sequence. See 96020-96121

96127   Code is out of numerical sequence. See 96020-96121

Clinical Example (96116)

A 68-year-old female is referred by her physician because of family reports of changes in her behavior including attention difficulties, memory problems, and difficulties with problem solving. A neurobehavioral status examination is completed.

Description of Procedure (96116)

Meet with patient and, if appropriate, significant others. Perform neurobehavioral status examination, which involves clinical assessment for impairments in acquired knowledge, attention, language, learning, memory, problem solving, and visual-spatial abilities. Observe behavior and record responses. Develop clinical impression.

Clinical Example (96121)

A 68-year-old female is referred by her physician because of family reports of changes in her behavior including attentional difficulties, memory problems, and difficulties with problem solving. A neurobehavioral status examination is completed. Patient requires an additional hour of neurobehavioral status examination beyond the first hour.

Description of Procedure (96121)

Meet with patient and, if appropriate, significant others. Perform neurobehavioral status examination, which involves clinical assessment for impairments in acquired knowledge, attention, language, learning, memory, problem solving, and visual-spatial abilities. Observe behavior and record responses. Develop clinical impression.

▶Testing Evaluation Services◀

● **96130**   Psychological testing evaluation services by physician or other qualified health care professional, including integration of patient data, interpretation of standardized test results and clinical data, clinical decision making, treatment planning and report, and interactive feedback to the patient, family member(s) or caregiver(s), when performed; first hour

+● **96131**   each additional hour (List separately in addition to code for primary procedure)

● **96132**   Neuropsychological testing evaluation services by physician or other qualified health care professional, including integration of patient data, interpretation of standardized test results and clinical data, clinical decision making, treatment planning and report, and interactive feedback to the patient, family member(s) or caregiver(s), when performed; first hour

+● **96133**   each additional hour (List separately in addition to code for primary procedure)

Clinical Example (96130)

A 35-year-old female, who is experiencing depressive symptoms, social withdrawal, and substantial fatigue, presents with a positive medical history of autoimmune disorder and recent emotional trauma. Her primary care physician refers her for psychological testing.

Description of Procedure (96130)

Interpret tests; integrate patient data; make clinical decision; diagnose and/or create treatment planning; provide interactive feedback, when performed; and create report.

Medicine 90281-99607

Clinical Example (96131)

A 35-year-old female who is experiencing depressive symptoms, social withdrawal, and substantial fatigue presents with a positive medical history of autoimmune disorder and recent emotional trauma. Her primary care physician refers her for psychological testing. Patient requires an additional hour of psychological testing beyond the first hour.

Description of Procedure (96131)

Interpret tests; integrate patient data; make clinical decision; diagnose and/or create treatment planning; provide interactive feedback, when performed; and create report.

Clinical Example (96132)

A 58-year-old male with a history of diabetes and hypertension presents with a six-month change in behavior, personality, and cognition and a positive family history of Alzheimers disease. His physician refers him for neuropsychological testing.

Description of Procedure (96132)

Interpret tests; integrate patient data; make clinical decision; diagnose and/or create treatment planning; provide interactive feedback, when performed; and create report.

Clinical Example (96133)

A 58-year-old male with a history of diabetes and hypertension presents with a six-month change in behavior, personality, and cognition and a positive family history of Alzheimers disease. His physician refers him for neuropsychological testing. Patient requires an additional hour of neuropsychological testing beyond the first hour.

Description of Procedure (96133)

Interpret tests; integrate patient data; make clinical decision; diagnose and/or create treatment planning; provide interactive feedback, when performed; and create report.

▶Test Administration and Scoring◀

● 96136   Psychological or neuropsychological test administration and scoring by physician or other qualified health care professional, two or more tests, any method; first 30 minutes

+● 96137   each additional 30 minutes (List separately in addition to code for primary procedure)

▶(96136, 96137 may be reported in conjunction with 96130, 96131, 96132, 96133 on the same or different days)◀

● 96138   Psychological or neuropsychological test administration and scoring by technician, two or more tests, any method; first 30 minutes

+● 96139   each additional 30 minutes (List separately in addition to code for primary procedure)

▶(96138, 96139 may be reported in conjunction with 96130, 96131, 96132, 96133 on the same or different days)◀

▶(For 96136, 96137, 96138, 96139, do not include time for evaluation services [eg, integration of patient data or interpretation of test results]. This time is included in 96130, 96131, 96132, 96133)◀

Clinical Example (96136)

A 46-year-old male with a history of coronary artery disease and recent myocardial infarction with reported symptoms of memory loss, anxiety, and depression. His primary care physician refers him for psychological or neuropsychological testing.

Description of Procedure (96136)

Administer a series of tests (standardized, rating scales, and/or projective). Record behavioral observations made during the testing. Score test protocol(s) according to the latest methods for each test.

Clinical Example (96137)

A 46-year-old male with a history of coronary artery disease and recent myocardial infarction with reported symptoms of memory loss, anxiety, and depression. His primary care physician refers him for psychological or neuropsychological testing. Patient requires an additional 30 minutes of psychological or neuropsychological test administration beyond the first 30 minutes.

Description of Procedure (96137)

Administer a series of tests (standardized, rating scales, and/or projective). Record behavioral observations made during the testing. Score test protocol(s) according to the latest methods for each test.

Clinical Example (96138)

A 46-year-old male with a history of coronary artery disease and recent myocardial infarction with reported symptoms of memory loss, anxiety, and depression. His primary care physician refers him for psychological or neuropsychological testing.

★ = Telemedicine   ✚ = Add-on code   ✔ = FDA approval pending   # = Resequenced code   ⊘ = Modifier 51 exempt

Description of Procedure (96138)

Technician gathers tests as ordered by the physician or other qualified health care professional; administers a series of tests (standardized, rating scales, and/or projective); records behavioral observations made during the testing; scores test protocol(s) according to the latest methods for each test; and transcribes all test scores onto data summary sheet.

Clinical Example (96139)

A 46-year-old male with a history of coronary artery disease and recent myocardial infarction with reported symptoms of memory loss, anxiety, and depression. His primary care physician refers him for psychological/ neuropsychological testing. Patient requires an additional 30 minutes of psychological or neuropsychological test administration beyond the first hour.

Description of Procedure (96139)

Technician gathers tests as ordered by the physician or other qualified health care professional; administers a series of tests (standardized, rating scales, and/or projective); records behavioral observations made during the testing; scores test protocol(s) according to the latest methods for each test; and transcribes all test scores onto data summary sheet.

►Automated Testing and Result◄

● **96146** Psychological or neuropsychological test administration, with single automated, standardized instrument via electronic platform, with automated result only

▶(If test is administered by physician, other qualified health care professional, or technician, do not report 96146. To report, see 96127, 96136, 96137, 96138, 96139)◄

Rationale

The Central Nervous System Assessments/Tests (eg, Neuro-Cognitive, Mental Status, Speech Testing) subsection has had substantial revisions. Specifically, codes 96101, 96102, 96103, 96111, 96118, 96119, and 96120 have been deleted; 12 codes (96112-96146) have been established to differentiate technician administration of neuropsychiatric testing from physician/ psychologist administration and assessment of testing; addition and revision of guidelines; revision of the exclusionary parenthetical note following the Central Nervous System Assessments/Tests guidelines; and revisions to code 96116.

The AMA RUC RAW identified codes 96101, 96102, 96103, 96111, 96118, 96119, and 96120 for high-volume growth, and a recommendation was made for revision to reflect current practice. As a result, it was determined that if such extensive revisions were needed, a new family of codes and guidelines should be added and codes 96101, 96102, 96103, 96111, 96118, 96119, and 96120 should be deleted. It is important to note that the addition of the new series of codes is not a one-to-one transition from the deleted codes.

The revisions made to this subsection now allow the reporting of services provided during testing of cognitive and neurobehavioral functions of the central nervous system. The new and revised codes in this subsection describe: (1) developmental/behavioral screening and testing services and (2) psychological/neuropsychological testing services. The family of codes has been divided by the type of testing performed (eg, Assessment of Aphasia and Cognitive Performance Testing). Key terms (cognitive performance testing; interactive feedback; interpretation and report; neurobehavioral status examination; neuropsychological testing evaluation services; psychological testing evaluation services; standardized instruments; and testing) have been added and defined within the guidelines to assist users with the new terminology used.

Codes 96112 and 96113 have been established to report developmental test administration including assessments.

Code 96116 has been revised to indicate that these services may be reported by a physician/QHP for the first hour. Code 96121 is an add-on code to code 96116, which can be reported for each additional hour of a neurobehavioral status examination.

Codes 96130-96133 may be reported for testing evaluation services. Codes 96130 and 96131 are for psychological testing and codes 96132 and 96133 are for neuropsychological testing evaluation services. These services include interactive feedback to the patient, family members, or caregivers.

Codes 96136-96139 may be reported for test administration and scoring. Codes 96136 and 96137 are reported when a physician/QHP is performing the service; while codes 96138 and 96139 are reported when a technician is performing the service. Code 96146 is reported when a single automated psychological or neuropsychological test that includes results is performed.

In support of the establishment of codes 97151-97158 (adaptive behavior services) and the deletion of codes 0359T-0361T, 0363T-0372T, and 0374T, the exclusionary parenthetical note following the central nervous system assessments/tests (eg, neurocognitive, mental status, speech testing) guidelines has been revised to reflect these changes. Refer to the codebook and the Rationale for codes 97151-97158, 0362T, and 0373T for a full discussion of these changes.

Clinical Example (96146)

A 70-year-old female presents with a history of failing memory. Her physician arranges for the administration of a single automated cognitive test handed to her by the clinical staff.

Description of Procedure (96146)

N/A

Health and Behavior Assessment/Intervention

Health and behavior assessment procedures are used to identify the psychological, behavioral, emotional, cognitive, and social factors important to the prevention, treatment, or management of physical health problems.

The focus of the assessment is not on mental health but on the biopsychosocial factors important to physical health problems and treatments. The focus of the intervention is to improve the patient's health and well-being utilizing cognitive, behavioral, social, and/or psychophysiological procedures designed to ameliorate specific disease-related problems.

Codes 96150-96155 describe services offered to patients who present with primary physical illnesses, diagnoses, or symptoms and may benefit from assessments and interventions that focus on the biopsychosocial factors related to the patient's health status. These services do not represent preventive medicine counseling and risk factor reduction interventions.

For patients that require psychiatric services (90785-90899) as well as health and behavior assessment/intervention (96150-96155), report the predominant service performed. Do not report 96150-96155 in conjunction with 90785-90899 on the same date.

▶Evaluation and management services codes (including counseling risk factor reduction and behavior change intervention [99401-99412]), should not be reported on the same day as health and behavior assessment/intervention codes 96150, 96151, 96152, 96153, 96154, 96155.◀

▶(For health and behavior assessment and/or intervention services [96150, 96151, 96152, 96153, 96154, 96155] performed by a physician or other qualified health care professional who may report evaluation and management services, see **Evaluation and Management** or **Preventive Medicine Services** codes)◀

▶(Do not report 96150, 96151, 96152, 96153, 96154, 96155 in conjunction with 97151, 97152, 97153, 97154, 97155, 97156, 97157, 97158, 0362T, 0373T)◀

★ **96150**   Health and behavior assessment (eg, health-focused clinical interview, behavioral observations, psychophysiological monitoring, health-oriented questionnaires), each 15 minutes face-to-face with the patient; initial assessment

★ **96151**   re-assessment

Rationale

The health and behavior assessment guidelines have been revised to clarify separate reporting of evaluation and management (E/M) services. This revision specifies that E/M services may not be reported on the same day as health and behavior assessment/intervention codes (96150, 96151, 96152, 96153, 96154, 96155).

In support of the establishment of codes 97151-97158 (adaptive behavior services) and the deletion of codes 0359T-0361T, 0363T-0372T, and 0374T, the exclusionary parenthetical note following the health and behavior assessment/intervention guidelines has been revised to reflect these changes.

Refer to the codebook and the Rationale for codes 97151-97158, 0362T, and 0373T for a full discussion of the changes.

Photodynamic Therapy

Codes 96573, 96574 should be used to report nonsurgical treatment of cutaneous lesions using photodynamic therapy by external application of light to destroy premalignant lesion(s) of the skin and adjacent mucosa (eg, face, scalp) by activation of photosensitizing drug(s).

A treatment session is defined as an application of photosensitizer to all lesions within an anatomic area (eg, face, scalp), with or without debridement of all premalignant hyperkeratotic lesions in that area, followed by illumination/activation with an appropriate light source to the same area.

★ = Telemedicine   ✚ = Add-on code   ⟋ = FDA approval pending   # = Resequenced code   ⊘ = Modifier 51 exempt

►Do not report codes for debridement (11000, 11001, 11004, 11005), lesion shaving (11300-11313), biopsy (11102, 11103, 11104, 11105, 11106, 11107), or lesion excision (11400-11471) within the treatment area(s) on the same day as photodynamic therapy (96573, 96574).◄

(To report ocular photodynamic therapy, use 67221)

96567 Photodynamic therapy by external application of light to destroy premalignant lesions of the skin and adjacent mucosa with application and illumination/activation of photosensitive drug(s), per day

(Use 96567 for reporting photodynamic therapy when physician or other qualified health care professional is not directly involved in the delivery of the photodynamic therapy service)

Rationale

In support of the establishment of codes for tangential, punch, and incisional biopsies (11102, 11103, 11104, 11105, 11106, 11107), the guidelines for photodynamic therapy have been revised.

Refer to the codebook and the Rationale for codes 11102, 11103, 11104, 11105, 11106, and 11107 for a full discussion of these changes.

Physical Medicine and Rehabilitation

Codes 97010-97763 should be used to report each distinct procedure performed. Do not append modifier 51 to 97010-97763.

The work of the physician or other qualified health care professional consists of face-to-face time with the patient (and caregiver, if applicable) delivering skilled services. For the purpose of determining the total time of a service, incremental intervals of treatment at the same visit may be accumulated.

The meanings of terms in the Physical Medicine and Rehabilitation section are not the same as those in the Evaluation and Management Services section (99201-99350). Do not use the Definitions of Commonly Used Terms in the Evaluation and Management (E/M) Guidelines for Physical Medicine and Rehabilitation services.

(For muscle testing, range of joint motion, electromyography, see 95831 et seq)

(For biofeedback training by EMG, use 90901)

►(For transcutaneous nerve stimulation [TENS], use 97014 for electrical stimulation requiring supervision only, or use 97032 for electrical stimulation requiring constant attendance)◄

Rationale

In support of the deletion of code 64550, a parenthetical note has been added to direct users to the appropriate codes for reporting electrical stimulation services.

Refer to the codebook and the Rationale for deleted code 64550 for a full discussion of these changes.

Therapeutic Procedures

97127 Therapeutic interventions that focus on cognitive function (eg, attention, memory, reasoning, executive function, problem solving, and/or pragmatic functioning) and compensatory strategies to manage the performance of an activity (eg, managing time or schedules, initiating, organizing and sequencing tasks), direct (one-on-one) patient contact

(Report 97127 only once per day)

►(Do not report 97127 in conjunction with 97153, 97155)◄

Rationale

In support of the establishment of codes 97153 and 97155 (adaptive behavior services) and the deletion of codes 0364T, 0365T, 0368T, and 0369T, the exclusionary parenthetical note following code 97127 has been revised to reflect these changes. Refer to the codebook and the Rationale for codes 97151-97158, 0362T, and 0373T for a full discussion of these changes.

97150   Therapeutic procedure(s), group (2 or more individuals)

(Report 97150 for each member of group)

(Group therapy procedures involve constant attendance of the physician or other qualified health care professional [ie, therapist], but by definition do not require one-on-one patient contact by the same physician or other qualified health care professional)

(For manipulation under general anesthesia, see appropriate anatomic section in **Musculoskeletal System**)

(For osteopathic manipulative treatment [OMT], see 98925-98929)

▶(Do not report 97150 in conjunction with 97154, 97158)◀

Rationale

In support of the establishment of codes 97151-97158 (adaptive behavior services) and the deletion of codes 0359T-0361T, 0363T-0372T, and 0374T, the exclusionary parenthetical note following code 97150 (group therapeutic procedure) has been revised with the removal of codes 0366T, 0367T, and 0372T and the addition of codes 97154 and 97158 (group adaptive behavior service).

Refer to the codebook and the Rationale for codes 97151-97158, 0362T, and 0373T for a full discussion of the changes.

97151   Code is out of numerical sequence. See 96020-96112

97152   Code is out of numerical sequence. See 96020-96112

97153   Code is out of numerical sequence. See 96020-96112

97154   Code is out of numerical sequence. See 96020-96112

97155   Code is out of numerical sequence. See 96020-96112

97156   Code is out of numerical sequence. See 96020-96112

97157   Code is out of numerical sequence. See 96020-96112

97158   Code is out of numerical sequence. See 96020-96112

Special Services, Procedures and Reports

▶The procedures with code numbers 99000 through 99082 provide the reporting physician or other qualified health care professional with the means of identifying the completion of special reports and services that are an adjunct to the basic services rendered. The specific number assigned indicates the special circumstances under which a basic procedure is performed.◀

Codes 99050-99060 are reported in addition to an associated basic service. Do not append modifier 51 to 99050-99060. Typically only a single adjunct code from among 99050-99060 would be reported per patient encounter. However, there may be circumstances in which reporting multiple adjunct codes per patient encounter may be appropriate.

Miscellaneous Services

▶(99090 has been deleted)◀

99091   Code is out of numerical sequence. See 99448-99455

Rationale

Code 99091 has been resequenced and moved to the new Digitally Stored Data Services/Remote Physiologic Monitoring subsection within the E/M section. Code 99090 has been deleted due to extremely low utilization.

Refer to the codebook and the Rationale for Digitally Stored Data Services/Remote Physiologic Monitoring subsection in the E/M section for a full discussion of these changes.

★=Telemedicine   ✚=Add-on code   ✎=FDA approval pending   #=Resequenced code   ⊘=Modifier 51 exempt

Category III Codes

Changes in the Category III section include the addition of 38 codes; revision of three codes; and deletion or conversion of 28 codes to Category I codes.

Two new subsections have been added: Wireless Cardiac Stimulation System for Left Ventricular Pacing and Cellular and Gene Therapy. In the Wireless Cardiac Stimulation System for Left Ventricular Pacing subsection, eight new codes have been added. In addition, introductory and exclusionary parenthetical notes to preclude reporting the new cardiac stimulators and device evaluation codes in conjunction with other codes in this subsection have been added.

The other additions to Category III include revision to the subsection title of "Adaptive Behavior" to "Adaptive Behavior Assessment and Treatment" and its following introductory guidelines and definitions. The introductory guidelines and definitions have been revised to address the differences between behavior-identification assessments and protocol-modification services. In addition, an exclusionary parenthetical note to preclude reporting the new adaptive behavior services codes in conjunction with other codes in the Medicine section has been added.

Summary of Additions, Deletions, and Revisions

The summary of changes shows the actual changes that have been made to the code descriptors.

New codes appear with a bullet (●) and are indicated as "Code added." Revised codes are preceded with a triangle (▲). Within revised codes, or if a code symbol has been deleted, the deleted language and code symbol appears with a ~~strikethrough~~ (⊖), while new text appears underlined.

The ✗ symbol is used to identify codes for vaccines that are pending FDA approval. The # symbol is used to identify codes that have been resequenced. CPT add-on codes are annotated by the + symbol. The ⊘ symbol is used to identify codes that are exempt from the use of modifier 51. The ★ symbol is used to identify codes that may be used for reporting telemedicine services. The ✕ is used to identify proprietary laboratory analyses (PLA) test that has an identical descriptor as another PLA test.

Code	Description
#●0512T	Code added
#+●0513T	Code added
0159T	~~Computer-aided detection, including computer algorithm analysis of MRI image data for lesion detection/characterization, pharmacokinetic analysis, with further physician review for interpretation, breast MRI (List separately in addition to code for primary procedure)~~
0188T	~~Remote real-time interactive video-conferenced critical care, evaluation and management of the critically ill or critically injured patient; first 30-74 minutes~~
0189T	~~each additional 30 minutes (List separately in addition to code for primary service)~~
0190T	~~Placement of intraocular radiation source applicator (List separately in addition to primary procedure)~~
0195T	~~Arthrodesis, pre-sacral interbody technique, disc space preparation, discectomy, without instrumentation, with image guidance, includes bone graft when performed; L5-S1 interspace~~

Code	Description
0196T	L4-L5 interspace (List separately in addition to code for primary procedure)
▲0335T	Insertion of sinus tarsi implantExtra-osseous subtalar joint implant for talotarsal stabilization
#●0510T	Code added
#●0511T	Code added
0337T	Endothelial function assessment, using peripheral vascular response to reactive hyperemia, non-invasive (eg, brachial artery ultrasound, peripheral artery tonometry), unilateral or bilateral
0346T	Ultrasound, elastography (List separately in addition to code for primary procedure)
0359T	**Behavior identification assessment,** by the physician or other qualified health care professional, face-to-face with patient and caregiver(s), includes administration of standardized and non-standardized tests, detailed behavioral history, patient observation and caregiver interview, interpretation of test results, discussion of findings and recommendations with the primary guardian(s)/caregiver(s), and preparation of report
0360T	**Observational behavioral follow-up assessment,** includes physician or other qualified health care professional direction with interpretation and report, administered by one technician; first 30 minutes of technician time, face-to-face with the patient
0361T	each additional 30 minutes of technician time, face-to-face with the patient (List separately in addition to code for primary service)
▲0362T	**Exposure behavioral follow-upBehavior identification supporting assessment,** includes physician or other qualified health care professional direction with interpretation and report, administered by physician or other qualified health care professional with the assistance of one or more technicianseach 15 minutes of technicians' time face-to-face with a patient, requiring the following components: ■ administration by the physician or other qualified health care professional who is on site; ■ with the assistance of two or more technicians; ■ for a patient who exhibits destructive behavior; ■ completion in an environment that is customized to the patient's behavior. first 30 minutes of technician(s) time, face-to-face with the patient
0363T	each additional 30 minutes of technician(s) time, face-to-face with the patient (List separately in addition to code for primary procedure)
0364T	Adaptive behavior treatment by protocol, administered by technician, face-to-face with one patient; first 30 minutes of technician time
0365T	each additional 30 minutes of technician time (List separately in addition to code for primary procedure)
0366T	Group adaptive behavior treatment by protocol, administered by technician, face-to-face with two or more patients; first 30 minutes of technician time
0367T	each additional 30 minutes of technician time (List separately in addition to code for primary procedure
0368T	Adaptive behavior treatment with protocol modification administered by physician or other qualified health care professional with one patient; first 30 minutes of patient face-to-face time
0369T	each additional 30 minutes of patient face-to-face time (List separately in addition to code for primary procedure)
0370T	Family adaptive behavior treatment guidance, administered by physician or other qualified health care professional (without the patient present)
0371T	Multiple-family group adaptive behavior treatment guidance, administered by physician or other qualified health care professional (without the patient present)

★ = Telemedicine   ✚ = Add-on code   ✔ = FDA approval pending   # = Resequenced code   ⊘ = Modifier 51 exempt

Code	Description
0372T	~~Adaptive behavior treatment social skills group, administered by physician or other qualified health care professional face-to-face with multiple patients~~
▲0373T	~~Exposure adaptive behavior treatment with protocol modification~~**Adaptive behavior treatment with protocol modification,** each 15 minutes of technicians' time face-to-face with a patient, requiring ~~two or more technicians for severe maladaptive behavior(s)~~the following components: ■ administration by the physician or other qualified health care professional who is on site; ■ with the assistance of two or more technicians; ■ for a patient who exhibits destructive behavior; ■ completion in an environment that is customized to the patient's behavior. ~~first 60 minutes of technicians' time, face-to-face with patient~~
0374T	~~each additional 30 minutes of technicians' time face-to-face with patient (List separately in addition to code for primary procedure)~~
0387T	~~Transcatheter insertion or replacement of permanent leadless pacemaker, ventricular~~
0388T	~~Transcatheter removal of permanent leadless pacemaker, ventricular~~
0389T	~~Programming device evaluation (in person) with iterative adjustment of the implantable device to test the function of the device and select optimal permanent programmed values with analysis, review and report, leadless pacemaker system~~
0390T	~~Peri-procedural device evaluation (in person) and programming of device system parameters before or after a surgery, procedure or test with analysis, review and report, leadless pacemaker system~~
0391T	~~Interrogation device evaluation (in person) with analysis, review and report, includes connection, recording and disconnection per patient encounter, leadless pacemaker system~~
0406T	~~Nasal endoscopy, surgical, ethmoid sinus, placement of drug eluting implant~~
0407T	~~with biopsy, polypectomy or debridement~~
#+●0523T	Code added
●0505T	Code added
●0506T	Code added
●0507T	Code added
●0508T	Code added
●0509T	Code added
+●0514T	Code added
●0515T	Code added
●0516T	Code added
●0517T	Code added
●0518T	Code added
●0519T	Code added
●0520T	Code added
●0521T	Code added

Category III 0042T-0542T

Code	Description
●0522T	Code added
●0524T	Code added
●0525T	Code added
●0526T	Code added
●0527T	Code added
●0528T	Code added
●0529T	Code added
●0530T	Code added
●0531T	Code added
●0532T	Code added
●0533T	Code added
●0534T	Code added
●0535T	Code added
●0536T	Code added
●0537T	Code added
●0538T	Code added
●0539T	Code added
●0540T	Code added
●0541T	Code added
●0542T	Code added

Category III 0042T-0542T

★ = Telemedicine ✚ = Add-on code ✐ = FDA approval pending # = Resequenced code ⊘ = Modifier 51 exempt

Category III Codes

►Services and procedures described in this section make use of alphanumeric characters. These codes have an alpha character as the 5th character in the string (ie, four digits followed by the letter T). The digits are not intended to reflect the placement of the code in the Category I section of CPT nomenclature. Codes in this section may or may not eventually receive a Category I CPT code. In either case, in general, a given Category III code will be archived five years from the date of initial publication or extension unless a modification of the archival date is specifically noted at the time of a revision or change to a code (eg, addition of parenthetical instructions, reinstatement). Services and procedures described by Category III codes which have been archived after five years, without conversion, must be reported using the Category I unlisted code unless another specific cross-reference is established at the time of archiving. New codes or revised codes in this section are released semi-annually via the AMA CPT website to expedite dissemination for reporting. Codes approved for deletion are published annually with the full set of temporary codes for emerging technology, services, procedures, and service paradigms in the CPT code set. Go to www.ama-assn.org/go/cpt for the most current listing.◄

Rationale

New and/or revised Category III codes are published semi-annually on the CPT website. Therefore, the introductory guidelines for the Category III section in the code set have been revised to clarify that Category III codes accepted for deletion will be published annually with the full set of temporary codes.

0101T   Extracorporeal shock wave involving musculoskeletal system, not otherwise specified, high energy

►(For extracorporeal shock wave therapy involving integumentary system not otherwise specified, see 0512T, 0513T)◄

►(Do not report 0101T in conjunction 0512T, 0513T, when treating same area)◄

0102T   Extracorporeal shock wave, high energy, performed by a physician, requiring anesthesia other than local, involving lateral humeral epicondyle

#● 0512T   Extracorporeal shock wave for integumentary wound healing, high energy, including topical application and dressing care; initial wound

#+● 0513T   each additional wound (List separately in addition to code for primary procedure)

►(Use 0513T in conjunction with 0512T)◄

Rationale

Two new Category III codes (0512T, 0513T) have been established to report high-energy extracorporeal shock wave for integumentary wound healing. In addition, related instructional parenthetical notes have been added throughout the code set to provide instruction regarding the appropriate codes to use for reporting applicable services related to shock-wave therapy.

Codes 0512T and 0513T identify integumentary wound healing that is different from extracorporeal shock-wave treatment identified in other CPT codes. These two new codes are differentiated from other Category I codes for extracorporeal shock-wave treatment by the anatomy treated.

In support of the establishment of new Category III codes 0512T and 0513T, parenthetical notes have been added following other extracorporeal shock-wave treatment codes 28890 and 0101T.

Clinical Example (0512T)

A 58-year-old female with type II diabetes mellitus presents with a stage II ulcer of greater than 30-day duration on the plantar aspect of the right foot. The ulcer measures 3 x 4 cm (12 cm^2). Comorbidities include hypertension, peripheral vascular disease, sensory neuropathy, and cardiovascular disease. Dorsalis pedis and posterior tibial pulses are palpable.

Description of Procedure (0512T)

Perform standard wound cleansing and examination on the patient. Perform standard of care treatment, including possible debridement as determined by the treating clinician. Take wound measurements, and shock-count delivery is determined based on wound volume and comorbidities. Prepare the device for treatment. Deliver high-energy shock impulses to the wound and at least 1 cm of the peri-wound. Clean the wound post-application, and perform a final examination of the wound and apply wet-to-moist dressings. A complete course of treatment includes as many as eight applications, typically performed in a ten-week period.

Clinical Example (0513T)

A 68-year-old male with type II diabetes mellitus presents with a stage II ulcer of one-year duration on the left foot. The ulcer measures 8 x 14 cm (112 cm^2). Medical history includes peripheral vascular disease, peripheral neuropathy, osteomyelitis, and hypothyroidism. The ulcer has shown resistance to multiple treatments, including surgical debridement, advanced dressings, and advanced wound therapies.

Description of Procedure (0513T)

Perform standard wound cleansing and examination on the patient. Perform standard of care treatment, including possible debridement as determined by the treating clinician. Take wound measurements, and shock-count delivery is determined based on wound volume and comorbidities. Prepare the device for treatment. High-energy shock impulses are delivered to the wound and at least 1 cm of the peri-wound. Clean the wound post-application, and perform a final examination of the wound and apply wet-to-moist dressings. A complete course of treatment includes as many as eight applications, typically performed in a ten-week period.

▶(0159T has been deleted. To report, see 77048, 77049)◀

+ 0163T   Total disc arthroplasty (artificial disc), anterior approach, including discectomy to prepare interspace (other than for decompression), each additional interspace, lumbar (List separately in addition to code for primary procedure)

(Use 0163T in conjunction with 22857)

Rationale

Code 0159T has been deleted from Category III codes and converted to Category I codes 77048 and 77049 to report magnetic resonance imaging of the breast, with or without contrast materials, including computer-aided detection (CAD), when performed.

Refer to the codebook and the Rationale for codes 77048 and 77049 for a full discussion of these changes.

Remote Real-Time Interactive Video-conferenced Critical Care Services

▶(0188T, 0189T have been deleted)◀

▶(For remote real-time interactive video-conferenced critical care, evaluation and management of the critically ill or critically injured patient, use 99499)◀

Rationale

In accordance with the CPT guidelines for archiving Category III codes, codes 0188T and 0189T (remote real-time interactive video-conferenced critical care) have been deleted. Report code 99499, *Unlisted evaluation and management service,* if remote real-time interactive video-conferenced critical care services are performed.

To reflect this change, the guidelines for critical care services and initial neonatal and pediatric critical care in Category I have been revised and the guidelines for remote real-time interactive video-conferenced critical care services in Category III have been deleted accordingly.

▶(0190T has been deleted)◀

▶(For placement of intraocular radiation source applicator, use 67299)◀

(For application of the source by radiation oncologist, see Clinical Brachytherapy section)

Rationale

In accordance with CPT guidelines for archiving Category III codes, code 0190T (placement of an intraocular radiation source applicator) has been deleted. Report code 67299, *Unlisted procedure, posterior segment,* if placement of an intraocular radiation source applicator is performed.

▶(0195T, 0196T have been deleted)◀

▶(For arthrodesis, pre-sacral interbody technique, disc space preparation, discectomy, without instrumentation, with image guidance, includes bone graft when performed, L4-L5 interspace, L5-S1 interspace, use 22899)◀

★ = Telemedicine   ✚ = Add-on code   ✒ = FDA approval pending   # = Resequenced code   ⊘ = Modifier 51 exempt

Rationale

In accordance with CPT guidelines for archiving Category III codes, codes 0195T and 0196T (arthrodesis, pre-sacral interbody technique, disc space preparation, discectomy, without instrumentation, with image guidance, includes bone graft, when performed) have been deleted. Report code 22899, *Unlisted procedure, spine,* if arthrodesis, pre-sacral interbody technique, disc-space preparation, discectomy, without instrumentation, with image guidance, includes bone graft (when performed), is performed. To reflect the change, all related parenthetical notes have been revised as well.

0312T Vagus nerve blocking therapy (morbid obesity); laparoscopic implantation of neurostimulator electrode array, anterior and posterior vagal trunks adjacent to esophagogastric junction (EGJ), with implantation of pulse generator, includes programming

0313T laparoscopic revision or replacement of vagal trunk neurostimulator electrode array, including connection to existing pulse generator

0314T laparoscopic removal of vagal trunk neurostimulator electrode array and pulse generator

0315T removal of pulse generator

0316T replacement of pulse generator

(Do not report 0315T in conjunction with 0316T)

0317T neurostimulator pulse generator electronic analysis, includes reprogramming when performed

(For implantation, revision, replacement, and/or removal of vagus [cranial] nerve neurostimulator electrode array and/or pulse generator for vagus nerve stimulation performed other than at the EGJ [eg, epilepsy], see 64568-64570)

▶(For electronic analysis with programming, when performed, of vagal nerve neurostimulators, see 95970, 95976, 95977. Test stimulation to confirm correct target site placement of the electrode array[s] and/or to confirm the functional status of the system is inherent to placement, and is not separately reported as electronic analysis or programming of the neurostimulator system. Electronic analysis [95970] at the time of implantation is not separately reported.)◀

Rationale

The parenthetical note following code 0317T has been revised in conjunction with reporting changes made to neurostimulator services codes in the Medicine section. The revisions to the parenthetical note include the addition of terms to match other neurostimulator

guidelines, the removal of deleted codes 95974 and 95975, and addition of codes 95976 and 95977. In addition, it also includes the inclusion of language that specifies that test stimulation for the purpose of confirming target placement and functional status of the system is inherently included as part of placement and not separately reported.

Refer to the codebook and the Rationale for codes 95970-95972 and 95976-95984 for a full discussion of the changes.

▲ **0335T** Insertion of sinus tarsi implant

▶(Do not report 0335T in conjunction with 28585, 28725, 29907)◀

#● **0510T** Removal of sinus tarsi implant

#● **0511T** Removal and reinsertion of sinus tarsi implant

Rationale

Code 0335T has been revised and two new codes (0510T, 0511T) have been added to better identify the insertion, removal, and removal and reinsertion services of a sinus tarsi implant device. An exclusionary parenthetical note has been added with instructions not to report code 0335T in conjunction with codes 28585, 28725, and 29907 (other talotarsal joint procedures).

Originally set to sundown as part of the CPT 2019 code set, code 0335T's sundown date has been extended to December 31, 2023, which means it will not be in the CPT 2024 code set. In addition, it has been revised to better specify the placement of a sinus tarsi implant without surgical attachment of the device (with the addition of the word "insertion").

The revised language also provides more specific identification of where the device is inserted (ie, into the sinus tarsi). The previous language in the code descriptor was "Extra-osseous subtalar joint implant for talotarsal stabilization," which was not as specific regarding the location of the implant insertion and how the device was used (ie, as an insert). The new language more specifically identifies the procedure by identifying the **insertion** of an implant to stabilize the sinus tarsi (the space between the calcaneus and the tarsus bones). Device implantation is accomplished by making a small incision and placing the implant into the cavity where it is held in place by soft tissue. The device is not anchored into bone or other osseous structures.

Insertion of a sinus tarsi implant may be performed as a stand-alone procedure or in combination with other surgical procedures performed on the foot bones. As a result, reporting in conjunction with other procedures may vary according to the procedures performed and may require use of appropriate modifiers to identify specific circumstances (eg, use of modifier 51 to identify multiple surgical procedures performed through the same incision). The exception to this is included in the exclusionary parenthetical note following code 0335T. The codes (28585, 28725, 29907) listed identify other talotarsal joint procedures (open treatment of talotarsal joint dislocation, includes internal fixation [28585]; arthrodesis, subtalar [28725]; and arthroscopy, subtalar joint, surgical; with subtalar arthrodesis [29907]), which would inherently include the insertion of the sinus tarsi device. As a result, code 0335T would not be separately reported when these codes are used.

Reversal (removal) of the procedure (insertion of the sinus tarsi device) may be reported with either code 0510T or 0511T. The procedures represented by codes 0510T and 0511T are differentiated by whether a sinus tarsi implant will be replaced into the space.

Code 0510T is used to identify the removal of the implant without replacement and code 0511T is used to identify the removal with the intent of replacing the device, such as to enable the correction of the insertion due to migration.

Clinical Example (0335T)

A 45-year-old female suffers discomfort as a result of excessive subtalar joint motion. The patient is a candidate for the insertion of a sinus tarsi implant because of documented reducibility of the deformity and the persistence of reoccurrence.

Description of Procedure (0335T)

Administer anesthesia and make an incision over the sinus tarsi. Dissect the soft tissues and perform trial sizing to determine the best size of sinus tarsi implant to restore a normal amount of subtalar joint motion. Place the appropriate implant within the sinus tarsi and use intraoperative radiographic imaging to confirm the desired placement. Suture the deep and superficial tissues.

Clinical Example (0510T)

A 22-year-old male received a sinus tarsi implant one year earlier. He complains of persistent pain that is attributed to the implant. No displacement of the implant can be seen on radiographic imaging. The patient is advised to have the implant removed permanently and to proceed with an alternative form of treatment.

Description of Procedure (0510T)

Administer anesthesia and make an incision over the sinus tarsi. Dissect the soft tissues. Identify the lateral end of the sinus tarsi implant and remove the entire implant. Suture the deep and superficial tissues.

Clinical Example (0511T)

A 38-year-old female received a sinus tarsi implant eight months earlier. She complains of persistent pain to the sinus tarsi area. Radiographs show a partially displaced sinus tarsi implant. The patient is scheduled to have the implant removed and a smaller-sized implant placed deeper within the sinus tarsi.

Description of Procedure (0511T)

Administer anesthesia and make an incision over the sinus tarsi. Dissect the soft tissues. Identify the lateral end of the sinus tarsi implant and remove the entire implant. Perform re-trial sizing to determine the optimal-sized implant to achieve the desired correction. Place the appropriate implant within the sinus tarsi and confirm the desired placement with intraoperative radiographic imaging. Suture the deep and superficial tissues.

▶(0337T has been deleted)◀

▶(For unilateral or bilateral endothelial function assessments, using peripheral vascular response to reactive hyperemia, noninvasive [eg, brachial artery ultrasound, peripheral artery tonometry], use 93998)◀

Rationale

In accordance with CPT guidelines for archiving Category III codes, code 0337T (endothelial function assessment, using peripheral vascular response to reactive hyperemia, non-invasive, unilateral or bilateral) has been deleted. Report code 93998, *Unlisted noninvasive vascular diagnostic study,* if endothelial function assessment, using peripheral vascular response to reactive hyperemia, non-invasive, unilateral or bilateral, is performed. To reflect the change, all related parenthetical notes have been revised as well.

0342T   Therapeutic apheresis with selective HDL delipidation and plasma reinfusion

▶Fluoroscopy (76000) and radiologic supervision and interpretation are inherent to the transcatheter mitral valve repair (TMVR) procedure and are not separately reportable. Diagnostic cardiac catheterization (93451, 93452, 93453, 93454, 93455, 93456, 93457, 93458,

93459, 93460, 93461, 93530, 93531, 93532, 93533) should **not** be reported with transcatheter mitral valve repair (0345T) for:◄

- Contrast injections, angiography, roadmapping, and/or fluoroscopic guidance for the transcatheter mitral valve repair (TMVR),

- Left ventricular angiography to assess mitral regurgitation, for guidance of TMVR, or

- Right and left heart catheterization for hemodynamic measurements before, during, and after TMVR for guidance of TMVR.

Rationale

In accordance with the deletion of code 76001, the guidelines following code 0342T have been revised with the removal of this code.

Refer to the codebook and the Rationale for code 76001 for a full discussion of these changes.

Diagnostic right and left heart catheterization (93451, 93452, 93453, 93456, 93457, 93458, 93459, 93460, 93461, 93530, 93531, 93532, 93533), and diagnostic coronary angiography (93454, 93455, 93456, 93457, 93458, 93459, 93460, 93461, 93563, 93564) not inherent to the TMVR, may be reported with 0345T, appended with modifier 59 if:

1. No prior study is available and a full diagnostic study is performed, or

2. A prior study is available, but as documented in the medical record:

   a. There is inadequate visualization of the anatomy and/or pathology, or

   b. The patient's condition with respect to the clinical indication has changed since the prior study, or

   c. There is a clinical change during the procedure that requires new evaluation.

Percutaneous coronary interventional procedures may be reported separately, when performed.

Other cardiac catheterization services may be reported separately, when performed for diagnostic purposes not intrinsic to the TMVR.

When transcatheter ventricular support is required, the appropriate code may be reported with the appropriate ventricular assist device (VAD) procedure (33990, 33991, 33992, 33993) or balloon pump insertion (33967, 33970, 33973).

0345T   Transcatheter mitral valve repair percutaneous approach via the coronary sinus

(For transcatheter mitral valve repair percutaneous approach including transseptal puncture when performed, see 33418, 33419)

(Do not report 0345T in conjunction with 93451, 93452, 93453, 93456, 93457, 93458, 93459, 93460, 93461 for diagnostic left and right heart catheterization procedures intrinsic to the valve repair procedure)

(Do not report 0345T in conjunction with 93453, 93454, 93563, 93564 for coronary angiography intrinsic to the valve repair procedure)

(For transcatheter mitral valve implantation/replacement [TMVI], see 0483T, 0484T)

►(0346T has been deleted. To report, see 76981, 76982, 76983)◄

Rationale

Code 0346T (ultrasound, elastography) has been deleted as three new Category I codes (76981, 76982, 76983) have been established to report ultrasound elastography. In addition, a parenthetical note to instruct users to use codes 76981, 76982, and 76983 has been added.

Refer to the codebook and the Rationale for codes 76981, 76982, and 76983 for a full discussion of these changes.

►Adaptive Behavior Assessments and Treatment◄

►**Behavior identification supporting assessment** (0362T) and **adaptive behavior treatment with protocol modification** (0373T) include the following required components:

- administration by the physician or other qualified health care professional who is on-site but not necessarily face-to-face with the patient;

- with the assistance of two or more technicians;

- for a patient with destructive behavior that requires the presence of a team;

- completion in an environment that is customized to the patient's behavior.

"On-site" is defined as immediately available and interruptible to provide assistance and direction throughout the performance of the procedure, however, the physician or other qualified health care professional does not need to be present in the room when the procedure is performed.

Category III 0042T-0542T

Typical patients for 0362T and 0373T present with one or more specific destructive behavior(s) (ie, maladaptive behaviors associated with high risk of medical consequences or property damage [eg, elopement, pica, or self-injury requiring medical attention, aggression with injury to other{s}, or breaking furniture, walls, or windows]). Code 0362T may include functional behavior assessment, functional analysis, other structured observations, and standardized and/or nonstandardized instruments and procedures to determine levels of adaptive and maladaptive behavior as well as other impairments in functioning.

Only count the time of one technician when two or more are present. For assistance with code selection of 97152, 0362T, see the Guide to Selection of Codes 97152 and 0362T on page 711. For assistance with code selection of 97153, 97155, 0373T, see Guide to Selection of Codes 97153, 97155, 0373T on page 712.◀

►(0359T, 0360T, 0361T have been deleted. To report, see 97151, 97152)◀

▲ **0362T**   **Behavior identification supporting assessment,** each 15 minutes of technicians' time face-to-face with a patient, requiring the following components:

- administration by the physician or other qualified health care professional who is on site;

- with the assistance of two or more technicians;

- for a patient who exhibits destructive behavior;

- completion in an environment that is customized to the patient's behavior.

►(0362T is reported based on a single technician's face-to-face time with the patient and not the combined time of multiple technicians [eg, one hour with three technicians equals one hour of service])◀

►(0362T may be repeated on different days until the behavior identification assessment [97151] and, if necessary, supporting assessment[s] [97152, 0362T], is complete)◀

►(For psychiatric diagnostic evaluation, see 90791, 90792)◀

►(For speech evaluations, see 92521, 92522, 92523, 92524)◀

►(For occupational therapy evaluation, see 97165, 97166, 97167, 97168)◀

►(For medical team conference, see 99366, 99367, 99368)◀

►(For health and behavior assessment/intervention, see 96150, 96151, 96152, 96153, 96154, 96155)◀

►(For neurobehavioral status examination, see 96116, 96121)◀

►(For neuropsychological testing, see 96132, 96133, 96136, 96137, 96138, 96139, 96146)◀

►(0363T, 0364T, 0365T, 0366T, 0367T, 0368T, 0369T, 0370T, 0371T, 0372T have been deleted. To report, see 97153, 97154, 97155, 97156, 97157, 97158, 0373T)◀

▲ **0373T**   **Adaptive behavior treatment with protocol modification,** each 15 minutes of technicians' time face-to-face with a patient, requiring the following components:

- administration by the physician or other qualified health care professional who is on site;

- with the assistance of two or more technicians;

- for a patient who exhibits destructive behavior;

- completion in an environment that is customized to the patient's behavior.

►(0373T is reported based on a single technician's face-to-face time with the patient and not the combined time of multiple technicians)◀

►(Do not report 0373T in conjunction with 90785-90899, 96105, 96110, 96116, 96121, 96150, 96151, 96152, 96153, 96154, 96155)◀

►(0374T has been deleted. To report, use 0373T)◀

Rationale

Many changes have been made to adaptive behavior services codes and guidelines, which coincide with the adaptive behavior services–related changes in Category I.

Refer to the codebook and the Rationale for codes 97151-97158 for a full discussion of these changes.

Codes 0359T-0361T, 0363T-0372T, and 0374T have been deleted and the services described by these deleted codes are now described by the converted Category I code (97151-97158). The two remaining adaptive behavior service codes (0362T, 0373T) have been revised. The Adaptive Behavior Assessments and the Adaptive Behavior Treatment subsections have been consolidated under one subsection entitled "Adaptive Behavior Assessments and Treatments." In accordance with the changes, the guidelines have been revised to reflect the revisions to codes 0362T and 0373T.

Codes 0362T (behavior assessment) and 0373T (behavior treatment with protocol modification) have been revised to reflect current practice by removing the term "exposure," revision of the time component to 15 minutes, and the addition of four required components that must be met in order to report the codes. The term "exposure" has been removed due to confusion among individuals providing the service about its meaning in the context of these services. For code 0362T, the term "functional

★ = Telemedicine   ✦ = Add-on code   ✗ = FDA approval pending   # = Resequenced code   ⊘ = Modifier 51 exempt

analysis" is synonymous with the term "exposure" and is more commonly used among providers. As such, a definition of functional analysis has been added to the adaptive behavior services guidelines in the Medicine section. Functional analysis may be performed as part of the behavior identification supporting assessment described in code 0362T, which is stated in the revised adaptive behavior assessments and treatment guidelines in Category III.

Services described in codes 0362T and 0373T involve the assistance of two or more technicians; however, time spent on these services is calculated based on the time spent by a single technician, not the combined time of multiple technicians, when reporting codes 0362T and 0373T. For example, one hour of face-to-face time spent with the patient by three technicians equals one hour of service. In addition, code 0362T has been further revised to describe a *supporting* assessment rather than a *follow-up* assessment, as the intent of the services is for supportive rather than follow-up purposes. It is important to note that new code 97152 has been added to the Medicine section, which also describes behavior identification supporting assessment. The difference between codes 0362T and 97152 is that code 97152 describes the assistance of one technician rather than multiple technicians, which has different reporting requirements than code 0362T.

In accordance with the deletion of code 96101 (psychological testing) in the Medicine section, the exclusionary parenthetical note following code 0374T has been revised to remove this code from its listing and to include several new central nervous system assessments/ tests codes from the Medicine section.

Refer to the codebook and the Rationale for codes 96112-96146 for a full discussion of these changes.

In accordance with the addition and revisions of codes in the Central Nervous System Assessments/Tests (eg, Neuro-Cognitive, Mental Status, Speech Testing) subsection, the parenthetical notes following code 0362T have been revised. Refer to the codebook and the Rationale for the Central Nervous System Assessments/ Tests (eg, Neuro-Cognitive, Mental Status, Speech Testing) subsection (96112-96146) for a full discussion of these changes.

Clinical Example (0362T)

A 26-year-old male requires additional assessment of a behavior—hitting his head with his fists—that is at risk of becoming self-injurious. Initial direct observation and measurement show that the behavior occurs more than 50 times per hour on average.

Description of Procedure (0362T)

To ensure the patient's safety during sessions, the protocol for the functional analysis specifies that:

■ sessions be conducted in a room devoid of any objects that might cause injury;

■ sessions be terminated immediately and medical treatment sought, if a fist-to-head hit causes tissue damage; and

■ qualified health care professional will observe all sessions via a one-way window.

The qualified health care professional directs two behavior technicians to implement the functional analysis procedures and record data. The qualified health care professional reviews and analyzes all graphed data from all sessions to identify the environmental event(s) in whose presence the level of behavior was highest and lowest.

Clinical Example (0373T)

A 16-year-old male has had two surgeries to relieve esophageal blockages due to pica involving repeated ingestion of small metal objects (eg, paper clips, push pins). The patient's pica behavior has not responded to previous treatment.

Description of Procedure (0373T)

The qualified health care professional supervising the patient's treatment plan has previously developed written protocols for reducing the patient's pica based on previous medical evaluation, functional analysis of the pica behavior, and other assessment data. A technician presents the patient with a series of trials in the patient's treatment plan. On each trial, place one small, preferred food item and another that resembles a pica item, which is not dangerous if ingested, on a table in front of the patient. Position a second technician directly behind the patient to provide the patient with a gentle physical prompt to pick up and eat the food item. If the patient tries to pick up the pica item, the second technician gently blocks that response and removes the pica item from the patient's line of sight. All protocols include procedures for recording the patient's responses on each trial (consuming the food item and/or attempting to pick up the pica item). The qualified health care professional directs the technicians in the implementation of the treatment and data-collection procedures. Before the session, a technician carefully inspects the room to ensure there are no potential pica items on the floor. The qualified health care professional is available to observe and/or assist with sessions, as needed.

Category III 0042T-0542T

Pacemaker-Leadless and Pocketless System

►(0387T, 0388T have been deleted. To report, see 33274, 33275)◄

►(0389T, 0390T, 0391T have been deleted. To report, see 33274, 33275, 93279, 93286, 93288, 93294, 93296)◄

Rationale

Codes 0387T (leadless pacemaker insertion or replacement), 0388T (leadless pacemaker removal), and 0389T, 0390T, and 0391T (leadless pacemaker device evaluation) have been deleted and the procedures described by these deleted codes have been converted to Category I codes (33274, 33275). A parenthetical note has been added to this section to refer users to the appropriate Category I codes.

Refer to the codebook and the Rationale for codes 33274, 33275, 93279, 93286, 93288, 93294, and 93296 for a full discussion of these changes.

0405T   Oversight of the care of an extracorporeal liver assist system patient requiring review of status, review of laboratories and other studies, and revision of orders and liver assist care plan (as appropriate), within a calendar month, 30 minutes or more of non-face-to-face time

►(0406T, 0407T have been deleted)◄

►(To report endoscopic placement of a drug-eluting implant in the ethmoid sinus without any other nasal/sinus endoscopic surgical service, use 31299. To report endoscopic placement of a drug-eluting implant in the ethmoid sinus in conjunction with biopsy, polypectomy, or debridement, use 31237)◄

Rationale

Codes 0406T and 0407T and all their related references have been deleted from the CPT code set. In their place, a deletion parenthetical note has been added.

In support of the deletion of codes 0406T and 0407T, existing parenthetical notes have been updated with the deletion of codes 0406T and 0407T. The two identical parenthetical notes included in the Surgery/Endoscopy subsection and Category III section direct users to report code 31299 for endoscopic placement of a drug-eluting implant in the ethmoid sinus without any other nasal/sinus endoscopic surgical service. In addition, code 31237 should be reported for endoscopic placement of a drug-eluting implant in the ethmoid sinus in conjunction with biopsy, polypectomy, or debridement.

0463T   Interrogation device evaluation (in person) with analysis, review and report, includes connection, recording and disconnection per patient encounter, implantable aortic counterpulsation ventricular assist system, per day

(Do not report 0463T in conjunction with 0451T-0462T)

►(Do not report 0451T-0463T in conjunction with 36000, 36002, 36005, 36010, 36200-36228, 75600-75774, 76000, 76936, 76937, 77001, 77002, 77011, 77012, 77021, 93451-93533, 93561-93572)◄

Rationale

In accordance with the deletion of code 76001 in the Radiology section, the parenthetical note following code 0463T has been revised with the removal of this code.

Refer to the codebook and the Rationale for code 76001 for a full discussion of these changes.

0501T   Noninvasive estimated coronary fractional flow reserve (FFR) derived from coronary computed tomography angiography data using computation fluid dynamics physiologic simulation software analysis of functional data to assess the severity of coronary artery disease; data preparation and transmission, analysis of fluid dynamics and simulated maximal coronary hyperemia, generation of estimated FFR model, with anatomical data review in comparison with estimated FFR model to reconcile discordant data, interpretation and report

0502T   data preparation and transmission

0503T   analysis of fluid dynamics and simulated maximal coronary hyperemia, and generation of estimated FFR model

0504T   anatomical data review in comparison with estimated FFR model to reconcile discordant data, interpretation and report

►(Do not report 0501T in conjunction with 0502T, 0503T, 0504T, 0523T)◄

Rationale

In accordance with the addition of code 0523T, the parenthetical note that follows code 0504T has been revised to preclude the use of code 0501T with code 0523T.

Refer to the codebook and the Rationale for code 0523T for a full discussion of these changes.

★ = Telemedicine   ✚ = Add-on code   ✗ = FDA approval pending   # = Resequenced code   ⊘ = Modifier 51 exempt

Category III 0042T-0542T

#+● **0523T**   Intraprocedural coronary fractional flow reserve (FFR) with 3D functional mapping of color-coded FFR values for the coronary tree, derived from coronary angiogram data, for real-time review and interpretation of possible atherosclerotic stenosis(es) intervention (List separately in addition to code for primary procedure)

> ►(Use 0523T in conjunction with 93454, 93455, 93456, 93457, 93458, 93459, 93460, 93461)◄

> ►(Do not report 0523T more than once per session)◄

> ►(Do not report 0523T in conjunction with 76376, 76377, 93571, 93572, 0501T, 0502T, 0503T, 0504T)◄

Rationale

Code 0523T has been established to report noninvasive intraprocedural coronary fractional flow reserve (FFR) derived from angiogram data. Before the addition of code 0523T, no codes described intraprocedural coronary FFR derived from angiogram data. Codes 93571 and 93572 in Category I describe invasive FFR procedures. Also, in comparison, codes 0501T-0504T describe FFR that utilize coronary computed tomography (CT) angiography data.

Compared to the technology represented in the other FFR codes, the new technology represented in code 0523T was developed to allow noninvasive measurement of FFR through the processing of angiography data. This technology provides real-time, intraprocedural information to the physician and allows the physician to make medical decisions on cardiac interventions. FFR produced with a three-dimensional (3D) image of the entire cardiac tree allows the physician to review and analyze multiple individual coronary lesions for FFR. Code 0523T is an add-on code that may be reported with codes 93454, 93455, 93456, 93457, 93458, 93459, 93460, and 93461 (coronary angiography). In addition, it may be reported only once per session.

Clinical Example (0523T)

During an angiography procedure for a 67-year-old male with abnormal EKG and chest pain, the physician notes narrowing of one or more of the coronary arteries. Coronary fractional flow reserve (FFR) mapping is ordered to determine the degree of blockage to decide whether percutaneous coronary intervention (PCI) is indicated, and if so, to use as a guide for that PCI procedure.

Description of Procedure (0523T)

Following the angiography procedure (separately reported), while the patient remains on the table, the physician selects the clinically appropriate angiographic views and imports the data into the FFR mapping software, which is present in the laboratory connected directly to the angiography system. Enter the mean arterial pressure into the FFR mapping software. The data are processed through an algorithm that analyzes anatomy, topology, pathology, and lumen extraction. The system calculates pressure-flow distribution, taking measured aortic pressure into account as a boundary condition. The computed noninvasive FFR values are displayed on a monitor in a color-coded model of the coronary tree. A three-dimensional (3D) viewer allows the physician to further interrogate specific areas of interest at each point along the coronary arteries and system. The data are processed during the procedure in the catheterization laboratory while the patient is on the table, allowing the physician to review and interpret the entire coronary tree model with FFR values in real time and decide whether PCI is required, and to guide the intervention. (**Note:** PCI is reported separately.) Prepare, notate, and document a final report in the patient's record. Communicate the study's results to the patient and the referring physician to facilitate appropriate patient management.

● **0505T**   Endovenous femoral-popliteal arterial revascularization, with transcatheter placement of intravascular stent graft(s) and closure by any method, including percutaneous or open vascular access, ultrasound guidance for vascular access when performed, all catheterization(s) and intraprocedural roadmapping and imaging guidance necessary to complete the intervention, all associated radiological supervision and interpretation, when performed, with crossing of the occlusive lesion in an extraluminal fashion

> ►(0505T includes all ipsilateral selective arterial and venous catheterization, all diagnostic imaging for ipsilateral, lower extremity arteriography, and all related radiological supervision and interpretation)◄

> ►(Do not report 0505T in conjunction with 37224, 37225, 37226, 37227, 37238, 37239, 37248, 37249, within the femoral-popliteal segment)◄

> ►(Do not report 0505T in conjunction with 76937, for ultrasound guidance for vascular access)◄

Rationale

Code 0505T has been added and numerous exclusionary and instructional parenthetical notes have been added in various sections of the CPT code set to identify endovenous femoral-popliteal arterial revascularization using intravascular stent grafts in an extraluminal fashion.

Revascularization procedures previously listed in the CPT code set treat clogged vessels in a number of ways. The occlusion may be treated directly from within the vessel by catheterizing the clogged vessel and breaking through the clog by punching a hole through it (atherectomy), by widening the constricted space by inflating a balloon within the clogged lumen of the vessel (angioplasty), or by surgically exposing the clog for treatment. A stent may be used to keep the newly opened pathway patent. The vessel can also be bypassed, ie, an alternate route can be made to circumvent blood flow around the occlusion. Usually the bypass is created by harvesting a vessel and connecting it above and below the clogged area to form the bypass around the occlusion.

Code 0505T includes (1) access of the treatment site/vessels; (2) all selective catheterization (arterial and venous) necessary to access the site for completion of the procedure; (3) closure by any method; and (4) ultrasound guidance, intraprocedural road mapping, and imaging needed to complete the procedure, and all associated radiological supervision and interpretation. As a result, parenthetical notes that contain all related codes within this section and in other sections of the CPT code set provide either instructions regarding all services that are inherently included (ie, imaging, catheterization, access) as part of the femoral-popliteal revascularization or exclusionary instructions indicating the codes that may not be reported in conjunction with code 0505T.

Clinical Example (0505T)

A 68-year-old male former smoker with known history of peripheral arterial disease presents with lifestyle-limiting intermittent claudication of the left leg. Prior diagnostic angiography demonstrated an occlusion of the left superficial femoral artery. The patient was determined to be a candidate for endovenous femoral-popliteal artery revascularization.

Description of Procedure (0505T)

Using standard technique, obtain arterial access to the contralateral femoral artery. After placement of a standard sheath, advance a guidewire over the aortic bifurcation and to the site of occlusion in the ipsilateral superficial femoral artery. Separately, obtain a second venous access in the ipsilateral posterior tibial vein.

Advance the snare (venous locator) through the venous sheath to the femoral vein at the level adjacent to the ipsilateral superficial femoral artery occlusion. Expand the snare/cage within the femoral vein. At this point, advance the crossing device (percutaneous anastomotic device) through the arterial access over the guidewire up to just above the level of the occlusion in the ipsilateral superficial femoral artery. Orient the crossing device in the superficial femoral artery under fluoroscopic guidance toward the snare cages in the femoral vein. "Fire" the needle of the crossing device through the sidewall of the superficial femoral artery above the occlusion, through the sidewall of the adjacent femoral vein, and direct into upper snare cage in the femoral vein. Advance a guidewire through the lumen of the needle and into the upper snare cage. Withdraw the needle and collapse the venous snare/cage, capturing the guidewire. Advance the venous sheath over the collapsed cage. Withdraw the snare/cage from the body via the posterior tibial vein sheath along with the guidewire until the wire is externalized. Also, withdraw the crossing device in the superficial femoral artery, enabling the guidewire to create a circuit running through the arterial sheath into the proximal superficial femoral artery, through the anastomosis into the femoral vein, and out of the body via the venous sheath.

Dilate the proximal anastomosis using standard angioplasty technique. Then, reintroduce the crossing device into the superficial femoral artery from the arterial sheath, through the proximal anastomosis, and place it into the femoral vein distal to the femoral artery occlusion. Advance the snare/cage through the venous sheath into the popliteal vein below the level of the occlusion. Expand the snare/cages.

Advance the crossing device through the arterial sheath until its tip is directly above the snare/cage tip. "Fire" the needle of the crossing device through the sidewall of the popliteal vein and through the sidewall of the adjacent popliteal artery just below the level of the occlusion. Advance a guidewire through the needle of the crossing device into the true lumen of the popliteal artery and distally into the tibial artery. Remove the crossing device. Collapse and remove the snare cages. Dilate the distal anastomosis over the guidewire from the arterial sheath using standard angioplasty technique.

Category III 0042T-0542T

Then use an exchange catheter to convert from a 0.014-in to a 0.035-in guidewire to facilitate stent graft delivery. In a continuous, overlapping fashion, deliver and deploy multiple stent grafts from the popliteal artery, through the distal anastomosis into the popliteal vein, up through the femoral vein, then through the proximal anastomosis into the proximal superficial femoral artery. The stent grafts are post-dilated, creating a percutaneous bypass around the superficial femoral artery occlusion utilizing the femoral vein as a conduit. Following the completion of angiography, remove the vascular access sheaths, which concludes the procedure.

● **0506T** Macular pigment optical density measurement by heterochromatic flicker photometry, unilateral or bilateral, with interpretation and report

Rationale

New code 0506T has been added to report macular pigment optical density measurement by heterochromatic flicker photometry, unilateral or bilateral, with interpretation and report. Measurement of macular pigment optical density by heterochromatic flicker photometry is a noninvasive, psychophysical assessment typically of patients at risk for visual disability or catastrophic vision loss. Before 2019, no code specifically described this procedure.

Clinical Example (0506T)

A 55-year-old male has reported difficulty reading with spots in his central vision. A retinal examination reveals soft drusen in both eyes. A measurement of macular pigment optical density with heterochromatic flicker photometry is ordered to determine if there is a deficiency in macular pigment.

Description of Procedure (0506T)

Position the patient at the instrument in a darkened room for measurement of macular pigment optical density (MPOD) and give him a response button. The patient may wear corrective lenses while one eye is occluded and the nonoccluded eye is tested. Instruct the patient to fixate on a small circular stimulus that alternates between a test wavelength (460 nm) and a reference wavelength (540 nm). Also instruct the patient to press the response button when he observes the stimulus flickering. Issue an interpretation and generate a report.

● **0507T** Near infrared dual imaging (ie, simultaneous reflective and transilluminated light) of meibomian glands, unilateral or bilateral, with interpretation and report

▶(For external ocular photography, use 92285)◀

▶(For tear film imaging, use 0330T)◀

Rationale

Code 0507T has been added to report near-infrared dual imaging of meibomian glands. In accordance with the addition of a new code, parenthetical notes have been added after code 0507T to direct users to the correct code for reporting external ocular photography (92285) or tear film imaging (0330T). Similarly, parenthetical notes with the same instructions have been added after code 92285 in the Medicine section.

Code 0507T describes an infrared imaging technique for evaluating the functioning of the meibomian glands. Meibomian glands are the glands in the eyelids that secrete lipids and keep tears from evaporating too quickly. This procedure involves the use of a portable lid everter, which acts as a source of near-infrared light to generate 3D images, and software that permits image manipulation and review. This produces two types of visualization— reflective and trans-illuminated light (ie, dual imaging)— which, when combined, can be used to create the 3D image. This results in a high-resolution image of the glands for diagnosis.

This procedure differs from other services that may be used to diagnose low levels of meibomian gland production of lipids. The procedure described in code 0330T (tear film imaging) uses digital interferometry to quantify lipid-layer thickness through image recording of the ocular surface. The imaging device converts the image recording of the lipid-layer thickness into a numerical value, which the physician uses to interpret and assess if the patient has a lipid deficiency. The procedure represented by code 92285 (external ocular photography) measures lipids with the use of a slit lamp-based technology. External ocular photography does not differentiate between film and digital media or between still and video images.

Code 0507T includes language that specifies inclusion of performance unilaterally and bilaterally, as well as the interpretation and report.

Clinical Example (0507T)

A 65-year-old male presents with burning sensation and dry eyes by Schirmer testing.

Description of Procedure (0507T)

The physician positions the patient and centers the eyelid for proper imaging. The physician uses the lid everter, which provides the near-infrared light, to evert the lower eyelids, flipping the lids over to clearly see the meibomian glands of the eyelids with even illumination. After proper focusing, the physician performs infrared meibomian gland imaging with portable device to capture the image, preview images, and archive images or re-record as needed.

● **0508T**   Pulse-echo ultrasound bone density measurement resulting in indicator of axial bone mineral density, tibia

Rationale

Code 0508T has been established to report pulse-echo ultrasound bone density measurements for bone mineral density (BMD) analysis. As this is a new technology to measure bone density, existing CPT codes do not accurately describe this procedure. Currently, codes 76977, 77080, and 77081 are used to report bone density measurements, in particular only peripheral bone mineral density measurements and/or using X-ray technology. In contrast, new code 0508T reports the measurements of axial bone mineral density using ultrasound technology.

Clinical Example (0508T)

A 70-year-old female is identified as at risk for osteoporosis and referred for screening by her physician.

Description of Procedure (0508T)

Enter ethnicity, age, weight, and height of the patient into measurement-device software. For the duration of the measurement, the patient should be lying (eg, on a bed). Alternatively, the patient may be sitting with one leg extended and supported (eg, with a chair). Clothing must be removed from ankle up to the knee.

Operator determines measurement location by locating the proximal head of tibia and marking it on the skin. Then the operator measures the distance from the distal head of tibia (on the medial malleolus) to proximal head of tibia. The measurement site is one-third the length of the tibia from the proximal head.

Before the pulse-echo ultrasound measurements, ultrasound gel is applied to the skin at the measurement location. The operator places the transducer on the skin beside the measurement location and moves it slowly over medial one-third proximal tibia site. When two ultrasound echo spikes are seen the operator is at the correct site. The operator may need to adjust the angle of the transducer to maximize the reflections. The measurement is accepted when two clear echoes are seen.

After the measurement, the pulse-echo device software will analyze the apparent cortical bone thickness and a density-index value, which is an estimation of proximal femur mineral density. After analysis, a report is prepared, which includes density index value with classification (green, yellow, and red) that is based on a 90% sensitivity and specificity thresholds for osteoporosis. The interpretation of the yellow and red results will require the clinical evaluation of a physician to determine whether a referral to the dual-energy X-ray absorptiometry (DXA) measurement or treatment of osteoporosis is appropriate.

▶Electroretinography (ERG) is used to evaluate function of the retina and optic nerve of the eye, including photoreceptors and ganglion cells. A number of techniques that target different areas of the eye, including full field (flash and flicker) (92273) for a global response of photoreceptors of the retina, multifocal (92274) for photoreceptors in multiple separate locations in the retina, including the macula, and pattern (0509T) for retinal ganglion cells, are used. Multiple additional terms and techniques are used to describe various types of ERG. If the technique used is not specifically named in the code descriptors for 92273, 92274, 0509T, use the unlisted procedure code 92499.◀

● **0509T**   Electroretinography (ERG) with interpretation and report, pattern (PERG)

▶(For full-field ERG, use 92273)◀

▶(For multifocal ERG, use 92274)◀

Rationale

Code 0509T has been added to describe pattern electroretinography (PERG). New guidelines and parenthetical notes have been added regarding the reporting of electroretinography (ERG) testing.

The addition of code 0509T is a result of a Centers for Medicare & Medicaid Services (CMS) analysis, which identified code 92275 (ERG) as potentially misvalued due to a sharp increase in utilization. This increase was due to the use of code 92275 to report PERG testing, which is a different procedure from ERG as described by code 92275. In order to accommodate appropriate coding and tracking of PERG testing, code 0509T has been added.

★ = Telemedicine   ✚ = Add-on code   ✎ = FDA approval pending   # = Resequenced code   ⊘ = Modifier 51 exempt

PERG evaluates retinal ganglion cells, which are located in the center of the retina. PERG testing may be performed for detection of conditions such as glaucoma. Interpretation and report are included in code 0509T; therefore, it must be performed in order to report code 0509T. Note that two additional types of ERG testing (full field ERG [ffERG] and multifocal ERG [mfERG]) are described in the Medicine section of the CPT code set. The new guidelines in Category III provide definitions for all three types of ERG and the parenthetical notes provide instructions on how to report these tests.

Refer to the codebook and the Rationale for codes 92273 and 92274 for a full discussion of these codes.

Clinical Example (0509T)

A 66-year-old female presents with possible mild optic disc cupping and possible glaucoma.

Description of Procedure (0509T)

Take patient un-dilated and wearing best correction into testing room. Position patient in a chair in front of the instrument display with a reversing pattern of light and dark fields. Topical anesthesia may be administered. Place electrodes on patient's forehead and on the inferior corneal surface of each eye or transcutaneously. Select a testing protocol. Record a pooled electrical response of retinal ganglion cells from the macular region. Physician evaluates the tracings and prepares a report.

0510T	Code is out of numerical sequence. See 0332T-0339T
0511T	Code is out of numerical sequence. See 0332T-0339T
0512T	Code is out of numerical sequence. See 0101T-0107T
0513T	Code is out of numerical sequence. See 0101T-0107T
+● 0514T	Intraoperative visual axis identification using patient fixation (List separately in addition to code for primary procedure)

▶(Use 0514T in conjunction with 66982, 66984)◀

Rationale

Code 0514T has been established to report intraoperative visual axis identification. This add-on code should be reported in conjunction with codes 66982 and 66984 (services related to removal of extracapsular cataract).

Prior to 2019, there was no CPT code to report visual-access alignment. Visual-access alignment enables physicians to align a permanent mark on the patient's unique visual access, which is preserved throughout the surgery. The location of the visual axis is highly variable among patients, which is dictated by individual anatomical differences of the eye. Those with large visual axis deviations have a greater chance of developing undesired visual phenomena.

Intraoperative visual axis identification enables the physician to obtain the precise location of the patient's visual axis intraoperatively before initiating any cataract surgical manipulations that disrupt the visual axis. The obtained location of the patient's visual axis is preserved for later use in surgery to create a reference marker for intraocular lenses positioning on the visual axis. It is anticipated that code 0514T will be used initially in associated conditions, such as age-related cataract treatment.

Clinical Example (0514T)

A 67-year-old female patient, who is scheduled to undergo cataract surgery with intraocular lens implantation, also requires visual axis identification using patient fixation.

Description of Procedure (0514T)

Prior to cataract extraction, the surgeon and the patient review how to perform fixation on the surgeon's command and the need to keep the patient more awake at the beginning of surgery to allow the patient to better fixate during the procedure. The surgeon then guides the patient to voluntary fixate on a designated microscope light as the patient is looking through a transparent visual axis alignment device within the anterior chamber. Concurrently, the surgeon looks through the coaxial eyepiece to view the reflections of that fixation light on the patient's eye to identify the P1 Purkinje image and the patient's visual axis.

▶Wireless Cardiac Stimulation System for Left Ventricular Pacing◀

▶A wireless cardiac stimulator system provides biventricular pacing by sensing right ventricular pacing output from a previously implanted conventional device (pacemaker or defibrillator, with univentricular or biventricular leads), and then transmitting an ultrasound pulse to a wireless electrode implanted on the endocardium of the left ventricle, which then emits a left ventricular pacing pulse.

The complete system consists of two components: a wireless endocardial left ventricle electrode and a pulse generator. The pulse generator has two components: a transmitter and a battery. The electrode is implanted transarterially into the left ventricular wall and powered wirelessly using ultrasound delivered by a subcutaneously implanted transmitter. Two subcutaneous pockets are created on the chest wall, one for the battery and one for the transmitter, and these two components are connected by a subcutaneously tunneled cable.

Patients with a wireless cardiac stimulator require programming/interrogation of their existing conventional device, as well as the wireless device. The wireless cardiac stimulator is programmed and interrogated with its own separate programmer and settings.

Code 0515T describes insertion of a complete wireless cardiac stimulator system (electrode and pulse generator, which includes transmitter and battery), including interrogation, programming, pocket creation, revision and repositioning, and all echocardiography and other imaging to guide the procedure, when performed. Use 0516T only when insertion of the electrode is a stand-alone procedure. For insertion of only a new generator or generator component (battery and/or transmitter), use 0517T.

For removal of only the generator or a generator component (battery and/or transmitter) without replacement, use 0518T. For removal and replacement of a generator or a generator component (battery and/or transmitter), use 0519T. For battery and/or generator removal and reinsertion performed together with a new electrode insertion, use 0520T.

All catheterization and imaging guidance (including transthoracic or transesophageal echocardiography) required to complete a wireless cardiac stimulator procedure is included in 0515T, 0516T, 0517T, 0518T, 0519T, 0520T. Do not report 76000, 76998, 93303-93355 in conjunction with 0515T, 0516T, 0517T, 0518T, 0519T, 0520T.

Do not report left heart catheterization codes (93452, 93453, 93458, 93459, 93460, 93461, 93531, 93532, 93533) for delivery of a wireless cardiac stimulator electrode into the left ventricle.◄

● **0515T** Insertion of wireless cardiac stimulator for left ventricular pacing, including device interrogation and programming, and imaging supervision and interpretation, when performed; complete system (includes electrode and generator [transmitter and battery])

● **0516T** electrode only

● **0517T** pulse generator component(s) (battery and/or transmitter) only

►(Do not report 0515T, 0516T, 0517T in conjunction with 0518T, 0519T, 0520T, 0521T, 0522T)◄

● **0518T** Removal of only pulse generator component(s) (battery and/or transmitter) of wireless cardiac stimulator for left ventricular pacing

►(Do not report 0518T in conjunction with 0515T, 0516T, 0517T, 0519T, 0520T, 0521T, 0522T)◄

● **0519T** Removal and replacement of wireless cardiac stimulator for left ventricular pacing; pulse generator component(s) (battery and/or transmitter)

● **0520T** pulse generator component(s) (battery and/or transmitter), including placement of a new electrode

►(Do not report 0519T, 0520T in conjunction with 0515T, 0516T, 0517T, 0518T, 0521T, 0522T)◄

● **0521T** Interrogation device evaluation (in person) with analysis, review and report, includes connection, recording, and disconnection per patient encounter, wireless cardiac stimulator for left ventricular pacing

►(Do not report 0521T in conjunction with 0515T, 0516T, 0517T, 0518T, 0519T, 0520T, 0522T)◄

● **0522T** Programming device evaluation (in person) with iterative adjustment of the implantable device to test the function of the device and select optimal permanent programmed values with analysis, including review and report, wireless cardiac stimulator for left ventricular pacing

►(Do not report 0522T in conjunction with 0515T, 0516T, 0517T, 0518T, 0519T, 0520T, 0521T)◄

Rationale

A new Category III subsection titled "Wireless Cardiac Stimulation System for Left Ventricular Pacing" and eight new Category III codes with guidelines and parenthetical notes have been established to report insertion; removal, removal with replacement; interrogation; and programming for a wireless cardiac stimulator system (electrode, transmitter, and battery) used for resynchronization of the heart. Existing parenthetical notes following codes 76000 and 76998 have been revised to accommodate the addition of the new Category III codes and section.

Wireless cardiac stimulation is accomplished using components from a previously implanted conventional device (which may have uni- or biventricular leads) that are activated by a wireless cardiac stimulator system. The wireless system consists of a wireless endocardiac left ventricular electrode and a pulse generator (which

Category III 0042T-0542T

consists of a transmitter and a battery source). The wireless components communicate with the previously implanted conventional pacemaker or defibrillator device using ultrasonic signals to activate the conventional device's implanted components. This results in the stimulation of the ventricular cardiac tissue (a "beat") via univentricular or biventricular leads according to the cadence of the wireless device.

Because imaging procedures are necessary for appropriate placement of the electrode used for the pacing and battery placement, they are inherently included as part of the procedure. Exclusionary parenthetical notes that follow codes 76000 (fluoroscopy) and 76998 (ultrasound guidance) in the Radiology section have been revised to prohibit reporting these codes in conjunction with the wireless cardiac stimulation procedure codes (0515T, 0516T, 0517T, 0518T, 0519T, 0520T). The guidelines associated with this new section provide additional instruction regarding inclusion of imaging, as well as catheterization and programming or interrogation needed for the placement and use of the device. This includes specific instruction that restricts reporting echocardiographic catheterizations (93303-93355) and left heart cardiac catheterization (93452-93461, 93531-93533) performed for the delivery of the wireless cardiac stimulator electrode into the left ventricle.

The guidelines for this new subsection also provide specific instructions regarding how to report the complete service (ie, insertion, imaging, interrogation/programming), as well as reporting for individual components when provided as separate services. This includes specific instructions regarding the use of code 0519T to identify removal and replacement of a generator/generator component and how to report generator removal with reinsertion performed with new electrode insertion (0520T).

Parenthetical notes within the section also provide additional instruction regarding the correct codes to use to report combined elements of these procedures (eg, removal and replacement of the generator components).

Clinical Example (0515T)

A 65-year-old female has ischemic cardiomyopathy, ejection fraction (EF) 28%, QRS 165ms (intrinsic), left bundle branch block and New York Heart Association (NYHA) Class III congestive heart failure. The patient meets Class I indications for cardiac resynchronization therapy (CRT) with conventional CRT-D device with no improvement. The patient is a nonresponder to CRT presenting for wireless cardiac stimulator system for left ventricular (LV) pacing.

Description of Procedure (0515T)

Obtain informed consent from the patient. Bring the patient to the electrophysiology laboratory and anesthetize to achieve deep sedation. Perform transthoracic echocardiography (TTE) imaging to verify the appropriate intercostal location to implant the transmitter. Prepare and drape the skin and make a 4-cm vertical skin incision. Using sharp and blunt technique, create pockets. Use a tunneling tool to place a drain from the battery pocket to the medial incision. Insert the transmitter's cable into the drain and pull through the tunnel to the battery pocket. Position the transmitter medially in the channel and secure. Connect the device battery to the cable and then secure in the battery pocket. Fill the pockets with saline and close suture incisions in two layers.

Prepare and drape the left groin in the usual sterile manner and administer anticoagulant. Obtain femoral arterial access. Utilizing a long sheath and a pigtail dilator, place the LV electrode within the LV. Verify appropriate positioning utilizing electrophysiologic evaluation. Then secure the electrode in place. Withdraw the placement sheath and achieve vascular hemostasis. Evaluate the system for biventricular capture functionality with the programmer.

Clinical Example (0516T)

A 65-year-old female has ischemic cardiomyopathy, EF 28%, QRS 165ms, left bundle branch block, and New York Heart Association Class III congestive heart failure. The patient meets Class I indications for CRT with a conventional CRT-D device with no improvement. The patient is a nonresponder to CRT presenting for insertion of a wireless cardiac stimulator electrode only for LV pacing.

Description of Procedure (0516T)

Obtain informed consent from the patient. Bring the patient to the electrophysiology laboratory and anesthetize to achieve deep sedation. Prepare and drape the left groin in the usual sterile manner and administer anticoagulant. Obtain femoral arterial access. Utilizing a long sheath and a pigtail dilator, place the LV electrode within the LV. Verify appropriate positioning utilizing electrophysiologic evaluation. Then secure the electrode in place. Withdraw the placement sheath and achieve vascular hemostasis.

Evaluate the system for biventricular capture functionality with the programmer. Perform the evaluation only when the transmitter and battery are implanted before the time of electrode insertion.

Clinical Example (0517T)

A 65-year-old female has ischemic cardiomyopathy, EF 28%, QRS 165ms, left bundle branch block, and New York Heart Association Class III congestive heart failure. The patient meets Class I indications for CRT with a conventional CRT-D device with no improvement. The patient is a nonresponder to CRT presenting for insertion of a wireless cardiac stimulator transmitter and battery for left ventricular pacing.

Description of Procedure (0517T)

Obtain informed consent from the patient. Bring the patient to the electrophysiology laboratory and anesthetize to achieve deep sedation. Perform TTE imaging to verify the appropriate intercostal location to implant the transmitter. Prepare and drape the skin and make a 4-cm vertical skin incision.

Using sharp and blunt technique, create pockets. Utilize a tunneling tool to place a drain from the battery pocket to the medial incision. Insert the transmitter's cable into the drain and pull through the tunnel to the battery pocket. Position the transmitter medially in the channel and secure. Connect the battery to the cable and then secure in the battery pocket. Fill the pockets with saline and close suture incisions in two layers. Then evaluate the system for biventricular capture functionality with the programmer. Perform the evaluation only when the electrode is implanted before the time of transmitter and battery insertion.

Clinical Example (0518T)

A 65-year-old female with a wireless cardiac stimulator system for LV pacing implanted previously develops a mild infection of the subcutaneous pocket. The pulse generator is removed followed by antibiotic treatment. A new pulse generator insertion will be performed after the infection has been resolved.

Description of Procedure (0518T)

Make an incision along the previous implant incision scar. Access the existing pocket and take care to remove the battery from the pocket. Using a torque wrench, disconnect the transmitter cable. Fill the pocket with saline and close the suture incision.

Clinical Example (0519T)

A 65-year-old female came in for a four-year follow-up with a low-battery voltage warning. At follow-up, the device exhibited biventricular pacing and the patient reported feeling well. After discussions with patient, it was agreed to proceed with battery replacement.

Description of Procedure (0519T)

Obtain informed consent from the patient. Bring the patient to the electrophysiology laboratory and anesthetize to achieve deep sedation. For the battery replacement, make an incision along the previous implant incision scar. Access the existing pocket and take care to remove the battery from the pocket. Using a torque wrench, disconnect the transmitter cable. Inspect the transmitter cable connector and battery header connection for any fluid or material inside; no issues noted. Then insert the transmitter cable into the new battery and tighten the set screws. Then place the battery into the existing pocket and secure with two sutures. Fill the pocket with saline and close the suture incision. Then evaluate the system for biventricular capture functionality with the programmer. Confirm biventricular pacing with previous settings.

Clinical Example (0520T)

A 65-year-old female came in for a four-year follow-up with a low-battery voltage warning. A device evaluation is performed to assess device, battery, and electrode function. Based on the diagnostics, the pulse generator, and programmer testing, it was found that the electrode was not functioning properly. After discussions with the patient, it was agreed to proceed with battery replacement and insertion of a new electrode.

Description of Procedure (0520T)

Obtain informed consent from the patient. Bring the patient to the electrophysiology laboratory and anesthetize to achieve deep sedation. For the battery replacement, make an incision along the previous implant incision scar. Access the existing pocket and take care to remove the battery from the pocket. Using a torque wrench, disconnect the transmitter cable. Inspect the transmitter cable connector and battery header connection for any fluid or material inside; no issues noted. Insert the transmitter cable into the new battery and tighten set screws. Then place the battery into the existing pocket and secure with two sutures. Fill the pocket with saline and close the suture incision.

Prepare and drape the left groin in the usual sterile manner and administer anticoagulant. Obtain femoral arterial access. Utilizing a long sheath and a pigtail dilator, place the LV electrode within the LV. Verify appropriate positioning utilizing electrophysiologic evaluation, then secure the electrode in place. Withdraw the placement sheath and obtain vascular hemostasis. Evaluate the system for biventricular capture functionality with the programmer. Confirm biventricular pacing with previous settings.

Category III   0042T-0542T

Clinical Example (0521T)

A 65-year-old female has ischemic cardiomyopathy, EF 28%, QRS 165ms, ! bundle branch block, and New York Heart Association Class III congestive heart failure. The patient meets Class I indications for CRT with a conventional CRT device with no improvement. The patient is a nonresponder to CRT with a wireless cardiac stimulator for LV pacing. The patient presents to the clinic for in-person follow-up to assess device function.

Description of Procedure (0521T)

Physician reviews the existing information and relevant clinical data to clarify the indications for the interrogation device evaluation (in person). Review patient records to identify the manufacturer and model of the wireless cardiac stimulation system pulse generator and electrode. Review prior records of the pulse generator and electrode and the programmed parameters too. In addition, review prior assessments of sensing characteristics and the patient's arrhythmia history, including any recent clinical events.

Interrogate the wireless cardiac stimulation system for information. Perform a critical review of the interrogated data with assessment of the appropriateness of the function of system and assessment of device function. Data-review includes: (1) testing to verify appropriateness of sensing of the coimplant right ventricular (RV) pacing signal and wireless cardiac stimulation system sensing vectors; (2) ultrasound/ pacing threshold testing; (3) alerts generated from the device; (4) battery status; and (5) evaluation of diagnostics, including the RV-pacing detection, RV-pacing spikes within rate limit, and LV-pacing attempts. Prepare, review, approve, sign, and distribute a final report.

Clinical Example (0522T)

A 65-year-old female has ischemic cardiomyopathy, EF 28%, QRS 165ms, left bundle branch block, and New York Heart Association Class III congestive heart failure. The patient meets Class I indications for CRT with a conventional CRT device with no improvement. The patient is a nonresponder to CRT with a wireless cardiac stimulator. A device evaluation is performed to assess device, function, and programming to the diagnostic parameters based on the patient's interrogated data.

Description of Procedure (0522T)

Assess patient history for indications and for changes in, or development of, interval symptoms or clinical episodes of arrhythmia or heart failure events. Review prior diagnostic history and previous programmed settings of the device. Query changes in anti-arrhythmic medications since the last device evaluation. Establish a communication link between the pulse generator and the programmer.

Make a detailed physician analysis of the following: (1) full interrogation of the stored pulse generator parameters obtained to verify appropriateness of sensing of the coimplant RV pacing signal and wireless cardiac stimulation system sensing vectors; (2) ultrasound/ pacing threshold testing; (3) alerts generated from the device; (4) battery status; and (5) evaluation of diagnostics, including the RV-pacing detection, RV-pacing spikes with rate limit, and LV-pacing attempts. Based on these analyzed information, the physician determines the appropriate settings and make detailed analyses on the sensing characteristics. If abnormal sensing is observed, then a change in the sense vector is made.

0523T	Code is out of numerical sequence. See 0503T-0506T
● 0524T	Endovenous catheter directed chemical ablation with balloon isolation of incompetent extremity vein, open or percutaneous, including all vascular access, catheter manipulation, diagnostic imaging, imaging guidance and monitoring

Rationale

Code 0524T has been added to report endovenous catheter directed chemical ablation with balloon isolation of incompetent extremity vein. This endovenous ablation procedure differs from mechanical occlusion chemical ablation (36473, 36474) in that this procedure uses a balloon to isolate the incompetent vein from other veins in the deep system when delivering the embolizing or sclerosing agent.

The procedure described in code 0524T employs a multi-lumen catheter with the inflatable balloon located at the distal tip. The distal lumen may be used to insert a guidewire for catheter placement in the event that there is difficulty threading the device, or it may be used for delivery of contrast agents during the procedure. The inflatable balloon is used to isolate the incompetent vein from the nontreated veins and for delivery of the embolizing or sclerosing agent to the incompetent vein. Code 0524T includes diagnostic imaging and imaging guidance performed in support of the procedure. Monitoring of vascular access and catheter manipulation is also included. The catheter may be introduced via percutaneous or cutdown approach.

Clinical Example (0524T)

A 46-year-old active female, whose mother had varicose vein surgery, presents with lower-extremity swelling and fatigue related to prolonged activity. A venous Doppler ultrasound demonstrates superficial venous reflux of the great saphenous vein. There was also noted loss of phasic flow in the common femoral vein.

Description of Procedure (0524T)

Place the patient in reverse-Trendelenburg position. Under sterile ultrasound guidance, access the great saphenous vein, either percutaneously or via cutdown. Insert a sheath (9 Fr) and insert the balloon catheter to the level of the saphenofemoral junction. With the device in the appropriate position, take the patient out of reverse-Trendelenburg position. Inflate the distal occlusion balloon and deliver the sclerosing solution. After delivery of the appropriate amount of solution, use the ultrasound probe to milk the solution proximally and distally in the vessel and allow to stand for two to four minutes. The solution is aspirated while milking the vessel from distal (sheath) to proximal (balloon site) with the probe. The balloon is then deflated and the catheter is retracted while aspiration continues. Place a suture at the access site. Wrap the leg in a compression dressing.

● **0525T** Insertion or replacement of intracardiac ischemia monitoring system, including testing of the lead and monitor, initial system programming, and imaging supervision and interpretation; complete system (electrode and implantable monitor)

● **0526T** electrode only

● **0527T** implantable monitor only

▶(Do not report 0525T, 0526T, 0527T in conjunction with 93000, 93005, 93010, 0528T, 0529T)◀

▶(For removal and replacement of intracardiac ischemia monitoring system or its components, see 0525T, 0526T, 0527T in conjunction with 0530T, 0531T, 0532T, as appropriate)◀

● **0528T** Programming device evaluation (in person) of intracardiac ischemia monitoring system with iterative adjustment of programmed values, with analysis, review, and report

▶(Do not report 0528T in conjunction with 93000, 93005, 93010, 0525T, 0526T, 0527T, 0529T, 0530T, 0531T, 0532T)◀

● **0529T** Interrogation device evaluation (in person) of intracardiac ischemia monitoring system with analysis, review, and report

▶(Do not report 0529T in conjunction with 93000, 93005, 93010, 0525T, 0526T, 0527T, 0528T, 0530T, 0531T, 0532T)◀

● **0530T** Removal of intracardiac ischemia monitoring system, including all imaging supervision and interpretation; complete system (electrode and implantable monitor)

● **0531T** electrode only

● **0532T** implantable monitor only

▶(Do not report 0530T, 0531T, 0532T in conjunction with 0528T, 0529T)◀

Rationale

Codes 0525T, 0526T, 0527T, 0528T, 0529T, 0530T, 0531T, and 0532T have been established to report intracardiac ischemia monitoring services. In addition, parenthetical notes have been added in the Medicine and Category III sections to provide instruction on the appropriate reporting of these services in conjunction with other services.

An intracardiac ischemic monitoring device system may be used to detect and alert patients during a major ischemic coronary event, such as ST-elevation myocardial infarction (STEMI) or non-STEMI. The device can detect and alert patients to both symptomatic and asymptomatic ischemic coronary events. Further, the function of this entire device (generator and transvenous lead) is to detect repeat ischemic coronary events in patients that are at high risk for a repeat ischemic coronary event.

Codes 0525T, 0526T, and 0527T include both insertion or replacement. To further clarify, code 0525T describes insertion or replacement of the complete system (electrode and implantable monitor). The insertion or replacement of only the electrode is described by code 0526T. Code 0527T describes insertion or replacement of the implantable monitor only. Code 0528T describes the programming device evaluation of the monitoring system with iterative adjustments to capture programmed values, analysis, review, and report. The interrogation of the intracardiac ischemia monitoring system with analysis, review, and report is described by code 0529T.

Codes 0530T, 0531T, and 0532T includes removal of the monitoring system, including all imaging, supervision, and interpretation. To further clarify, code 0530T describes the removal of the complete system (electrode and implantable monitor). The removal of only electrode is described by code 0531T. Code 0532T describes the removal of the implantable monitor only.

Clinical Example (0525T)

A postmenopausal 62-year-old female with prior myocardial infarction (MI), diabetes mellitus, hypertension, and hyperlipidemia presents with unstable angina due to a 70% stenosis of the right coronary artery. Medical management is optimized. In order to manage potential subsequent ischemic events, an intracardiac ischemic monitoring system is implanted.

Description of Procedure (0525T)

Transport the patient to the cardiac catheterization laboratory in a fasting state. Provide moderate sedation. Prepare and drape the region of the left deltopectoral groove. Prior to the incision, the patient undergoes moderate sedation with local anesthesia. An electrophysiologist, cardiologist, or cardiovascular surgeon then performs the percutaneous access of the left axillary vein. Locate the vein under fluoroscopy after administering 5 cc of contrast in the left peripheral intravenously (IV). Advance a wire in the left axillary vein using fluoroscopy. Following this, make a transverse incision through the skin and subcutaneous tissue, exposing the pectoral fascia and muscle beneath. Fashion a pocket in the medial direction. Using the previously placed guidewire, advance a peel-away sheath over the wire into the vein. Remove the dilator and wire. Under fluoroscopy, pass an active pacing lead across the tricuspid valve and position in the apex of the right ventricle. Remove the peel-away sheath. Establish adequate sensing function. Perform both unipolar and bipolar lead testing to confirm proper placement and fixation. Then advance the suture sleeve to the entry point of the tissue and connect securely to the tissue. Wash the pocket with antibiotic-impregnated saline. Obtain and connect an ischemia-monitoring device (IMD) securely to the lead. Coil any excess lead within the pocket. Initiate a data retrieval session using the data retrieval instructions. Upon successful data retrieval, pass a suture through the holes in the IMD to secure the device, and flush and close the device pocket in layers to reduce dead space. Transport the patient to the recovery room. Prior to discharge, interrogate the IMD, adjust the settings to allow the device to collect sample data (minimal programming), and obtain and record electrogram readings. Generate a procedure report.

Clinical Example (0526T)

At a one-year follow-up of a previously placed IMD in a 61-year-old female, it is determined that the transvenous lead is not adequately capturing the intracardiac electrocardiographic (ECG) signal and the cardiologist/electrophysiologist determines that this lead requires replacement/revision.

Description of Procedure (0526T)

An interventional electrophysiologist, cardiologist, or cardiovascular surgeon performs the procedure in a catheterization or electrophysiology laboratory. Prior to the incision, the patient undergoes moderate sedation. Local anesthetic is administered. The device pocket is surgically entered. Using a combination of blunt and

sharp dissection, free the device from the fascia. Under fluoroscopy, extract the old active-fixation pacing lead. Using a guidewire placed in the axillary vein, advance a peel-away sheath over the wire into the vein. Disconnect the device from the old transvenous lead. Remove the dilator and wire. Then pass the new active pacing lead across the tricuspid valve and position in the apex of the right ventricle. Remove the peel-away sheath. Establish adequate sensing function. Connect the new lead to the existing device. Again, verify adequate sensing function. Coil any excess lead within the pocket. Initiate a data retrieval session using the data-retrieval instructions. Upon successful data retrieval, pass a suture through the holes in the IMD to secure the device, and flush and close the device pocket in layers. Apply a sterile pressure dressing. Prior to recovery, interrogate the IMD, record the electrogram readings, and generate a report. Transport the patient to the recovery room.

Clinical Example (0527T)

At the seven-year follow-up appointment of a 68-year-old female, who has a previously placed ischemia monitoring system, it is determined that the device's battery is depleted and replacement is indicated. The old device is replaced with a new monitor, which is connected to the previously implanted lead.

Description of Procedure (0527T)

An interventional cardiologist, electrophysiologist, or a cardiovascular surgeon performs the procedure in an operating room. Prior to the incision, the patient undergoes moderate sedation. Provide local anesthetic over the palpable region of previously implanted ischemia monitor. Enter the device pocket surgically. Using a combination of blunt and sharp dissection, free the indwelling device from the fascia. Detach and explant the device from the lead. Interrogate the current lead to ensure appropriate sensing thresholds. Once this IMD has been explanted, place a new device either in the same pocket created in the left pectoral tissue dorsal to the skin incision or in an alternate site. Then connect the existing lead to the new IMD. Coil any excess lead within the pocket. Initiate a data retrieval session using the data-retrieval instructions. Upon successful data retrieval, pass a suture through the holes in the IMD to secure the device, and then flush and close the incision in layers to reduce dead space. Prior to recovery, interrogate the IMD and record the electrogram readings. Generate a procedure report. Transport the patient to the recovery room.

Clinical Example (0528T)

A 55-year-old female with a previously placed intracardiac ischemia monitoring system presents for programming of the device.

Description of Procedure (0528T)

Obtain a brief examination and directed history. Obtain a 12-lead EKG. Physician programmer interrogates the implantable device. A cardiologist, electrophysiologist, or qualified health care professional uses physician programmer to obtain data for the patient in a physician office or hospital outpatient setting. The clinician establishes the implantable device alarm and alert-configuration settings for patient's use. The ST-thresholds for all subjects are initially set using a feature of the physician programmer, which analyzes ST-deviation histogram data. Using a software feature termed "Autopick," a threshold for acute coronary syndrome (ACS) detection is set for the patient's normal heart-rate range with thresholds for demand ischemia to set in up to four elevated heart-rate ranges. The patient undergoes training on and review of the meaning of the alarms and the appropriate action to take upon occurrence of a device alarm.

Clinical Example (0529T)

A postmenopausal, 60-year-old female with a previously placed intracardiac ischemia monitoring system presents at the cardiologist's/electrophysiologist's office for evaluation of device status and function.

Description of Procedure (0529T)

Obtain a brief examination and directed history. The cardiologist or qualified health care professional uses physician programmer to retrieve the ischemia, threshold, and event data from the implanted intracardiac ischemia monitor in a physician office or hospital outpatient setting. The physician then reviews the data and generates a report. When interrogation occurs at the scheduled six-month visits, the physician also checks parameter settings and saves any parameter changes based on review, reviews medications taken and records any changes, provides reinforcement training on alarms, and checks the occurrence of any symptomatic adverse experiences. Update the threshold settings based on the up-to-14 days of ST-level data stored in five heart-rate ranges downloaded from the implantable device in histogram format. The programmer calculates the appropriate threshold levels for detection of transmural and sub-endocardial ischemic events and uploads those thresholds to the implantable device.

Clinical Example (0530T)

A 62-year-old female is scheduled for magnetic resonance imaging (MRI), which is medically necessary. A decision is made to remove the electrode lead and intracardiac ischemia-monitoring device.

Description of Procedure (0530T)

The procedure is performed by an interventional cardiologist or electrophysiologist in an interventional catheterization or electrophysiology laboratory. Before the incision, the patient undergoes moderate sedation. Enter the device pocket surgically. Using a combination of blunt and sharp dissection, free the device from the fascia. Disconnect the device from the transvenous lead and remove the device. Then anesthetize the patient. Under fluoroscopy, extract the active-fixation pacing lead. If the lead is over a year old, use laser if needed. Flush and close the device pocket. Apply sterile pressure dressing. Generate a procedure report. Transport the patient to the recovery room.

Clinical Example (0531T)

A 60-year-old diabetic female, who has had two prior heart attacks and who has an abandoned pacemaker lead (the ischemia monitor was removed a year or two previously), is scheduled for a medically necessary MRI, and the electrode lead must be removed.

Description of Procedure (0531T)

An interventional cardiologist or electrophysiologist in an interventional catheterization laboratory performs the procedure. Prior to the incision, the patient undergoes moderate sedation. Prepare and drape the region of the left deltopectoral groove. Administer general anesthetic and then perform percutaneous access of the left subclavian (or axillary/cephalic) vein. Locate the vein under fluoroscopy after administering 5 cc of contrast in the left peripheral IV. Then advance a sheath in the left axillary vein using fluoroscopy. Extract the active-fixation pacing lead and use laser to facilitate lead extraction, if needed. Flush and close the surgical incision. Apply a sterile pressure dressing. Generate a report. Transport the patient to the recovery room.

Clinical Example (0532T)

A 62-year-old female with progressing cardiovascular disease now needs a pacemaker.

Description of Procedure (0532T)

An interventional cardiologist, electrophysiologist, or a cardiovascular surgeon performs the procedure in an operating room. Prior to the incision, the patient undergoes moderate sedation. Administer local anesthesia over the palpable region of previously implanted ischemia monitor. Enter the device pocket surgically. Using a combination of blunt and sharp dissection, free the indwelling device from the fascia. Detach the device from the lead and explant the device. Connect a pacemaker to the lead and establish adequate sensing. Coil any excess lead within the pocket and

Category III 0042T-0542T

secure the pacemaker within the pocket. Flush and close the incision in layers to reduce dead space. Apply a sterile pressure dressing. Generate a report. Transport the patient to the recovery room.

● **0533T**   Continuous recording of movement disorder symptoms, including bradykinesia, dyskinesia, and tremor for 6 days up to 10 days; includes set-up, patient training, configuration of monitor, data upload, analysis and initial report configuration, download review, interpretation and report

● **0534T**   set-up, patient training, configuration of monitor

● **0535T**   data upload, analysis and initial report configuration

● **0536T**   download review, interpretation and report

Rationale

Four new Category III codes (0533T, 0534T, 0535T, 0536T) have been established to report the use of a noninvasive movement-recording device, which quantifies kinematics of movement disorder symptoms, including bradykinesia, dyskinesia, and tremor, by continuously recording gross motor movement over an extended period of time.

Code 0533T should be used to report set-up, patient training, configuration of monitor, data upload, analysis and initial report configuration, download review, interpretation and report. The additional codes (0534T, 0535T, 0536T) are used to report specific aspects of the entire service. For example, if only the download review and interpretation and report is performed, then code 0536T should be reported.

Prior to 2019, no code specifically described this procedure. These four new codes enable the use of a noninvasive movement-recording device to be reported. These services are usually used with patients with Parkinson's disease and patients with unspecified tremors.

Clinical Example (0533T)

A 65-year-old male presents with a five-year history of Parkinson's disease. Despite previous therapy management changes, the patient is not able to maintain gross motor control, which results in significant impact on daily activities. The clinician is unable to objectively identify movement disorder symptoms, including bradykinesia, dyskinesia, and tremor in order to adjust therapy and dosing. Personal kinetic recording is ordered.

Description of Procedure (0533T)

Refer the patient for a personal kinetigraph assessment. Give the patient the data logger and train him on how to use the device, about medication reminders, and on medication acknowledgments. The patient wears the device for seven days. The patient returns the device and the logger-movement recording data file is uploaded. Generate a patient record with analysis that includes Parkinson's symptomology charted via a summary over the course of the recording.

Clinical Example (0534T)

A 65-year-old male presents with a five-year history of Parkinson's disease. The clinician is unable to objectively identify movement disorder symptoms and a personal kinetic recording is ordered. Monitor is programmed for patient and patient is educated and trained on use of kinetic recording device, diary logging, and medication tracking.

Description of Procedure (0534T)

Refer the patient for a personal kinetigraph assessment and configure a patient-specific data logger based on information from patient's medical records. Train patient on how to use the device. Patient wears the device for seven days. Upon completion of prescribed wear time, patient returns the device for analysis.

Clinical Example (0535T)

A 65-year-old male with a five-year history of Parkinson's disease has completed the requested wear time of seven days with the personal kinetic recording device. The monitor is returned to the facility for data extraction, analysis, and report generation. An initial report is generated noting episodes of bradykinesia, dyskinesia, and tremor duration and intensity, and uploaded to HIPPA-compliant website for review and interpretation by physician or qualified health care professional.

Description of Procedure (0535T)

Patient returns the logger to the facility. Connect the logger and upload the raw data-recording file. The initial technical report includes a multipage document that includes Parkinson's symptomology charted via a summary over the course of the recording. An initial technical report consisting of graphic activity plots of symptoms over each day and total wear period, peri-dose response curves, as well as a summary data table of symptom scores, is generated.

Clinical Example (0536T)

A 65-year-old male with Parkinson's disease has a completed his seven-day use of personal kinetic recording.

Description of Procedure (0536T)

Physician downloads, reviews, and interprets the personal kinetic report with analysis, reviewing summary plots of all symptomology, daily plots of all symptomology, summary symptomology scores, and medication correlations. The physician communicates the findings of the final report to the patient and gives a copy to the referring physician, as necessary. The physician or other qualified health care professional creates a copy of the final report and stores it in the patient's file.

►Cellular and Gene Therapy◄

►Cellular and gene therapies involve the collection, processing and handling of cells or other tissues, genetic modification of those cells or tissues, and administration of the genetically modified cells or tissues with the intent to treat, modify, reverse or cure a serious or life-threatening disease or condition.

Codes 0537T, 0538T, 0539T, 0540T describe the various steps required to collect, prepare, transport, receive, and administer genetically modified T cells. The collection and handling code (0537T) may be reported only once per day, regardless of the number of collections or quantity of cells collected. Similarly, the administration code (0540T) may only be reported once per day, regardless of the number of units administered. The development of genetically modified cells is not reported with this family of codes.

Chimeric antigen receptor therapy (CAR-T) with genetically modified T cells begins with the collection of cells from the patient by peripheral blood leukocyte cell harvesting. The cells are then cryopreserved and/or otherwise prepared for processing or shipping to a manufacturing or cell processing facility, if applicable, where gene modification and expansion of the cells is performed. When gene modification and expansion of the cells by the manufacturer is complete, the genetically modified cells are returned to the physician or other qualified health care professional in which additional preparation occurs including thawing of the cryopreserved CAR-T cells, if necessary, before the cells are administered to the patient.

The procedure to administer CAR-T cells includes physician monitoring of multiple physiologic parameters,

physician verification of cell processing, evaluation of the patient during, as well as immediately before and after the administration of the CAR-T cells, physician presence during the administration and direct supervision of clinical staff, and management of any adverse events during the administration. Care on the same date of service that is not directly related to the service of administration of the CAR-T cells (eg, care provided after the administration is complete, care for the patient's underlying condition or for other medical problems) may be separately reported using the appropriate evaluation and management code with modifier 25. Management of uncomplicated adverse events (eg, nausea, urticaria) during the infusion is not reported separately.

The fluid used to administer the cells and other infusions for incidental hydration (eg, 96360, 96361) are not reported separately. Similarly, infusion(s) of any supportive medication(s) (eg, steroids) concurrently with the CAR-T cell administration are not reported separately. However, hydration or administration of medications (eg, antibiotics, opioids) unrelated to the CAR-T administration may be reported separately with modifier 59.◄

● **0537T** Chimeric antigen receptor T-cell (CAR-T) therapy; harvesting of blood-derived T lymphocytes for development of genetically modified autologous CAR-T cells, per day

● **0538T** preparation of blood-derived T lymphocytes for transportation (eg, cryopreservation, storage)

● **0539T** receipt and preparation of CAR-T cells for administration

● **0540T** CAR-T cell administration, autologous

Rationale

A new subsection titled "Cellular and Gene Therapy," new guidelines, and four new codes have been added to to identify chimeric antigen receptor T cell (CAR-T) therapy services.

As noted in the guidelines, the work identified by these codes includes services necessary to provide CAR-T treatment to a patient, in order to treat, modify, reverse, or cure a patient of a serious/life-threatening disease or condition. The work identified includes T-cells collection from the patient (includes the selection and separation of the appropriate cells for the procedure); all processing and handling of the cells (such as freezing in preparation for transport to and from the genetic modification facility); administration of genetically modified cells/tissue into the patient; and any treatment or services necessary to afford the patient comfort or to facilitate the administration of the cells to the patient. The guidelines direct users to

★ = Telemedicine   ✚ = Add-on code   ✗ = FDA approval pending   # = Resequenced code   ⊘ = Modifier 51 exempt

Category III 0042T-0542T

report handling of the cells and administration of the modified cells/tissue only once during the date of service. Included is specific language that notifies users that genetic modification of the cells/tissue to fight the disease/condition is not included as part of the services. Because modification of the T-cells by an outside facility/ laboratory is accomplished separately from the collection, processing, handling, and administration of the T-cells, it is not reported with these codes. Similarly, the expansion of the cells (ie, growing more of the cells/tissue to be used for treatment outside of the body) is not included in these codes.

The guidelines included for this section also provide specific instructions regarding how to report services that are not inherent to the CAR-T administration. Services that are typically part of the administration are included and not reported separately from the administration service identified by code 0540T.

Clinical Example (0537T)

A 67-year-old male with refractory diffuse large B-cell lymphoma is referred for treatment with autologous chimeric antigen receptor T cell (CAR-T) therapy.

Description of Procedure (0537T)

The physician or other qualified health care professional reviews the appropriate venous access with cell harvesting procedure personnel and assesses the clinical status of the patient during the cell harvesting procedure. The physician or other qualified health care professional reviews final hematological parameters and the patient's complete blood cell count (CBC) to determine if platelets need to be transfused (which is reported separately with code 36430). Quality assessment of the collected cell product is reviewed by the physician or other qualified health care professional, using assessment measures, such as cell counts, cell differentials, flow cytometry, infectious disease diagnostic and culture studies, antibody screen, and ABO-Rh results.

Clinical Example (0538T)

A 67-year-old male with refractory diffuse large B-cell lymphoma is referred for treatment with autologous CAR-T therapy.

Description of Procedure (0538T)

When required by product protocol, cryopreserve cells after collection and prior to transfer for genetic modification. Physician or other qualified health care professional performs quality measures that include assessment, review, and documentation of freezer curves

to ensure that the cells have been frozen in a manner safe for future cellular therapy use. Physician or other qualified health care professional documents unplanned deviations in standard operating procedures. Attach proper labeling to identify patient, date of collection, and assessment of risk of infectious disease transmission. Handle post-collection cell product appropriately, including placement in appropriate transport containers for shipment to site of genetic modification and relabeling for chain of custody, witnessed by two licensed professionals. Identify and record product characteristics, including infectious disease diagnostic and culture study results, which must be sent with the cells. Transfer the specimen to the manufacturer pursuant to process specifications.

Clinical Example (0539T)

A 67-year-old male with refractory diffuse large B-cell lymphoma is referred for treatment with autologous CAR-T therapy.

Description of Procedure (0539T)

Upon receipt of genetically modified cells by the center, the handling process is reversed, including facility relabeling the appropriate unique patient identifiers witnessed by two licensed professionals. Perform cell dose, sample purity, and quality assurance testing, and store cells to ensure safety and viability, and to minimize risk of product cross-contamination. Document any error in labeling. The physician or other qualified health care professional oversees the thawing of cryopreserved, genetically modified cells for cellular therapy. These cells must be thawed in a controlled manner to ensure viability and stored in containers to minimize risk of product cross-contamination. Problems or deviations must be documented.

Clinical Example (0540T)

A 67-year-old male with refractory diffuse large B-cell lymphoma is referred for treatment with autologous CAR-T therapy.

Description of Procedure (0540T)

The physician or other qualified health care professional evaluates the patient immediately before the autologous CAR-T infusion and monitors multiple physiologic parameters, including frequent monitoring of vital signs and clinical status. The physician or other qualified health care professional, nurse, and cell-processing technologist review the cell-product label, patient identification, sterility testing, and product characteristics. The physician or other qualified health care professional is present for 15 to 30 minutes to supervise the initiation of the product infusion and is immediately available to manage toxicities and complications occurring during and immediately following the infusion.

● **0541T**   Myocardial imaging by magnetocardiography (MCG) for detection of cardiac ischemia, by signal acquisition using minimum 36 channel grid, generation of magnetic-field time-series images, quantitative analysis of magnetic dipoles, machine learning–derived clinical scoring, and automated report generation, single study

● **0542T**   interpretation and report

Rationale

Two new Category III codes (0541T, 0542T) have been established to report myocardial imaging by magnetocardiography (MCG).

Code 0541T describes a single MCG study using signal acquisition, generation of magnetic-field time-series images, quantitative analysis of magnetic dipoles, machine learning-derived clinical scoring, and automated report generation. Code 0542T describes the work involved in interpreting and reporting the MCG study.

MCG is a new, noninvasive diagnostic procedure that leverages MCG technology. MCG is intended to assist in the rapid identification of cardiac ischemia that causes acute coronary syndrome (ACS), when other standard procedures for diagnosis of cardiac ischemia produce equivocal, nondiagnostic, or negative results, but ACS is still suspected or considered to be a possibility in the differential diagnosis.

Clinical Example (0541T)

A 67-year-old female with history of obesity, hypertension, and type II diabetes presents to a local emergency room with pressure over her left chest, nausea, and some mild dizziness. ECG shows nonspecific T-wave changes but is equivocal for ischemia. Initial troponin I levels are normal. Patient is referred for magnetocardiography (MCG) study.

Description of Procedure (0541T)

Place the patient supine on the device table and position a magnetic sensor grid over the chest. The technician confirms that sensor data is of adequate quality and obtains a 90-second image acquisition. Generate magnetic-field time-series images and generate an automated report with still-frame and time series magnetic images.

Clinical Example (0542T)

A 67-year-old female with history of obesity, hypertension, and type II diabetes presents to a local emergency room with pressure over her left chest, nausea, and some mild dizziness. ECG shows nonspecific T-wave changes but is equivocal for ischemia. Initial troponin I levels are normal. Patient is referred for MCG study.

Description of Procedure (0542T)

The physician or other qualified health care professional reviews the animated magnetic-field images, analytics platform results, and automated report with the patient's clinical information, and generates a final report.

★ = Telemedicine   + = Add-on code   ✗ = FDA approval pending   # = Resequenced code   ⊘ = Modifier 51 exempt

Appendix A

In Appendix A, the code range in the descriptor for modifier 63 has been revised to include code 20100. This revision comes in accordance with the deletion of code 20005.

Summary of Additions, Deletions, and Revisions

The summary of changes shows the actual changes that have been made to the code descriptors.

New codes appear with a bullet (●) and are indicated as "Code added." Revised codes are preceded with a triangle (▲). Within revised codes, or if a code symbol has been deleted, the deleted language and code symbol appears with a ~~strikethrough~~ (⊖), while new text appears <u>underlined</u>.

The ⚡ symbol is used to identify codes for vaccines that are pending FDA approval. The # symbol is used to identify codes that have been resequenced. CPT add-on codes are annotated by the + symbol. The ⊘ symbol is used to identify codes that are exempt from the use of modifier 51. The ★ symbol is used to identify codes that may be used for reporting telemedicine services. The ✖ is used to identify proprietary laboratory analyses (PLA) test that has an identical descriptor as another PLA test.

Modifier	Modifier Descriptor
63	▶**Procedure Performed on Infants less than 4 kg:** Procedures performed on neonates and infants up to a present body weight of 4 kg may involve significantly increased complexity and physician or other qualified health care professional work commonly associated with these patients. This circumstance may be reported by adding modifier 63 to the procedure number. **Note:** Unless otherwise designated, this modifier may only be appended to procedures/services listed in the 20100-69990 code series. Modifier 63 should not be appended to any CPT codes listed in the **Evaluation and Management Services, Anesthesia, Radiology, Pathology/Laboratory,** or **Medicine** sections.◀

Appendix A

Modifiers

63 ▶**Procedure Performed on Infants less than 4 kg:**
Procedures performed on neonates and infants up to a present body weight of 4 kg may involve significantly increased complexity and physician or other qualified health care professional work commonly associated with these patients. This circumstance may be reported by adding modifier 63 to the procedure number. **Note:** Unless otherwise designated, this modifier may only be appended to procedures/services listed in the 20100-69990 code series. Modifier 63 should not be appended to any CPT codes listed in the **Evaluation and Management Services, Anesthesia, Radiology, Pathology/Laboratory,** or **Medicine** sections.◀

Rationale

In support of the deletion of code 20005, the code range in the descriptor for modifier 63 has been revised to begin with code 20100, which is now the first code in that section.

Refer to the codebook and the Rationale for code 20005 for a full discussion of these changes.

★ = Telemedicine   ✚ = Add-on code   ✔ = FDA approval pending   # = Resequenced code   ⃠ = Modifier 51 exempt

Appendix L

The introductory guidelines to Appendix L have been revised to clarify the locations that can be the starting point of catheterization. In addition, the vascular charts have been revised to further clarify the order of vessels for arterial and vascular branching for catheterization procedures. In addition, multiple anatomical illustrations have been added to provide visual details of the arterial and venous vascular families.

Appendix L

Vascular Families

▶Appendix L is a vascular branching model that assumes the aorta, vena cava, pulmonary artery, or portal vein is the starting point of catheterization. Accordingly, branches have been categorized into first, second, third order, and beyond. (Note that this categorization does not apply, for instance, if a femoral or carotid artery were catheterized directly in an antegrade direction.) Common branching patterns of typical anatomy are shown in the charts and illustrations.

No specific coding instructions should be inferred from Appendix L. End-users must determine how best to code any specific procedure based on variant anatomy and different vascular access point relative to vessel(s) selectively catheterized (eg, antegrade femoral artery, radial artery, retrograde femoral to ipsilateral internal iliac artery catheterization, transsplenic splenic vein access to portal venous system, etc).◀

Reference: Standstring, S. *Gray's Anatomy: The Anatomical Basis of Clinical Practice.* 41st ed. New York: Elsevier Limited; 2016.

Rationale

The Appendix L guidelines for the vascular families have been revised to more specifically identify the base structure for the branching and to provide better directions regarding vascular access and the direction of the branching (antegrade vs retrograde). The vascular charts now reflect arterial anatomy information that more completely encompasses the vessels that would be catheterized and selected, as appropriate, when providing such services.

In accordance with the improved guidelines, new detailed arterial and venous anatomical charts have been included to provide better modeling and clarification regarding the order of vessels for arterial and venous vascular branching for catheterization procedures. In addition to the revised vascular charts, 16 new detailed illustrations of the vascular families have been added for an anatomical view of the arterial and venous vascular families.

★ = Telemedicine   ✚ = Add-on code   𝗡 = FDA approval pending   # = Resequenced code   ⃠ = Modifier 51 exempt

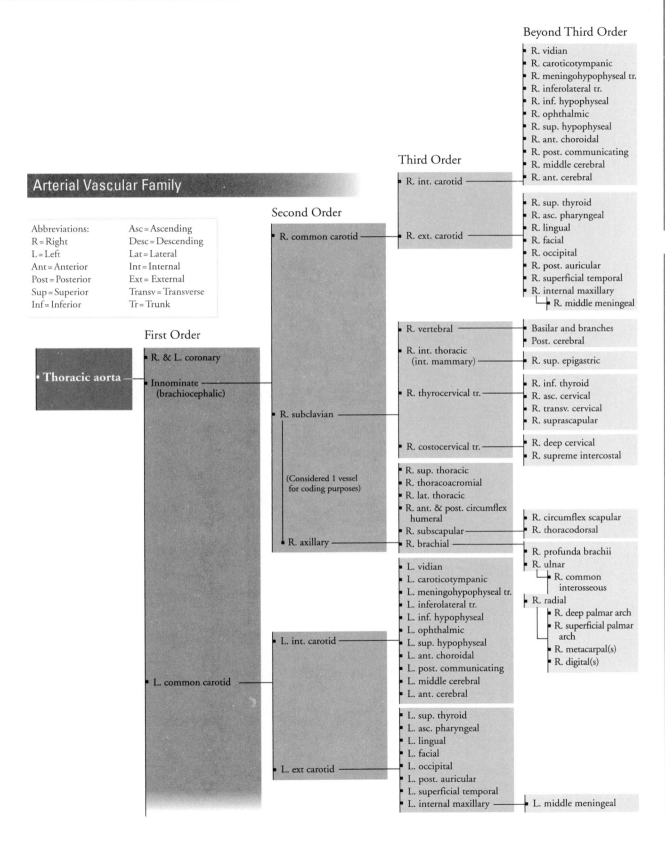

Beyond Third Order
- R. vidian
- R. caroticotympanic
- R. meningohypophyseal tr.
- R. inferolateral tr.
- R. inf. hypophyseal
- R. ophthalmic
- R. sup. hypophyseal
- R. ant. choroidal
- R. post. communicating
- R. middle cerebral
- R. ant. cerebral

Third Order
- R. int. carotid

- R. ext. carotid

  - R. sup. thyroid
  - R. asc. pharyngeal
  - R. lingual
  - R. facial
  - R. occipital
  - R. post. auricular
  - R. superficial temporal
  - R. internal maxillary
    - R. middle meningeal

Arterial Vascular Family

Second Order
- R. common carotid

Abbreviations:
R = Right   Asc = Ascending
L = Left   Desc = Descending
Ant = Anterior   Lat = Lateral
Post = Posterior   Int = Internal
Sup = Superior   Ext = External
Inf = Inferior   Transv = Transverse
                         Tr = Trunk

- R. vertebral ——— Basilar and branches / Post. cerebral
- R. int. thoracic (int. mammary) ——— R. sup. epigastric
- R. thyrocervical tr.
  - R. inf. thyroid
  - R. asc. cervical
  - R. transv. cervical
  - R. suprascapular
- R. costocervical tr.
  - R. deep cervical
  - R. supreme intercostal

First Order

- Thoracic aorta
  - R. & L. coronary
  - Innominate (brachiocephalic)

- R. subclavian

(Considered 1 vessel for coding purposes)

- R. sup. thoracic
- R. thoracoacromial
- R. lat. thoracic
- R. ant. & post. circumflex humeral
- R. subscapular
  - R. circumflex scapular
  - R. thoracodorsal
- R. axillary —— R. brachial
  - R. profunda brachii
  - R. ulnar
    - R. common interosseous
  - R. radial
    - R. deep palmar arch
    - R. superficial palmar arch
    - R. metacarpal(s)
    - R. digital(s)

- L. int. carotid
  - L. vidian
  - L. caroticotympanic
  - L. meningohypophyseal tr.
  - L. inferolateral tr.
  - L. inf. hypophyseal
  - L. ophthalmic
  - L. sup. hypophyseal
  - L. ant. choroidal
  - L. post. communicating
  - L. middle cerebral
  - L. ant. cerebral

- L. common carotid

- L. ext carotid
  - L. sup. thyroid
  - L. asc. pharyngeal
  - L. lingual
  - L. facial
  - L. occipital
  - L. post. auricular
  - L. superficial temporal
  - L. internal maxillary —— L. middle meningeal

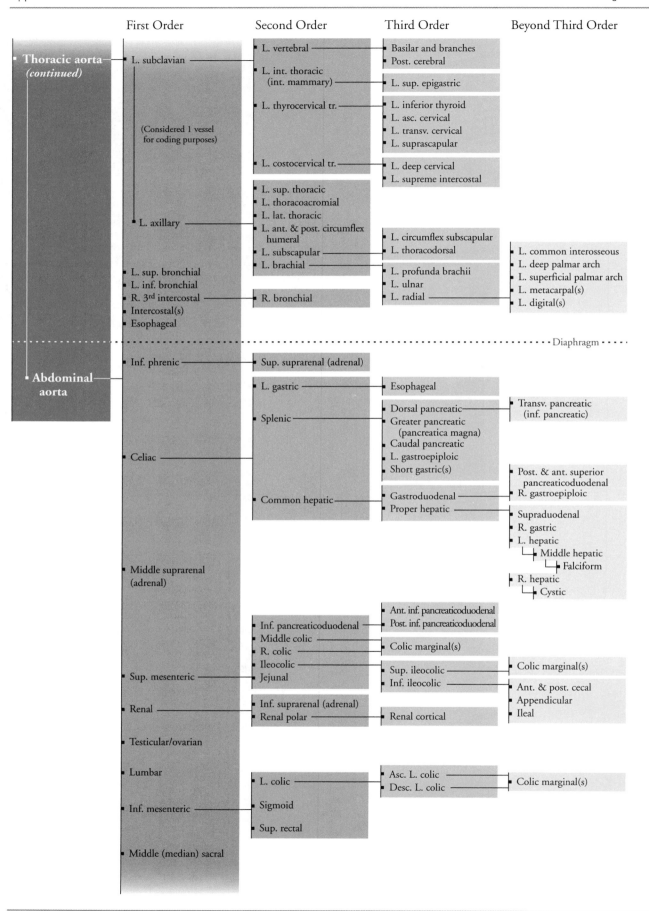

First Order | Second Order | Third Order | Beyond Third Order

Thoracic aorta *(continued)*

L. subclavian
- L. vertebral — Basilar and branches / Post. cerebral
- L. int. thoracic (int. mammary) — L. sup. epigastric
- L. thyrocervical tr. — L. inferior thyroid / L. asc. cervical / L. transv. cervical / L. suprascapular
- L. costocervical tr. — L. deep cervical / L. supreme intercostal

(Considered 1 vessel for coding purposes)

L. axillary
- L. sup. thoracic
- L. thoracoacromial
- L. lat. thoracic
- L. ant. & post. circumflex humeral
- L. subscapular — L. circumflex subscapular / L. thoracodorsal
- L. brachial — L. profunda brachii / L. ulnar / L. radial — L. common interosseous / L. deep palmar arch / L. superficial palmar arch / L. metacarpal(s) / L. digital(s)

- L. sup. bronchial
- L. inf. bronchial
- R. 3rd intercostal — R. bronchial
- Intercostal(s)
- Esophageal

· · · · · Diaphragm · · · · ·

Abdominal aorta

- Inf. phrenic — Sup. suprarenal (adrenal)

- Celiac
  - L. gastric — Esophageal
  - Splenic — Dorsal pancreatic — Transv. pancreatic (inf. pancreatic) / Greater pancreatic (pancreatica magna) / Caudal pancreatic / L. gastroepiploic / Short gastric(s)
  - Common hepatic — Gastroduodenal — Post. & ant. superior pancreaticoduodenal / R. gastroepiploic / Proper hepatic — Supraduodenal / R. gastric / L. hepatic — Middle hepatic — Falciform / R. hepatic — Cystic

- Middle suprarenal (adrenal)

- Sup. mesenteric
  - Inf. pancreaticoduodenal — Ant. inf. pancreaticoduodenal / Post. inf. pancreaticoduodenal
  - Middle colic — Colic marginal(s)
  - R. colic
  - Ileocolic — Sup. ileocolic — Colic marginal(s) / Inf. ileocolic — Ant. & post. cecal / Appendicular / Ileal
  - Jejunal

- Renal
  - Inf. suprarenal (adrenal)
  - Renal polar — Renal cortical

- Testicular/ovarian

- Lumbar

- Inf. mesenteric
  - L. colic — Asc. L. colic / Desc. L. colic — Colic marginal(s)
  - Sigmoid
  - Sup. rectal

- Middle (median) sacral

★ = Telemedicine   ✚ = Add-on code   ✒ = FDA approval pending   # = Resequenced code   ⊘ = Modifier 51 exempt

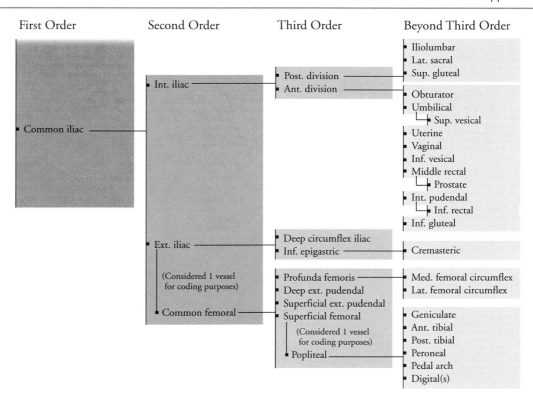

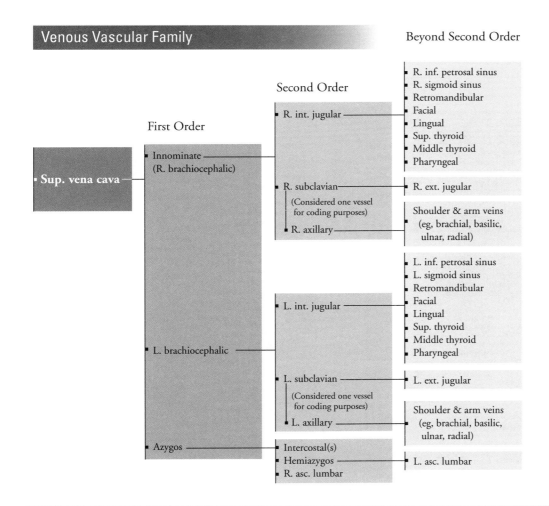

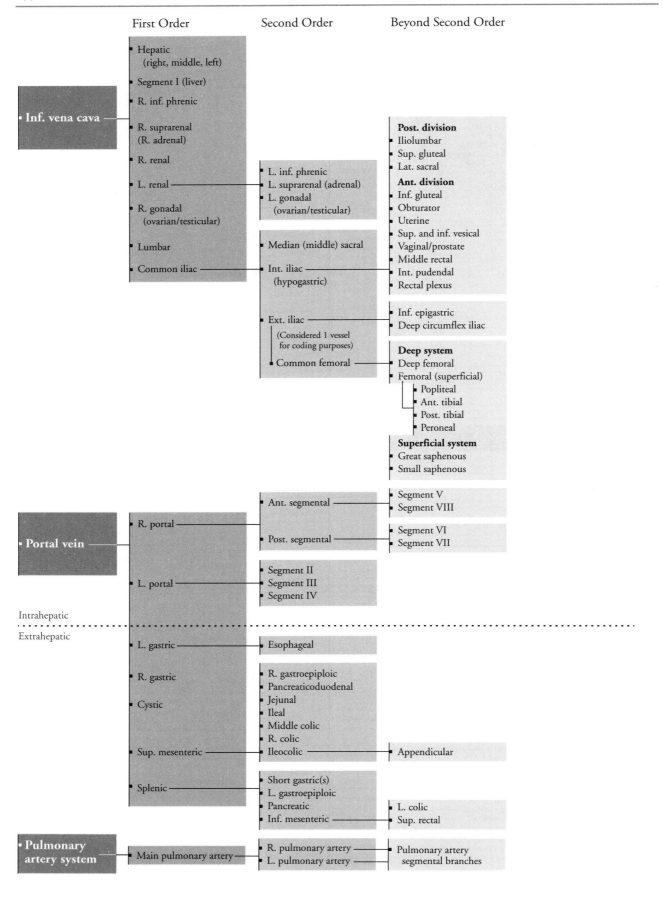

First Order   Second Order   Beyond Second Order

- **Inf. vena cava**
  - Hepatic (right, middle, left)
  - Segment I (liver)
  - R. inf. phrenic
  - R. suprarenal (R. adrenal)
  - R. renal
  - L. renal
    - L. inf. phrenic
    - L. suprarenal (adrenal)
    - L. gonadal (ovarian/testicular)
  - R. gonadal (ovarian/testicular)
  - Lumbar
    - Median (middle) sacral
  - Common iliac
    - Int. iliac (hypogastric)

      Post. division
      - Iliolumbar
      - Sup. gluteal
      - Lat. sacral

      Ant. division
      - Inf. gluteal
      - Obturator
      - Uterine
      - Sup. and inf. vesical
      - Vaginal/prostate
      - Middle rectal
      - Int. pudendal
      - Rectal plexus

    - Ext. iliac
      - Inf. epigastric
      - Deep circumflex iliac

      (Considered 1 vessel for coding purposes)

    - Common femoral

      Deep system
      - Deep femoral
      - Femoral (superficial)
        - Popliteal
        - Ant. tibial
        - Post. tibial
        - Peroneal

      Superficial system
      - Great saphenous
      - Small saphenous

- **Portal vein**
  - R. portal
    - Ant. segmental
      - Segment V
      - Segment VIII
    - Post. segmental
      - Segment VI
      - Segment VII
  - L. portal
    - Segment II
    - Segment III
    - Segment IV

Intrahepatic
· ·
Extrahepatic

  - L. gastric
    - Esophageal
  - R. gastric
    - R. gastroepiploic
    - Pancreaticoduodenal
    - Jejunal
    - Ileal
    - Middle colic
    - R. colic
  - Cystic
  - Sup. mesenteric
    - Ileocolic
      - Appendicular
  - Splenic
    - Short gastric(s)
    - L. gastroepiploic
    - Pancreatic
    - Inf. mesenteric
      - L. colic
      - Sup. rectal

- **Pulmonary artery system**
  - Main pulmonary artery
    - R. pulmonary artery
    - L. pulmonary artery
      - Pulmonary artery segmental branches

★ = Telemedicine   ✚ = Add-on code   ⊘ = FDA approval pending   # = Resequenced code   ⊘ = Modifier 51 exempt

Arterial Vascular Family: Thorax and Abdomen

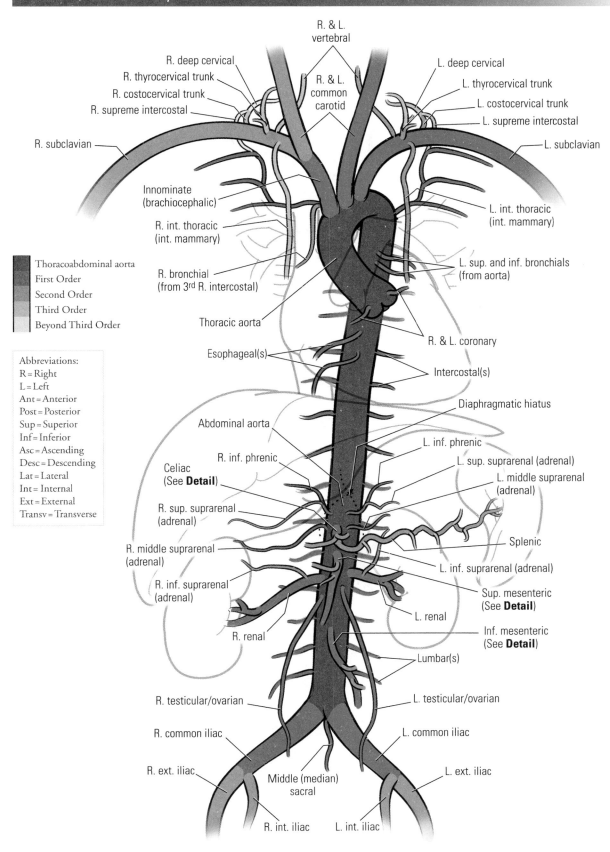

Thoracoabdominal aorta
First Order
Second Order
Third Order
Beyond Third Order

Abbreviations:
R = Right
L = Left
Ant = Anterior
Post = Posterior
Sup = Superior
Inf = Inferior
Asc = Ascending
Desc = Descending
Lat = Lateral
Int = Internal
Ext = External
Transv = Transverse

R. & L. vertebral
R. deep cervical
R. thyrocervical trunk
R. costocervical trunk
R. supreme intercostal
R. subclavian
Innominate (brachiocephalic)
R. int. thoracic (int. mammary)
R. bronchial (from 3rd R. intercostal)
Thoracic aorta
Esophageal(s)
Abdominal aorta
R. inf. phrenic
Celiac (See Detail)
R. sup. suprarenal (adrenal)
R. middle suprarenal (adrenal)
R. inf. suprarenal (adrenal)
R. renal
R. testicular/ovarian
R. common iliac
R. ext. iliac
Middle (median) sacral
R. int. iliac

R. & L. common carotid

L. deep cervical
L. thyrocervical trunk
L. costocervical trunk
L. supreme intercostal
L. subclavian
L. int. thoracic (int. mammary)
L. sup. and inf. bronchials (from aorta)
R. & L. coronary
Intercostal(s)
Diaphragmatic hiatus
L. inf. phrenic
L. sup. suprarenal (adrenal)
L. middle suprarenal (adrenal)
Splenic
L. inf. suprarenal (adrenal)
Sup. mesenteric (See Detail)
Inf. mesenteric (See Detail)
L. renal
Lumbar(s)
L. testicular/ovarian
L. common iliac
L. ext. iliac
L. int. iliac

Venous Vascular Family: Thorax and Abdomen

Appendix L

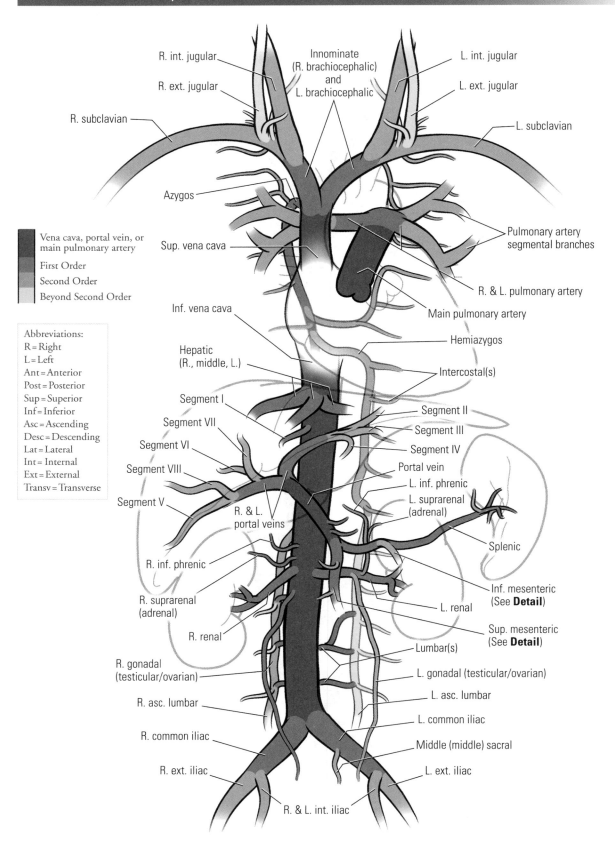

Vena cava, portal vein, or main pulmonary artery
First Order
Second Order
Beyond Second Order

Abbreviations:
R = Right
L = Left
Ant = Anterior
Post = Posterior
Sup = Superior
Inf = Inferior
Asc = Ascending
Desc = Descending
Lat = Lateral
Int = Internal
Ext = External
Transv = Transverse

R. int. jugular
R. ext. jugular
R. subclavian
Azygos
Sup. vena cava
Inf. vena cava
Hepatic (R., middle, L.)
Segment I
Segment VII
Segment VI
Segment VIII
Segment V
R. & L. portal veins
R. inf. phrenic
R. suprarenal (adrenal)
R. renal
R. gonadal (testicular/ovarian)
R. asc. lumbar
R. common iliac
R. ext. iliac
R. & L. int. iliac

Innominate (R. brachiocephalic) and L. brachiocephalic
L. int. jugular
L. ext. jugular
L. subclavian
Pulmonary artery segmental branches
R. & L. pulmonary artery
Main pulmonary artery
Hemiazygos
Intercostal(s)
Segment II
Segment III
Segment IV
Portal vein
L. inf. phrenic
L. suprarenal (adrenal)
Splenic
Inf. mesenteric (See **Detail**)
L. renal
Sup. mesenteric (See **Detail**)
Lumbar(s)
L. gonadal (testicular/ovarian)
L. asc. lumbar
L. common iliac
Middle (middle) sacral
L. ext. iliac

★ = Telemedicine ✚ = Add-on code ⚡ = FDA approval pending # = Resequenced code ⊘ = Modifier 51 exempt

Arterial Vascular Family: Abdomen, Detail

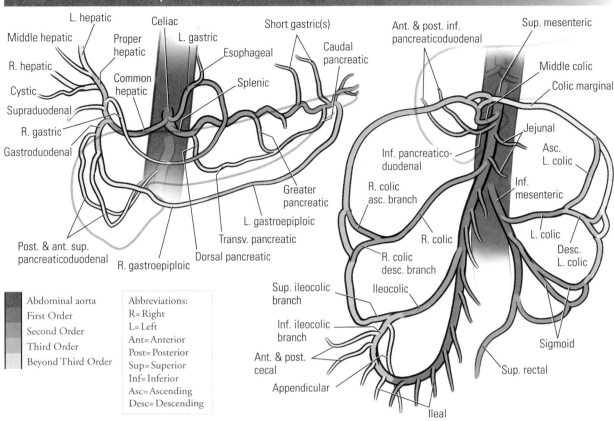

Abbreviations:
R = Right
L = Left
Ant = Anterior
Post = Posterior
Sup = Superior
Inf = Inferior
Asc = Ascending
Desc = Descending

Abdominal aorta
First Order
Second Order
Third Order
Beyond Third Order

Venous Vascular Family: Abdomen, Detail

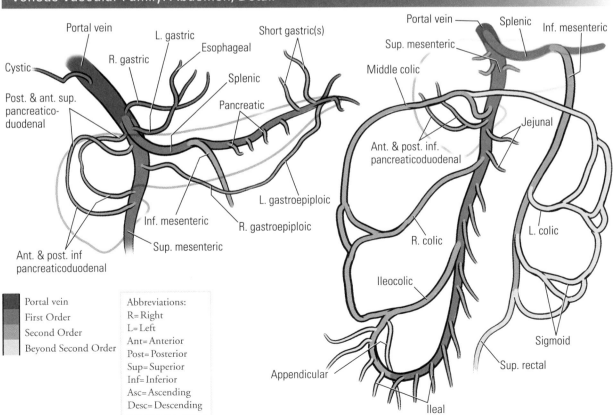

Portal vein
First Order
Second Order
Beyond Second Order

Abbreviations:
R = Right
L = Left
Ant = Anterior
Post = Posterior
Sup = Superior
Inf = Inferior
Asc = Ascending
Desc = Descending

Arterial Vascular Family: Upper Limb

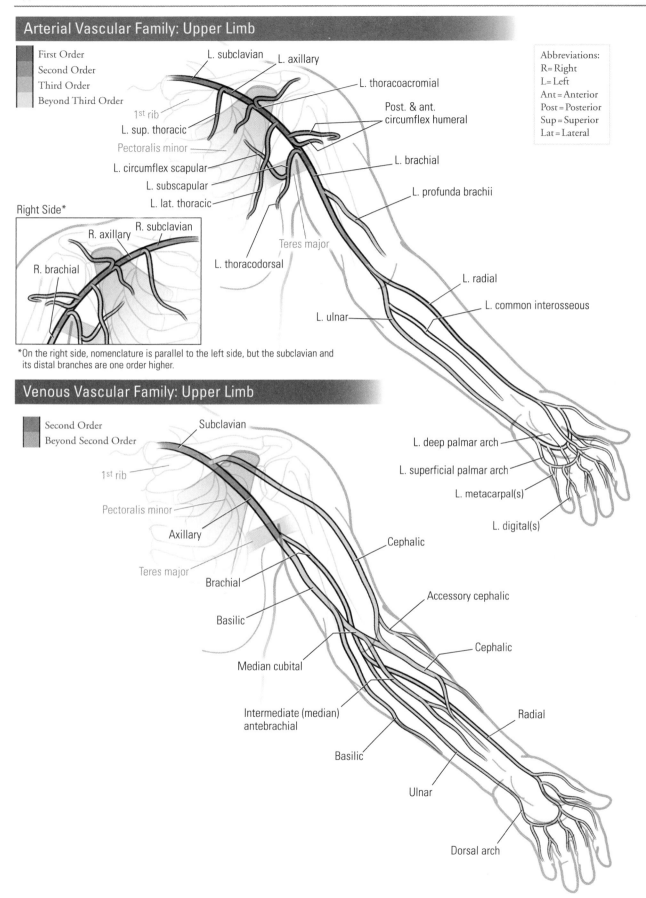

First Order
Second Order
Third Order
Beyond Third Order

Abbreviations:
R = Right
L = Left
Ant = Anterior
Post = Posterior
Sup = Superior
Lat = Lateral

L. subclavian
L. axillary
L. thoracoacromial
Post. & ant. circumflex humeral
1st rib
L. sup. thoracic
Pectoralis minor
L. brachial
L. circumflex scapular
L. subscapular
L. lat. thoracic
L. profunda brachii
Teres major
L. thoracodorsal
L. radial
L. ulnar
L. common interosseous

Right Side*
R. axillary
R. subclavian
R. brachial

*On the right side, nomenclature is parallel to the left side, but the subclavian and its distal branches are one order higher.

Venous Vascular Family: Upper Limb

Second Order
Beyond Second Order

Subclavian
1st rib
Pectoralis minor
Axillary
Teres major
Brachial
Basilic
Median cubital
Intermediate (median) antebrachial
Basilic

Cephalic
Accessory cephalic
Cephalic
Radial
Ulnar
Dorsal arch

L. deep palmar arch
L. superficial palmar arch
L. metacarpal(s)
L. digital(s)

★ = Telemedicine   ✚ = Add-on code   ✎ = FDA approval pending   # = Resequenced code   ⊘ = Modifier 51 exempt

Arterial Vascular Family: Lower Limb

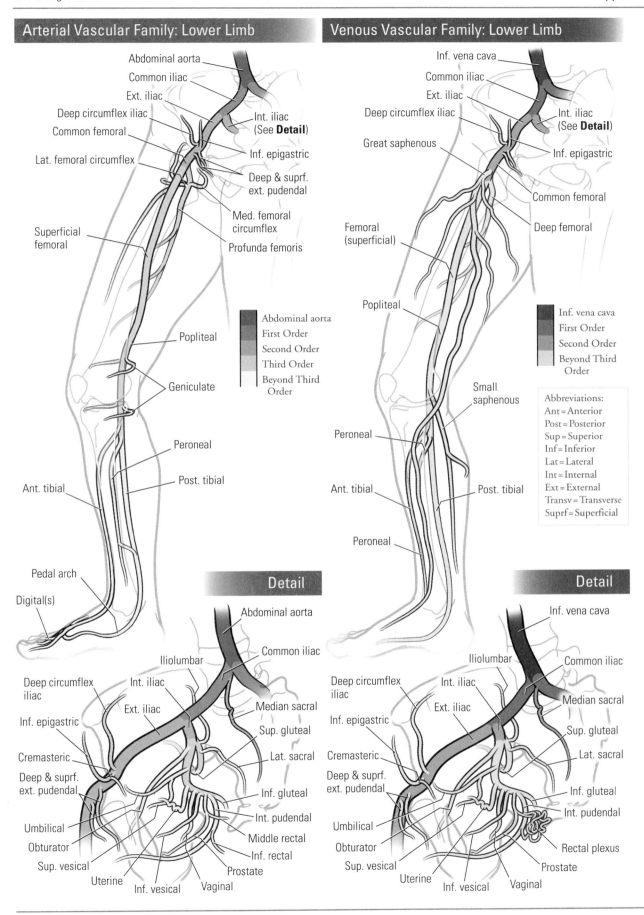

Abdominal aorta
Common iliac
Ext. iliac
Deep circumflex iliac
Common femoral
Lat. femoral circumflex
Superficial femoral
Int. iliac (See **Detail**)
Inf. epigastric
Deep & suprf. ext. pudendal
Med. femoral circumflex
Profunda femoris
Popliteal
Geniculate
Peroneal
Post. tibial
Ant. tibial
Pedal arch
Digital(s)

Abdominal aorta
First Order
Second Order
Third Order
Beyond Third Order

Detail

Abdominal aorta
Iliolumbar
Deep circumflex iliac
Int. iliac
Common iliac
Inf. epigastric
Ext. iliac
Median sacral
Sup. gluteal
Cremasteric
Lat. sacral
Deep & suprf. ext. pudendal
Inf. gluteal
Umbilical
Int. pudendal
Obturator
Middle rectal
Sup. vesical
Inf. rectal
Uterine
Prostate
Inf. vesical
Vaginal

Venous Vascular Family: Lower Limb

Inf. vena cava
Common iliac
Ext. iliac
Deep circumflex iliac
Great saphenous
Int. iliac (See **Detail**)
Inf. epigastric
Common femoral
Deep femoral
Femoral (superficial)
Popliteal
Small saphenous
Peroneal
Post. tibial
Ant. tibial
Peroneal

Inf. vena cava
First Order
Second Order
Beyond Third Order

Abbreviations:
Ant = Anterior
Post = Posterior
Sup = Superior
Inf = Inferior
Lat = Lateral
Int = Internal
Ext = External
Transv = Transverse
Suprf = Superficial

Detail

Inf. vena cava
Iliolumbar
Deep circumflex iliac
Int. iliac
Common iliac
Inf. epigastric
Ext. iliac
Median sacral
Sup. gluteal
Cremasteric
Lat. sacral
Deep & suprf. ext. pudendal
Inf. gluteal
Umbilical
Int. pudendal
Obturator
Rectal plexus
Sup. vesical
Prostate
Uterine
Vaginal
Inf. vesical

Arterial Vascular Family: Head and Neck

First Order
Second Order
Third Order
Beyond Third Order

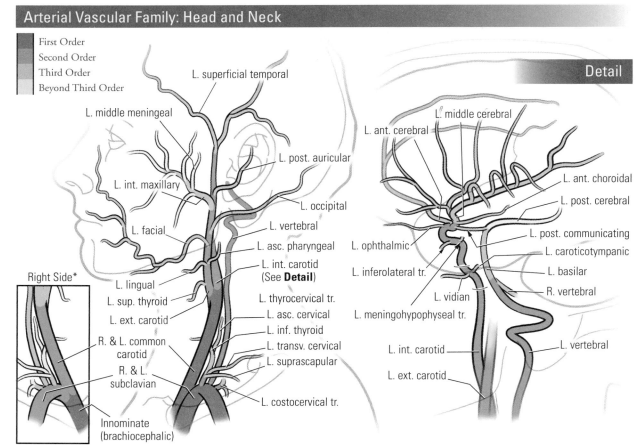

Detail

L. superficial temporal
L. middle meningeal
L. post. auricular
L. int. maxillary
L. occipital
L. facial
L. vertebral
L. asc. pharyngeal
L. int. carotid (See **Detail**)
L. lingual
L. thyrocervical tr.
L. sup. thyroid
L. asc. cervical
L. ext. carotid
L. inf. thyroid
L. transv. cervical
L. suprascapular
L. costocervical tr.

Right Side*
R. & L. common carotid
R. & L. subclavian
Innominate (brachiocephalic)

L. middle cerebral
L. ant. cerebral
L. ant. choroidal
L. post. cerebral
L. post. communicating
L. ophthalmic
L. caroticotympanic
L. inferolateral tr.
L. basilar
R. vertebral
L. vidian
L. meningohypophyseal tr.
L. int. carotid
L. vertebral
L. ext. carotid

*On the right side, nomenclature is parallel to the left side, but the subclavian and common carotid and their distal branches are one order higher.

Venous Vascular Family: Head and Neck

First Order
Second Order
Beyond Second Order

Abbreviations:	
R = Right	Inf = Inferior
L = Left	Asc = Ascending
Ant = Anterior	Int = Internal
Post = Posterior	Ext = External
Sup = Superior	Transv = Transverse
	Tr = Trunk

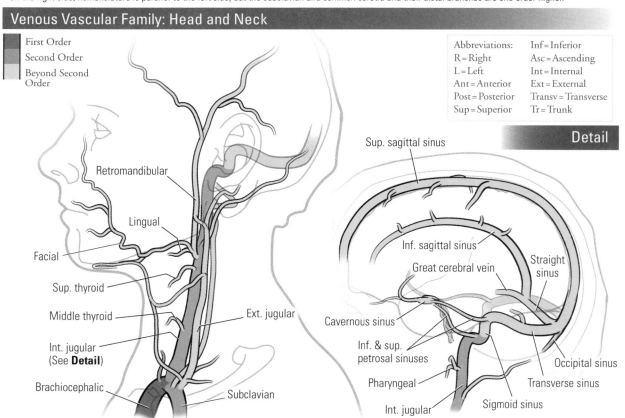

Detail

Retromandibular
Lingual
Facial
Sup. thyroid
Middle thyroid
Int. jugular (See **Detail**)
Brachiocephalic
Ext. jugular
Subclavian

Sup. sagittal sinus
Inf. sagittal sinus
Great cerebral vein
Straight sinus
Cavernous sinus
Inf. & sup. petrosal sinuses
Occipital sinus
Pharyngeal
Transverse sinus
Int. jugular
Sigmoid sinus

★ = Telemedicine   ✚ = Add-on code   ✔ = FDA approval pending   # = Resequenced code   ⊘ = Modifier 51 exempt

Appendix N

Appendix N has been revised to include updated, revised, and/or new resequenced codes with their corresponding ranges. These ranges provide a more efficient way of locating resequenced codes within the codebook.

Summary of Additions, Deletions, and Revisions

The summary of changes shows the actual changes that have been made to the code descriptors.

New codes appear with a bullet (●) and are indicated as "Code added." Revised codes are preceded with a triangle (▲). Within revised codes, or if a code symbol has been deleted, the deleted language and code symbol appears with a ~~strikethrough~~ (⊖), while new text appears <u>underlined</u>.

The ✔ symbol is used to identify codes for vaccines that are pending FDA approval. The # symbol is used to identify codes that have been resequenced. CPT add-on codes are annotated by the ✛ symbol. The ⊘ symbol is used to identify codes that are exempt from the use of modifier 51. The ★ symbol is used to identify codes that may be used for reporting telemedicine services. The ✕ is used to identify proprietary laboratory analyses (PLA) test that has an identical descriptor as another PLA test.

Resequenced Code	Corresponding Locations of Resequenced Code
<u>**10004**</u>	<u>10021-10035</u>
<u>**10005**</u>	<u>10021-10035</u>
<u>**10006**</u>	<u>10021-10035</u>
<u>**10007**</u>	<u>10021-10035</u>
<u>**10008**</u>	<u>10021-10035</u>
<u>**10009**</u>	<u>10021-10035</u>
<u>**10010**</u>	<u>10021-10035</u>
<u>**10011**</u>	<u>10021-10035</u>
<u>**10012**</u>	<u>10021-10035</u>
<u>**33274**</u>	<u>33244-33251</u>
<u>**33275**</u>	<u>33244-33251</u>
<u>**33440**</u>	<u>33406-33412</u>
<u>**36572**</u>	<u>36568-36571</u>
<u>**36573**</u>	<u>36568-36571</u>
~~**37211**~~	~~37197-37216~~
~~**37212**~~	~~37197-37216~~
~~**37213**~~	~~37197-37216~~

Resequenced Code	Corresponding Locations of Resequenced Code
~~**37214**~~	~~37197-37216~~
46947	4676<u>0</u>~~1~~-46910
50430	5039<u>0</u>5-50405
50431	5039<u>0</u>5-50405
50432	5039<u>0</u>5-50405
50433	5039<u>0</u>5-50405
50434	5039<u>0</u>5-50405
50435	5039<u>0</u>5-50405
<u>**50436**</u>	<u>50390-50405</u>
<u>**50437**</u>	<u>50390-50405</u>
81105	8125<u>5</u>7-8127<u>0</u>6~~1~~
81106	81255-81270<u>81257-81261</u>
81107	81255-81270<u>81257-81261</u>
81108	81255-81270<u>81257-81261</u>
81109	81255-81270<u>81257-81261</u>
81110	81255-81270<u>81257-81261</u>
81111	81255-81270<u>81257-81261</u>

Appendix N

Resequenced Code	Corresponding Locations of Resequenced Code
81112	81255-81270~~81257-81261~~
81120	81255-81270~~81257-81261~~
81121	81255-81270~~81257-81261~~
81161	81228~~10~~-81235
81162	81182~~210~~-81220~~35~~
81163	81182-81220
81164	81182-81220
81165	81182-81220
81166	81182-81220
81167	81182-81220
81173	81171-81176
81174	81171-81176
81184	81182-81220
81185	81182-81220
81186	81182-81220
81187	81223-81226
81188	81223-81226
81189	81223-81226
81190	81223-81226
81200	81171-81176
81201	81171-81176
81202	81171-81176
81203	81171-81176
81204	81171-81176
81205	81182-81220
81206	81182-81220
81207	81182-81220
81208	81182-81220
81209	81182-81220
81210	81182-81220
81219	81182-81220
81227	81223-81226

Resequenced Code	Corresponding Locations of Resequenced Code
81230	81225~~6~~-81229
81231	81225~~6~~-81229
81233	81182-81220
81234	81228-81235
81238	81240-81248~~3~~
81239	81228-81235
81245	81240-81248
81246	81240-81248
81250	81243-81248
81257	81253-81256
81258	81253-81256
81259	81253-81256
81261	81255-81270
81262	81255-81270
81263	81255-81270
81264	81255-81270
81265	81223-81226
81266	81223-81226
81267	81223-81226
81268	81223-81226
81269	81253~~7~~-81256~~61~~
81271	81255-81270
81274	81255-81270
81283	81255~~7~~-81270~~61~~
81284	81243-81248
81285	81243-81248
81286	81243-81248
81287	81276-81297~~4~~
81288	81276-81297~~4~~
81289	81243-81248
81291	81299-81310
81292	81276-81297

★ = Telemedicine   ✚ = Add-on code   ⊶ = FDA approval pending   # = Resequenced code   ⊘ = Modifier 51 exempt

Resequenced Code	Corresponding Locations of Resequenced Code
81293	81276-81297
81294	81276-81297
81295	81276-81297
81301	81276-81297
81302	81276-81297
81303	81276-81297
81304	81276-81297
81306	81310-81318
81312	81310-81318
81320	81310-81318
81324	81310-81318
81325	81310-81318
81326	81310-81318
81332	81318-81335
81334	81318~~25~~-81335~~28~~
81336	81318-81335
81337	81318-81335
81343	81318-81335
81344	81318-81335
81345	81318-81335
~~81448~~	~~81437-81440~~
81361	81253-81256
81362	81253-81256
81363	81253-81256
81364	81253-81256
81448	81437-81440
92558	92585-9258~~8607~~
92597	926~~03585~~-92607
92618	926~~03585~~-92607
93264	93272-93280
95829	95827-95832

Resequenced Code	Corresponding Locations of Resequenced Code
95836	95827-95832
95983	95976-95981
95984	95976-95981
96125	96020-96121
96127	96020-96121
97151	96020-96112
97152	96020-96112
97153	96020-96112
97154	96020-96112
97155	96020-96112
97156	96020-96112
97157	96020-96112
97158	96020-96112
99091	99448-99455
99451	99448-99455
99452	99448-99455
99453	99448-99455
99454	99448-99455
99457	99448-99455
99491	99480-99489
0253T	018~~491~~4T-~~0196T~~0200T
0376T	0184T-0200T~~0190T-0195T~~
0464T	0332T-0339~~7~~T
0488T	0402T-0405T
0510T	0332T-0339T
0511T	0332T-0339T
0512T	0101T-0107T
0513T	0101T-0107T
0523T	0503T-0506T

Appendix N

Summary of Resequenced Codes

This is a table of CPT codes that do not appear in numeric sequence in the listing of CPT codes and the code ranges with their corresponding locations. Rather than deleting and renumbering, resequencing allows existing codes to be relocated to an appropriate location for the code concept, regardless of the numeric sequence. The codes listed below are identified in the CPT 2019 code set with a # symbol for the location of the resequenced number within the family of related concepts. Numerically placed references (eg, **Code is out of numerical sequence. See...**) are used as navigational alerts to direct the user to the location of an out-of-sequence code.

Resequenced Code	Corresponding Locations of Resequenced Code	Resequenced Code	Corresponding Locations of Resequenced Code	Resequenced Code	Corresponding Locations of Resequenced Code	Resequenced Code	Corresponding Locations of Resequenced Code
10004	10021-10035	28039	28035-28047	33274	33244-33251	43211	43216-43227
10005	10021-10035	28041	28035-28047	33275	33244-33251	43212	43216-43227
10006	10021-10035	28295	28292-28298	33440	33406-33412	43213	43216-43227
10007	10021-10035	29914	29862-29867	33962	33958-33968	43214	43216-43227
10008	10021-10035	29915	29862-29867	33963	33958-33968	43233	43248-43251
10009	10021-10035	29916	29862-29867	33964	33958-33968	43266	43254-43261
10010	10021-10035	31253	31254-31267	33965	33958-33968	43270	43254-43261
10011	10021-10035	31257	31254-31267	33966	33958-33968	43274	43264-43279
10012	10021-10035	31259	31254-31267	33969	33958-33968	43275	43264-43279
11045	11012-11047	31551	31579-31587	33984	33958-33968	43276	43264-43279
11046	11012-11047	31552	31579-31587	33985	33958-33968	43277	43264-43279
21552	21550-21558	31553	31579-31587	33986	33958-33968	43278	43264-43279
21554	21550-21558	31554	31579-31587	33987	33958-33968	44381	44380-44385
22858	22853-22861	31572	31577-31580	33988	33958-33968	44401	44391-44402
22859	22853-22861	31573	31577-31580	33989	33958-33968	45346	45337-45341
23071	23066-23078	31574	31577-31580	34812	34712-34716	45388	45381-45385
23073	23066-23078	31651	31646-31649	34820	34712-34716	45390	45391-45397
24071	24066-24079	32994	32997-32999	34833	34712-34716	45398	45391-45397
24073	24066-24079	33221	33212-33215	34834	34712-34716	45399	45910-45999
25071	25066-25078	33227	33226-33244	36465	36470-36474	46220	46200-46255
25073	25066-25078	33228	33226-33244	36466	36470-36474	46320	46200-46255
26111	26110-26118	33229	33226-33244	36482	36478-36500	46945	46200-46255
26113	26110-26118	33230	33226-33244	36483	36478-36500	46946	46200-46255
27043	27041-27052	33231	33226-33244	36572	36568-36571	46947	46760-46910
27045	27041-27052	33262	33226-33244	36573	36568-36571	50430	50390-50405
27059	27041-27052	33263	33226-33244	37246	37234-37237	50431	50390-50405
27329	27358-27365	33264	33226-33244	37247	37234-37237	50432	50390-50405
27337	27326-27331	33270	33244-33251	37248	37234-37237	50433	50390-50405
27339	27326-27331	33271	33244-33251	37249	37234-37237	50434	50390-50405
27632	27616-27625	33272	33244-33251	38243	38240-38300	50435	50390-50405
27634	27616-27625	33273	33244-33251	43210	43254-43261	50436	50390-50405

★ = Telemedicine   ✚ = Add-on code   ⃥ = FDA approval pending   # = Resequenced code   ⊘ = Modifier 51 exempt

Resequenced Code	Corresponding Locations of Resequenced Code	Resequenced Code	Corresponding Locations of Resequenced Code	Resequenced Code	Corresponding Locations of Resequenced Code	Resequenced Code	Corresponding Locations of Resequenced Code
50437	50390-50405	80323	See Definitive Drug Testing subsection	80340	See Definitive Drug Testing subsection	80357	See Definitive Drug Testing subsection
51797	51728-51741						
52356	52352-52355	80324	See Definitive Drug Testing subsection	80341	See Definitive Drug Testing subsection	80358	See Definitive Drug Testing subsection
58674	58520-58542						
64461	64483-64487	80325	See Definitive Drug Testing subsection	80342	See Definitive Drug Testing subsection	80359	See Definitive Drug Testing subsection
64462	64483-64487						
64463	64483-64487						
64633	64617-64632	80326	See Definitive Drug Testing subsection	80343	See Definitive Drug Testing subsection	80360	See Definitive Drug Testing subsection
64634	64617-64632						
64635	64617-64632						
64636	64617-64632	80327	See Definitive Drug Testing subsection	80344	See Definitive Drug Testing subsection	80361	See Definitive Drug Testing subsection
67810	67710-67801						
77085	77080-77261	80328	See Definitive Drug Testing subsection	80345	See Definitive Drug Testing subsection	80362	See Definitive Drug Testing subsection
77086	77080-77261						
77295	77293-77301						
77385	77412-77427	80329	See Definitive Drug Testing subsection	80346	See Definitive Drug Testing subsection	80363	See Definitive Drug Testing subsection
77386	77412-77427						
77387	77412-77427	80330	See Definitive Drug Testing subsection	80347	See Definitive Drug Testing subsection	80364	See Definitive Drug Testing subsection
77424	77412-77427						
77425	77412-77427	80331	See Definitive Drug Testing subsection	80348	See Definitive Drug Testing subsection	80365	See Definitive Drug Testing subsection
80081	80053-80069						
80164	80200-80203	80332	See Definitive Drug Testing subsection	80349	See Definitive Drug Testing subsection	80366	See Definitive Drug Testing subsection
80165	80200-80203						
80171	80168-80173	80333	See Definitive Drug Testing subsection	80350	See Definitive Drug Testing subsection	80367	See Definitive Drug Testing subsection
80305	See Presumptive Drug Class Screening subsection	80334	See Definitive Drug Testing subsection	80351	See Definitive Drug Testing subsection	80368	See Definitive Drug Testing subsection
		80335	See Definitive Drug Testing subsection	80352	See Definitive Drug Testing subsection	80369	See Definitive Drug Testing subsection
80306	See Presumptive Drug Class Screening subsection	80336	See Definitive Drug Testing subsection	80353	See Definitive Drug Testing subsection	80370	See Definitive Drug Testing subsection
80307	See Presumptive Drug Class Screening subsection	80337	See Definitive Drug Testing subsection	80354	See Definitive Drug Testing subsection	80371	See Definitive Drug Testing subsection
80320	See Definitive Drug Testing subsection	80338	See Definitive Drug Testing subsection	80355	See Definitive Drug Testing subsection	80372	See Definitive Drug Testing subsection
80321	See Definitive Drug Testing subsection	80339	See Definitive Drug Testing subsection	80356	See Definitive Drug Testing subsection	80373	See Definitive Drug Testing subsection
80322	See Definitive Drug Testing subsection						

Resequenced Code	Corresponding Locations of Resequenced Code
80374	See Definitive Drug Testing subsection
80375	See Definitive Drug Testing subsection
80376	See Definitive Drug Testing subsection
80377	See Definitive Drug Testing subsection
81105	81255-81270
81106	81255-81270
81107	81255-81270
81108	81255-81270
81109	81255-81270
81110	81255-81270
81111	81255-81270
81112	81255-81270
81120	81255-81270
81121	81255-81270
81161	81228-81235
81162	81182-81220
81163	81182-81220
81164	81182-81220
81165	81182-81220
81166	81182-81220
81167	81182-81220
81173	81171-81176
81174	81171-81176
81184	81182-81220
81185	81182-81220
81186	81182-81220
81187	81223-81226
81188	81223-81226
81189	81223-81226
81190	81223-81226
81200	81171-81176
81201	81171-81176
81202	81171-81176
81203	81171-81176
81204	81171-81176
81205	81182-81220
81206	81182-81220
81207	81182-81220

Resequenced Code	Corresponding Locations of Resequenced Code
81208	81182-81220
81209	81182-81220
81210	81182-81220
81219	81182-81220
81227	81223-81226
81230	81225-81229
81231	81225-81229
81233	81182-81220
81234	81228-81235
81238	81240-81248
81239	81228-81235
81245	81240-81248
81246	81240-81248
81250	81243-81248
81257	81253-81256
81258	81253-81256
81259	81253-81256
81261	81255-81270
81262	81255-81270
81263	81255-81270
81264	81255-81270
81265	81223-81226
81266	81223-81226
81267	81223-81226
81268	81223-81226
81269	81253-81256
81271	81255-81270
81274	81255-81270
81283	81255-81270
81284	81243-81248
81285	81243-81248
81286	81243-81248
81287	81276-81297
81288	81276-81297
81289	81243-81248
81291	81299-81310
81292	81276-81297
81293	81276-81297
81294	81276-81297
81295	81276-81297
81301	81276-81297
81302	81276-81297
81303	81276-81297
81304	81276-81297

Resequenced Code	Corresponding Locations of Resequenced Code
81306	81310-81318
81312	81310-81318
81320	81310-81318
81324	81310-81318
81325	81310-81318
81326	81310-81318
81332	81318-81335
81334	81318-81335
81336	81318-81335
81337	81318-81335
81343	81318-81335
81344	81318-81335
81345	81318-81335
81361	81253-81256
81362	81253-81256
81363	81253-81256
81364	81253-81256
81448	81437-81440
81479	81407-81411
82042	82044-82085
82652	82300-82310
83992	See Definitive Drug Testing subsection
86152	86146-86155
86153	86146-86155
87623	87538-87541
87624	87538-87541
87625	87538-87541
87806	87802-87903
87906	87802-87903
87910	87802-87903
87912	87802-87903
88177	88172-88175
88341	88334-88372
88350	88334-88372
88364	88334-88372
88373	88334-88372
88374	88334-88372
88377	88334-88372
90620	90717-90739
90621	90717-90739
90625	90717-90739
90630	90653-90656
90644	90717-90739

Resequenced Code	Corresponding Locations of Resequenced Code
90672	90658-90664
90673	90658-90664
90674	90658-90664
90750	90717-90739
90756	90658-90664
92558	92585-92588
92597	92603-92607
92618	92603-92607
92920	92997-93005
92921	92997-93005
92924	92997-93005
92925	92997-93005
92928	92997-93005
92929	92997-93005
92933	92997-93005
92934	92997-93005
92937	92997-93005
92938	92997-93005
92941	92997-93005
92943	92997-93005
92944	92997-93005
92973	92997-93005
92974	92997-93005
92975	92997-93005
92977	92997-93005
92978	92997-93005
92979	92997-93005
93260	93283-93291
93261	93283-93291
93264	93272-93280
95249	95199-95803
95782	95805-95813
95783	95805-95813
95800	95805-95813
95801	95805-95813
95836	95827-95832
95885	95870-95874
95886	95870-95874
95887	95870-95874
95938	95912-95933
95939	95912-95933
95940	95912-95933
95941	95912-95933
95943	95912-95933

★ = Telemedicine   ✚ = Add-on code   ✔ = FDA approval pending   # = Resequenced code   ⃠ = Modifier 51 exempt

Resequenced Code	Corresponding Locations of Resequenced Code	Resequenced Code	Corresponding Locations of Resequenced Code
95983	95976-95981	97169	See Athletic Training Evaluations subsection
95984	95976-95981		
96125	96020-96121	97170	See Athletic Training Evaluations subsection
96127	96020-96121		
97151	96020-96112		
97152	96020-96112	97171	See Athletic Training Evaluations subsection
97153	96020-96112		
97154	96020-96112		
97155	96020-96112	97172	See Athletic Training Evaluations subsection
97156	96020-96112		
97157	96020-96112		
97158	96020-96112		
97161	See Physical Therapy Evaluations subsection	99091	99448-99455
		99177	99173-99183
97162	See Physical Therapy Evaluations subsection	99224	99219-99222
		99225	99219-99222
		99226	99219-99222
97163	See Physical Therapy Evaluations subsection	99415	99358-99366
		99416	99358-99366
		99451	99448-99455
		99452	99448-99455
97164	See Physical Therapy Evaluations subsection	99453	99448-99455
		99454	99448-99455
		99457	99448-99455
97165	See Occupational Therapy Evaluations subsection	99484	99497-99499
		99485	99466-99469
		99486	99466-99469
		99490	99480-99489
97166	See Occupational Therapy Evaluations subsection	99491	99480-99489
		0253T	0184T-0200T
		0357T	0055T-0072T
		0376T	0184T-0200T
97167	See Occupational Therapy Evaluations subsection	0464T	0332T-0339T
		0488T	0402T-0405T
		0510T	0332T-0339T
		0511T	0332T-0339T
97168	See Occupational Therapy Evaluations subsection	0512T	0101T-0107T
		0513T	0101T-0107T
		0523T	0503T-0506T

Appendix N

Rationale

Appendix N has been updated to include the addition of 51 codes, 34 revisions, and the deletion of five codes. The code ranges in the out-of-sequence cross-reference notes for resequenced codes located throughout the code set have been condensed by reducing the size of the ranges to provide more accurate cross-referenced ranges. These editorially revised code ranges are consolidated in Appendix N to provide additional assistance and ease in locating all resequenced codes.

Within every section, resequenced codes that are numerically out of sequence are identified with the # symbol as a navigational alert to inform users that the code is resequenced and to read the cross-reference note provided to find the location of the resequenced code. Resequencing is used to enable related concepts to be placed in appropriate locations within families of codes, regardless of sequential numerical placement.

★ = Telemedicine   ✚ = Add-on code   ✎ = FDA approval pending   # = Resequenced code   ⊘ = Modifier 51 exempt

Appendix O

In Appendix O, three new administrative multianalyte assay with algorithmic analyses (MAAA) codes (0011M, 0012M, and 0013M) have been added; one code (0001M) has been deleted; and two new codes (81518 and 81596) have been added to the Category I MAAA listing. In addition, all proprietary laboratory analyses (PLA) codes and their procedural proprietary names have also been added.

Summary of Additions, Deletions, and Revisions

The summary of changes shows the actual changes that have been made to the code descriptors.

New codes appear with a bullet (●) and are indicated as "Code added." Revised codes are preceded with a triangle (▲). Within revised codes, or if a code symbol has been deleted, the deleted language and code symbol appears with a strikethrough (⊖), while new text appears underlined.

The ✗ symbol is used to identify codes for vaccines that are pending FDA approval. The # symbol is used to identify codes that have been resequenced. CPT add-on codes are annotated by the ✚ symbol. The ⊘ symbol is used to identify codes that are exempt from the use of modifier 51. The ★ symbol is used to identify codes that may be used for reporting telemedicine services. The ✖ is used to identify proprietary laboratory analyses (PLA) test that has an identical descriptor as another PLA test.

Proprietary Name and Clinical Laboratory or Manufacturer	Alpha-Numeric Code	Code Descriptor
Administrative Codes for Multianalyte Assays with Algorithmic Analyses (MAAA)		
~~HCV FibroSURE™, LabCorp FibroTest™, Quest Diagnostics/ BioPredictive~~	▶(0001M has been deleted. To report, use 81596◀	~~Infectious disease, HCV, six biochemical assays (ALT, A2-macroglobulin, apolipoprotein A-1, total bilirubin, GGT, and haptoglobin) utilizing serum, prognostic algorithm reported as scores for fibrosis and necroinflammatory activity in liver~~
▶NeoLAB™ Prostate Liquid Biopsy, NeoGenomics Laboratories◀	●0011M	▶Oncology, prostate cancer, mRNA expression assay of 12 genes (10 content and 2 housekeeping), RT-PCR test utilizing blood plasma and/or urine, algorithms to predict high-grade prostate cancer risk◀
▶Cxbladder™ Detect, Pacific Edge Diagnostics USA, Ltd◀	●0012M	▶Oncology (urothelial), mRNA, gene expression profiling by real-time quantitative PCR of five genes *(MDK, HOXA13, CDC2 [CDK1], IGFBP5, and CXCR2)*, utilizing urine, algorithm reported as a risk score for having urothelial carcinoma◀
▶Cxbladder™ Monitor, Pacific Edge Diagnostics USA, Ltd◀	●0013M	▶Oncology (urothelial), mRNA, gene expression profiling by real-time quantitative PCR of five genes *(MDK, HOXA13, CDC2 [CDK1], IGFBP5, and CXCR2)*, utilizing urine, algorithm reported as a risk score for having recurrent urothelial carcinoma◀

(*Continued on page 226*)

Proprietary Name and Clinical Laboratory or Manufacturer	Alpha-Numeric Code	Code Descriptor
Category I Codes for Multianalyte Assays with Algorithmic Analyses (MAAA)		
~~Pathwork~~® Tissue of Origin Test <u>Kit-FFPE</u>, <u>Cancer Genetics, Inc</u> ~~Pathwork Diagnostics~~	81504	Oncology (tissue of origin), microarray gene expression profiling of >2000 genes, utilizing formalin-fixed paraffin-embedded tissue, algorithm reported as tissue similarity scores
▶Breast Cancer Index, Biotheranostics, Inc◀	●81518	▶Oncology (breast), mRNA, gene expression profiling by real-time RT-PCR of 11 genes (7 content and 4 housekeeping), utilizing formalin-fixed paraffin-embedded tissue, algorithms reported as percentage risk for metastatic recurrence and likelihood of benefit from extended endocrine therapy◀
▶HCV FibroSURE™, FibroTest™, BioPredictive S.A.S.◀	●81596	▶Infectious disease, chronic hepatitis C virus (HCV) infection, six biochemical assays (ALT, A2-macroglobulin, apolipoprotein A-1, total bilirubin, GGT, and haptoglobin) utilizing serum, prognostic algorithm reported as scores for fibrosis and necroinflammatory activity in liver◀
Proprietary Laboratory Analyses (PLA)		
	▶(0004U has been deleted)◀	
▶Drug-drug, Drug-substance Identification and Interaction, Aegis Sciences Corporation◀ ~~Aegis Drug-Drug Interaction Test~~	▲0006U	~~Prescription drug monitoring, 120 or more drugs and substances, definitive tandem mass spectrometry with chromatography, urine, qualitative report of presence (including quantitative levels, when detected) or absence of each drug or substance with description and severity of potential interactions, with identified substances, per date of service~~ ▶Detection of interacting medications, substances, supplements and foods, 120 or more analytes, definitive chromatography with mass spectrometry, urine, description and severity of each interaction identified, per date of service◀
ToxProtect, Genotox Laboratories Ltd	✂0007U	Drug test(s), presumptive, with definitive confirmation of positive results, any number of drug classes, urine, includes specimen verification including DNA authentication in comparison to buccal DNA, per date of service ▶(For additional PLA code with identical clinical descriptor, see 0020U. See Appendix O to determine appropriate code assignment)◀
	▶(0015U has been deleted)◀	
▶ThyraMIR™, Interface Diagnostics, Interface Diagnostics◀	●0018U	▶Oncology (thyroid), microRNA profiling by RT-PCR of 10 microRNA sequences, utilizing fine needle aspirate, algorithm reported as a positive or negative result for moderate to high risk of malignancy◀

★ = Telemedicine   ✚ = Add-on code   ✗ = FDA approval pending   # = Resequenced code   ⊘ = Modifier 51 exempt

Proprietary Name and Clinical Laboratory or Manufacturer	Alpha-Numeric Code	Code Descriptor
▶OncoTarget/OncoTreat, Columbia University Department of Pathology and Cell Biology, Darwin Health◀	●0019U	▶Oncology, RNA, gene expression by whole transcriptome sequencing, formalin-fixed paraffin embedded tissue or fresh frozen tissue, predictive algorithm reported as potential targets for therapeutic agents◀
▶ToxLok, InSource Diagnostics, InSource Diagnostics◀	�●0020U	▶Drug test(s), presumptive, with definitive confirmation of positive results, any number of drug classes, urine, with specimen verification including DNA authentication in comparison to buccal DNA, per date of service (For additional PLA code with identical clinical descriptor, see 0007U. See Appendix O to determine appropriate code assignment)◀
▶Apifiny®, Armune BioSience, Inc◀	●0021U	▶Oncology (prostate), detection of 8 autoantibodies (ARF 6, NKX3-1, 5'-UTR-BMI1, CEP 164, 3'-UTR-Ropporin, Desmocollin, AURKAIP-1, CSNK2A2), multiplexed immunoassay and flow cytometry serum, algorithm reported as risk score◀
▶Oncomine™ Dx Target Test, Thermo Fisher Scientific◀	●0022U	▶Targeted genomic sequence analysis panel, non-small cell lung neoplasia, DNA and RNA analysis, 23 genes, interrogation for sequence variants and rearrangements, reported as presence/absence of variants and associated therapy(ies) to consider◀
▶LeukoStrat® CDx FLT3 Mutation Assay, LabPMM LLC, an Invivoscribe Technologies, Inc Company, Invivoscribe Technologies, Inc◀	●0023U	▶Oncology (acute myelogenous leukemia), DNA, genotyping of internal tandem duplication, p. D835, p.I836, using mononuclear cells, reported as detection or non-detection of FLT3 mutation and indication for or against the use of midostaurin◀
▶GlycA, Laboratory Corporation of America, Laboratory Corporation of America◀	●0024U	▶Glycosylated acute phase proteins (GlycA), nuclear magnetic resonance spectroscopy, quantitative◀
▶UrSure Tenofovir Quantification Test, Synergy Medical Laboratories, UrSure Inc◀	●0025U	▶Tenofovir, by liquid chromatography with tandem mass spectrometry (LC-MS/MS), urine, quantitative◀
▶Thyroseq Genomic Classifier, CBLPath, Inc, University of Pittsburgh Medical Center◀	●0026U	▶Oncology (thyroid), DNA and mRNA of 112 genes, next-generation sequencing, fine needle aspirate of thyroid nodule, algorithmic analysis reported as a categorical result ("Positive, high probability of malignancy" or "Negative, low probability of malignancy")◀
▶JAK2 Exons 12 to 15 Sequencing, Mayo Clinic, Mayo Clinic◀	●0027U	▶JAK2 (Janus kinase 2) (eg, myeloproliferative disorder) gene analysis, targeted sequence analysis exons 12-15◀
▶CYP2D6 Genotype Cascade, Mayo Clinic, Mayo Clinic◀	●0028U	▶CYP2D6 (cytochrome P450, family 2, subfamily D, polypeptide 6) (eg, drug metabolism) gene analysis, copy number variants, common variants with reflex to targeted sequence analysis◀

(Continued on page 228)

▲=Revised code   ●=New code   ▶ ◀=Contains new or revised text   ✝=Duplicate PLA test

Proprietary Name and Clinical Laboratory or Manufacturer	Alpha-Numeric Code	Code Descriptor
▶Focused Pharmacogenomics Panel, Mayo Clinic, Mayo Clinic◀	●0029U	▶Drug metabolism (adverse drug reactions and drug response), targeted sequence analysis (ie, *CYP1A2, CYP2C19, CYP2C9, CYP2D6, CYP3A4, CYP3A5, CYP4F2, SLCO1B1, VKORC1* and rs12777823)◀
▶Warfarin Response Genotype, Mayo Clinic, Mayo Clinic◀	●0030U	▶Drug metabolism (warfarin drug response), targeted sequence analysis (ie, *CYP2C9, CYP4F2, VKORC1,* rs12777823)◀
▶Cytochrome P450 1A2 Genotype, Mayo Clinic, Mayo Clinic◀	●0031U	▶*CYP1A2 (cytochrome P450 family 1, subfamily A, member 2)* (eg, drug metabolism) gene analysis, common variants (ie, *1F, *1K, *6, *7)◀
▶Catechol-O-Methyltransferase *(COMT)* Genotype, Mayo Clinic, Mayo Clinic◀	●0032U	▶*COMT (catechol-O-methyltransferase)* (eg, drug metabolism) gene analysis, c.472G>A (rs4680) variant◀
▶Serotonin Receptor Genotype *(HTR2A* and *HTR2C)*, Mayo Clinic, Mayo Clinic◀	●0033U	▶*HTR2A (5-hydroxytryptamine receptor 2A), HTR2C (5-hydroxytryptamine receptor 2C)* (eg, citalopram metabolism) gene analysis, common variants (ie, *HTR2A* rs7997012 [c.614-2211T>C], *HTR2C* rs3813929 [c.-759C>T] and rs1414334 [c.551-3008C>G])◀
▶Thiopurine Methyltransferase *(TPMT)* and Nudix Hydrolase *(NUDT15)* Genotyping, Mayo Clinic, Mayo Clinic◀	●0034U	▶*TPMT (thiopurine S-methyltransferase), NUDT15 (nudix hydroxylase 15)* (eg, thiopurine metabolism) gene analysis, common variants (ie, *TPMT* *2, *3A, *3B, *3C, *4, *5, *6, *8, *12; *NUDT15* *3, *4, *5)◀
▶Real-time quaking-induced conversion for prion detection (RT-QuIC), National Prion Disease Pathology Surveillance Center◀	●0035U	▶Neurology (prion disease), cerebrospinal fluid, detection of prion protein by quaking-induced conformational conversion, qualitative◀
▶EXaCT-1 Whole Exome Testing, Lab of Oncology-Molecular Detection, Weill Cornell Medicine-Clinical Genomics Laboratory◀	●0036U	▶Exome (ie, somatic mutations), paired formalin-fixed paraffin-embedded tumor tissue and normal specimen, sequence analyses◀
▶FoundationOne CDx™ (F1CDx), Foundation Medicine, Inc, Foundation Medicine, Inc◀	●0037U	▶Targeted genomic sequence analysis, solid organ neoplasm, DNA analysis of 324 genes, interrogation for sequence variants, gene copy number amplifications, gene rearrangements, microsatellite instability and tumor mutational burden◀
▶Sensieva™ Droplet 25OH Vitamin D2/D3 Microvolume LC/MS Assay, InSource Diagnostics, InSource Diagnostics◀	●0038U	▶Vitamin D, 25 hydroxy D2 and D3, by LC-MS/MS, serum microsample, quantitative◀
▶Anti-dsDNA, High Salt/Avidity, University of Washington, Department of Laboratory Medicine, Bio-Rad◀	●0039U	▶Deoxyribonucleic acid (DNA) antibody, double stranded, high avidity◀
▶MRDx BCR-ABL Test, MolecularMD, MolecularMD◀	●0040U	▶*BCR/ABL1 (t(9;22))* (eg, chronic myelogenous leukemia) translocation analysis, major breakpoint, quantitative◀

★ = Telemedicine   ✚ = Add-on code   ✎ = FDA approval pending   # = Resequenced code   ⊘ = Modifier 51 exempt

Proprietary Name and Clinical Laboratory or Manufacturer	Alpha-Numeric Code	Code Descriptor
▶Lyme ImmunoBlot IgM, IGeneX Inc, ID-FISH Technology Inc (ASR) (Lyme ImmunoBlot IgM Strips Only)◀	●0041U	▶Borrelia burgdorferi, antibody detection of 5 recombinant protein groups, by immunoblot, IgM◀
▶Lyme ImmunoBlot IgG, IGeneX Inc, ID-FISH Technology Inc (ASR) (Lyme ImmunoBlot IgG Strips Only)◀	●0042U	▶Borrelia burgdorferi, antibody detection of 12 recombinant protein groups, by immunoblot, IgG◀
▶Tick-Borne Relapsing Fever (TBRF) Borrelia ImmunoBlots IgM Test, IGeneX Inc, ID-FISH Technology◀	●0043U	▶Tick-borne relapsing fever Borrelia group, antibody detection to 4 recombinant protein groups, by immunoblot, IgM◀
▶Tick-Borne Relapsing Fever (TBRF) Borrelia ImmunoBlots IgG Test, IGeneX Inc, ID-FISH Technology Inc (Provides TBRF ImmunoBlot IgG Strips)◀	●0044U	▶Tick-borne relapsing fever Borrelia group, antibody detection to 4 recombinant protein groups, by immunoblot, IgG◀
▶The Oncotype DX® Breast DCIS Score™ Test, Genomic Health, Inc, Genomic Health, Inc◀	●0045U	▶Oncology (breast ductal carcinoma in situ), mRNA, gene expression profiling by real-time RT-PCR of 12 genes (7 content and 5 housekeeping), utilizing formalin-fixed paraffin-embedded tissue, algorithm reported as recurrence score◀
▶*FLT3* ITD MRD by NGS, LabPMM LLC, an Invivoscribe Technologies, Inc Company◀	●0046U	▶*FLT3 (fms-related tyrosine kinase 3)* (eg, acute myeloid leukemia) internal tandem duplication (ITD) variants, quantitative◀
▶Oncotype DX Genomic Prostate Score, Genomic Health, Inc, Genomic Health, Inc◀	●0047U	▶Oncology (prostate), mRNA, gene expression profiling by real-time RT-PCR of 17 genes (12 content and 5 housekeeping), utilizing formalin-fixed paraffin-embedded tissue, algorithm reported as a risk score◀
▶MSK-IMPACT (Integrated Mutation Profiling of Actionable Cancer Targets), Memorial Sloan Kettering Cancer Center◀	●0048U	▶Oncology (solid organ neoplasia), DNA, targeted sequencing of protein-coding exons of 468 cancer-associated genes, including interrogation for somatic mutations and microsatellite instability, matched with normal specimens, utilizing formalin-fixed paraffin-embedded tumor tissue, report of clinically significant mutation(s)◀
▶NPM1 MRD by NGS, LabPMM LLC, an Invivoscribe Technologies, Inc Company◀	●0049U	▶*NPM1 (nucleophosmin)* (eg, acute myeloid leukemia) gene analysis, quantitative◀
▶MyAML NGS Panel, LabPMM LLC, an Invivoscribe Technologies, Inc Company◀	●0050U	▶Targeted genomic sequence analysis panel, acute myelogenous leukemia, DNA analysis, 194 genes, interrogation for sequence variants, copy number variants or rearrangements◀
▶UCompliDx, Elite Medical Laboratory Solutions, LLC, Elite Medical Laboratory Solutions, LLC (LDT)◀	●0051U	▶Prescription drug monitoring, evaluation of drugs present by LC-MS/MS, urine, 31 drug panel, reported as quantitative results, detected or not detected, per date of service◀

(*Continued on page 230*)

▲=Revised code ●=New code ▶ ◀=Contains new or revised text ✶=Duplicate PLA test

Proprietary Name and Clinical Laboratory or Manufacturer	Alpha-Numeric Code	Code Descriptor
▶VAP Cholesterol Test, VAP Diagnostics Laboratory, Inc, VAP Diagnostics Laboratory, Inc◀	●0052U	▶Lipoprotein, blood, high resolution fractionation and quantitation of lipoproteins including all five major lipoprotein classes and the subclasses of HDL, LDL, and VLDL by vertical auto profile ultracentrifugation◀
▶Prostate Cancer Risk Panel, Mayo Clinic, Laboratory Developed Test◀	●0053U	▶Oncology (prostate cancer), FISH analysis of 4 genes (ASAP1, HDAC9, CHD1 and PTEN), needle biopsy specimen, algorithm reported as probability of higher tumor grade◀
▶AssuranceRx Micro Serum, Firstox Laboratories, LLC, Firstox Laboratories, LLC◀	●0054U	▶Prescription drug monitoring, 14 or more classes of drugs and substances, definitive tandem mass spectrometry with chromatography, capillary blood, quantitative report with therapeutic and toxic ranges, including steady-state range for the prescribed dose when detected, per date of service◀
▶myTAIHEART, TAI Diagnostics, Inc, TAI Diagnostics, Inc◀	●0055U	▶Cardiology (heart transplant), cell-free DNA, PCR assay of 96 DNA target sequences (94 single nucleotide polymorphism targets and two control targets), plasma◀
▶MatePair Acute Myeloid Leukemia Panel, Mayo Clinic, Laboratory Developed Test◀	●0056U	▶Hematology (acute myelogenous leukemia), DNA, whole genome next-generation sequencing to detect gene rearrangement(s), blood or bone marrow, report of specific gene rearrangement(s)◀
▶RNA-Sequencing by NGS, OmniSeq, Inc, Life Technologies Corporation◀	●0057U	▶Oncology (solid organ neoplasia), mRNA, gene expression profiling by massively parallel sequencing for analysis of 51 genes, utilizing formalin-fixed paraffin-embedded tissue, algorithm reported as a normalized percentile rank◀
▶Merkel SmT Oncoprotein Antibody Titer, University of Washington, Department of Laboratory Medicine◀	●0058U	▶Oncology (Merkel cell carcinoma), detection of antibodies to the Merkel cell polyoma virus oncoprotein (small T antigen), serum, quantitative◀
▶Merkel Virus VP1 Capsid Antibody, University of Washington, Department of Laboratory Medicine◀	●0059U	▶Oncology (Merkel cell carcinoma), detection of antibodies to the Merkel cell polyoma virus capsid protein (VP1), serum, reported as positive or negative◀
▶Twins Zygosity PLA, Natera, Inc, Natera, Inc◀	●0060U	▶Twin zygosity, genomic-targeted sequence analysis of chromosome 2, using circulating cell-free fetal DNA in maternal blood◀
▶Transcutaneous multispectral measurement of tissue oxygenation and hemoglobin using spatial frequency domain imaging (SFDI), Modulated Imaging, Inc, Modulated Imaging, Inc◀	●0061U	▶Transcutaneous measurement of five biomarkers (tissue oxygenation [StO_2], oxyhemoglobin [$ctHbO_2$], deoxyhemoglobin [ctHbR], papillary and reticular dermal hemoglobin concentrations [ctHb1 and ctHb2]), using spatial frequency domain imaging (SFDI) and multi-spectral analysis◀

★ = Telemedicine   ✚ = Add-on code   ✗ = FDA approval pending   # = Resequenced code   ⊘ = Modifier 51 exempt

Appendix O

Multianalyte Assays with Algorithmic Analyses

The following list includes three types of CPT codes:

1. Multianalyte assays with algorithmic analyses (MAAA) administrative codes

2. Category I MAAA codes

3. Proprietary laboratory analyses (PLA) codes

1. Multianalyte assays with algorithmic analyses (MAAAs) are procedures that utilize multiple results derived from assays of various types, including molecular pathology assays, fluorescent in situ hybridization assays and non-nucleic acid based assays (eg, proteins, polypeptides, lipids, carbohydrates). Algorithmic analysis using the results of these assays as well as other patient information (if used) is then performed and reported typically as a numeric score(s) or as a probability. MAAAs are typically unique to a single clinical laboratory or manufacturer. The results of individual component procedure(s) that are inputs to the MAAAs may be provided on the associated laboratory report, however these assays are not reported separately using additional codes. MAAAs, by nature, are typically unique to a single clinical laboratory or manufacturer.

The list includes a proprietary name and clinical laboratory or manufacturer in the first column, an alpha-numeric code in the second column and code descriptor in the third column. The format for the code descriptor usually includes (in order): The list includes a proprietary name and clinical laboratory or manufacturer in the first column, an alpha-numeric code in the second column and code descriptor in the third column. The format for the code descriptor usually includes (in order):

- Disease type (eg, oncology, autoimmune, tissue rejection),

- Chemical(s) analyzed (eg, DNA, RNA, protein, antibody),

- Number of markers (eg, number of genes, number of proteins),

- Methodology(s) (eg, microarray, real-time [RT]-PCR, in situ hybridization [ISH], enzyme linked immunosorbent assays [ELISA]),

- Number of functional domains (if indicated),

- Specimen type (eg, blood, fresh tissue, formalin-fixed paraffin-embedded),

- Algorithm result type (eg, prognostic, diagnostic),

- Report (eg, probability index, risk score).

MAAA procedures that have been assigned a Category I code are noted in the list below and additionally listed in the Category I MAAA section (81500-81599). The Category I MAAA section introductory language and associated parenthetical instruction(s) should be used to govern the appropriate use for Category I MAAA codes. If a specific MAAA procedure has not been assigned a Category I code, it is indicated as a four-digit number followed by the letter M.

When a specific MAAA procedure is not included in either the list below or in the Category I MAAA section, report the analysis using the Category I MAAA unlisted code (81599). The codes below are specific to the assays identified in Appendix O by proprietary name. In order to report an MAAA code, the analysis performed must fulfill the code descriptor **and**, if proprietary, must be the test represented by the proprietary name listed in Appendix O. When an analysis is performed that may potentially fall within a specific descriptor, however the proprietary name is not included in the list below, the MAAA unlisted code (81599) should be used.

Additions in this section may be released tri-annually (or quarterly for PLA codes) via the AMA CPT website to expedite dissemination for reporting. The list will be published annually in the CPT codebook. Go to www.ama-assn.org/go/cpt for the most current listing.

These administrative codes encompass all analytical services required for the algorithmic analysis (eg, cell lysis, nucleic acid stabilization, extraction, digestion, amplification, hybridization and detection) in addition to the algorithmic analysis itself, when applicable. Procedures that are required prior to cell lysis (eg, micro-dissection, codes 88380 and 88381) should be reported separately.

The codes in this list are provided as an administrative coding set to facilitate accurate reporting of MAAA services. The minimum standard for inclusion in this list is that an analysis is generally available for patient care. The AMA has not reviewed procedures in the administrative coding set for clinical utility. The list is not a complete list of all MAAA procedures.

2. Category I MAAA codes are included below along with their proprietary names. These codes are also listed in the Pathology and Laboratory section of the CPT code set (81490-81599).

3. PLA codes created in response to the Protecting Access to Medicare Act (PAMA) of 2014 are listed along with their proprietary names. These codes are also located at the end of the Pathology and Laboratory section of the CPT code set. In some instances, the descriptor language of PLA codes may be identical, which are differentiated only by the listed propriety names.

Proprietary Name and Clinical Laboratory or Manufacturer	Alpha-Numeric Code	Code Descriptor
Administrative Codes for Multianalyte Assays with Algorithmic Analyses (MAAA)		
—	►(0001M has been deleted. To report, use 81596◄	—
ASH FibroSURE™, LabCorp	0002M	Liver disease, ten biochemical assays (ALT, A2-macroglobulin, apolipoprotein A-1, total bilirubin, GGT, haptoglobin, AST, glucose, total cholesterol and triglycerides) utilizing serum, prognostic algorithm reported as quantitative scores for fibrosis, steatosis and alcoholic steatohepatitis (ASH)
NASH FibroSURE™, LabCorp	0003M	Liver disease, ten biochemical assays (ALT, A2-macroglobulin, apolipoprotein A-1, total bilirubin, GGT, haptoglobin, AST, glucose, total cholesterol and triglycerides) utilizing serum, prognostic algorithm reported as quantitative scores for fibrosis, steatosis and nonalcoholic steatohepatitis (NASH)
ScoliScore™ Transgenomic	0004M	Scoliosis, DNA analysis of 53 single nucleotide polymorphisms (SNPs), using saliva, prognostic algorithm reported as a risk score
HeproDX™, GoPath Laboratories, LLC	0006M	Oncology (hepatic), mRNA expression levels of 161 genes, utilizing fresh hepatocellular carcinoma tumor tissue, with alpha-fetoprotein level, algorithm reported as a risk classifier
NETest, Wren Laboratories, LLC	0007M	Oncology (gastrointestinal neuroendocrine tumors), real-time PCR expression analysis of 51 genes, utilizing whole peripheral blood, algorithm reported as a nomogram of tumor disease index
—	(0008M has been deleted, use 81520)	—
VisibiliT test, Sequenom Center for Molecular Medicine, LLC	0009M	Fetal aneuploidy (trisomy 21, and 18) DNA sequence analysis of selected regions using maternal plasma, algorithm reported as a risk score for each trisomy
—	(0010M has been deleted, use 81539)	—
►NeoLAB™ Prostate Liquid Biopsy, NeoGenomics Laboratories◄	●0011M	►Oncology, prostate cancer, mRNA expression assay of 12 genes (10 content and 2 housekeeping), RT-PCR test utilizing blood plasma and/or urine, algorithms to predict high-grade prostate cancer risk◄
►Cxbladder™ Detect, Pacific Edge Diagnostics USA, Ltd◄	●0012M	►Oncology (urothelial), mRNA, gene expression profiling by real-time quantitative PCR of five genes (MDK, HOXA13, CDC2 [CDK1], IGFBP5, and CXCR2), utilizing urine, algorithm reported as a risk score for having urothelial carcinoma◄

★ = Telemedicine   ✚ = Add-on code   ✗ = FDA approval pending   # = Resequenced code   ⊘ = Modifier 51 exempt

Proprietary Name and Clinical Laboratory or Manufacturer	Alpha-Numeric Code	Code Descriptor
►Cxbladder™ Monitor, Pacific Edge Diagnostics USA, Ltd◄	●0013M	►Oncology (urothelial), mRNA, gene expression profiling by real-time quantitative PCR of five genes (*MDK, HOXA13, CDC2 [CDK1], IGFBP5,* and *CXCR2),* utilizing urine, algorithm reported as a risk score for having recurrent urothelial carcinoma◄
Category I Codes for Multianalyte Assays with Algorithmic Analyses (MAAA)		
Vectra® DA, Crescendo Bioscience, Inc	81490	Autoimmune (rheumatoid arthritis), analysis of 12 biomarkers using immunoassays, utilizing serum, prognostic algorithm reported as a disease activity score (Do not report 81490 in conjunction with 86140)
Corus® CAD, CardioDx, Inc	81493	Coronary artery disease, mRNA, gene expression profiling by real-time RT-PCR of 23 genes, utilizing whole peripheral blood, algorithm reported as a risk score
AlloMap®, CareDx, Inc	81595	Cardiology (heart transplant), mRNA, gene expression profiling by real-time quantitative PCR of 20 genes (11 content and 9 housekeeping), utilizing subfraction of peripheral blood, algorithm reported as a rejection risk score
Risk of Ovarian Malignancy Algorithm (ROMA)™, Fujirebio Diagnostics	81500	Oncology (ovarian), biochemical assays of two proteins (CA-125 and HE4), utilizing serum, with menopausal status, algorithm reported as a risk score
OVA1™, Vermillion, Inc	81503	Oncology (ovarian), biochemical assays of five proteins (CA-125, apolipoprotein A1, beta-2 microglobulin, transferrin, and pre-albumin), utilizing serum, algorithm reported as a risk score
Tissue of Origin Test Kit-FFPE, Cancer Genetics, Inc	81504	Oncology (tissue of origin), microarray gene expression profiling of >2000 genes, utilizing formalin-fixed paraffin-embedded tissue, algorithm reported as tissue similarity scores
PreDx Diabetes Risk Score™, Tethys Clinical Laboratory	81506	Endocrinology (type 2 diabetes), biochemical assays of seven analytes (glucose, HbA1c, insulin, hs-CRP, adiponectin, ferritin, interleukin 2-receptor alpha), utilizing serum or plasma, algorithm reporting a risk score
Harmony™ Prenatal Test, Ariosa Diagnostics	81507	Fetal aneuploidy (trisomy 21, 18, and 13) DNA sequence analysis of selected regions using maternal plasma, algorithm reported as a risk score for each trisomy

(*Continued on page 234*)

Proprietary Name and Clinical Laboratory or Manufacturer	Alpha-Numeric Code	Code Descriptor
No proprietary name and clinical laboratory or manufacturer. Maternal serum screening procedures are well-established procedures and are performed by many laboratories throughout the country. The concept of prenatal screens has existed and evolved for over 10 years and is not exclusive to any one facility.	81508	Fetal congenital abnormalities, biochemical assays of two proteins (PAPP-A, hCG [any form]), utilizing maternal serum, algorithm reported as a risk score
	81509	Fetal congenital abnormalities, biochemical assays of three proteins (PAPP-A, hCG [any form], DIA), utilizing maternal serum, algorithm reported as a risk score
	81510	Fetal congenital abnormalities, biochemical assays of three analytes (AFP, uE3, hCG [any form]), utilizing maternal serum, algorithm reported as a risk score
	81511	Fetal congenital abnormalities, biochemical assays of four analytes (AFP, uE3, hCG [any form], DIA) utilizing maternal serum, algorithm reported as a risk score (may include additional results from previous biochemical testing)
	81512	Fetal congenital abnormalities, biochemical assays of five analytes (AFP, uE3, total hCG, hyperglycosylated hCG, DIA) utilizing maternal serum, algorithm reported as a risk score
▶Breast Cancer Index, Biotheranostics, Inc◀	●81518	▶Oncology (breast), mRNA, gene expression profiling by real-time RT-PCR of 11 genes (7 content and 4 housekeeping), utilizing formalin-fixed paraffin-embedded tissue, algorithms reported as percentage risk for metastatic recurrence and likelihood of benefit from extended endocrine therapy◀
Oncotype DX®, Genomic Health	81519	Oncology (breast), mRNA, gene expression profiling by real-time RT-PCR of 21 genes, utilizing formalin-fixed paraffin-embedded tissue, algorithm reported as recurrence score
Prosigna® Breast Cancer Assay, NanoString Technologies, Inc	81520	Oncology (breast), mRNA gene expression profiling by hybrid capture of 58 genes (50 content and 8 housekeeping), utilizing formalin-fixed paraffin-embedded tissue, algorithm reported as a recurrence risk score
MammaPrint®, Agendia, Inc	81521	Oncology (breast), mRNA, microarray gene expression profiling of 70 content genes and 465 housekeeping genes, utilizing fresh frozen or formalin-fixed paraffin-embedded tissue, algorithm reported as index related to risk of distant metastasis
Oncotype DX® Colon Cancer Assay, Genomic Health	81525	Oncology (colon), mRNA, gene expression profiling by real-time RT-PCR of 12 genes (7 content and 5 housekeeping), utilizing formalin-fixed paraffin-embedded tissue, algorithm reported as a recurrence score

Proprietary Name and Clinical Laboratory or Manufacturer	Alpha-Numeric Code	Code Descriptor
Cologuard™, Exact Sciences, Inc	81528	Oncology (colorectal) screening, quantitative real-time target and signal amplification of 10 DNA markers (KRAS mutations, promoter methylation of NDRG4 and BMP3) and fecal hemoglobin, utilizing stool, algorithm reported as a positive or negative result (Do not report 81528 in conjunction with 81275, 82274)
ChemoFX®, Helomics, Corp	81535 +81536	Oncology (gynecologic), live tumor cell culture and chemotherapeutic response by DAPI stain and morphology, predictive algorithm reported as a drug response score; first single drug or drug combination 　each additional single drug or drug combination (List separately in addition to code for primary procedure) (Use 81536 in conjunction with 81535)
VeriStrat, Biodesix, Inc	81538	Oncology (lung), mass spectrometric 8-protein signature, including amyloid A, utilizing serum, prognostic and predictive algorithm reported as good versus poor overall survival
4Kscore test, OPKO Health, Inc	81539	Oncology (high-grade prostate cancer), biochemical assay of four proteins (Total PSA, Free PSA, Intact PSA and human kallikrein-2 [hK2]), utilizing plasma or serum, prognostic algorithm reported as a probability score
CancerTYPE ID, bioTheranostics, Inc	81540	Oncology (tumor of unknown origin), mRNA, gene expression profiling by real-time RT-PCR of 92 genes (87 content and 5 housekeeping) to classify tumor into main cancer type and subtype, utilizing formalin-fixed paraffin-embedded tissue, algorithm reported as a probability of a predicted main cancer type and subtype
Prolaris®, Myriad Genetic Laboratories, Inc	81541	Oncology (prostate), mRNA gene expression profiling by real-time RT-PCR of 46 genes (31 content and 15 housekeeping), utilizing formalin-fixed paraffin-embedded tissue, algorithm reported as a disease-specific mortality risk score
Afirma® Gene Expression Classifier, Veracyte, Inc	81545	Oncology (thyroid), gene expression analysis of 142 genes, utilizing fine needle aspirate, algorithm reported as a categorical result (eg, benign or suspicious)
ConfirmMDx® for Prostate Cancer, MDxHealth, Inc	81551	Oncology (prostate), promoter methylation profiling by real-time PCR of 3 genes (GSTP1, APC, RASSF1), utilizing formalin-fixed paraffin-embedded tissue, algorithm reported as a likelihood of prostate cancer detection on repeat biopsy

(Continued on page 236)

Appendix O

Proprietary Name and Clinical Laboratory or Manufacturer	Alpha-Numeric Code	Code Descriptor
▶HCV FibroSURE™, FibroTest™, BioPredictive S.A.S.◀	●81596	▶Infectious disease, chronic hepatitis C virus (HCV) infection, six biochemical assays (ALT, A2-macroglobulin, apolipoprotein A-1, total bilirubin, GGT, and haptoglobin) utilizing serum, prognostic algorithm reported as scores for fibrosis and necroinflammatory activity in liver◀
	81599	Unlisted multianalyte assay with algorithmic analysis
Proprietary Laboratory Analyses (PLA)		
PreciseType® HEA Test, Immucor, Inc	0001U	Red blood cell antigen typing, DNA, human erythrocyte antigen gene analysis of 35 antigens from 11 blood groups, utilizing whole blood, common RBC alleles reported
PolypDX™, Atlantic Diagnostic Laboratories, LLC, Metabolomic Technologies, Inc	0002U	Oncology (colorectal), quantitative assessment of three urine metabolites (ascorbic acid, succinic acid and carnitine) by liquid chromatography with tandem mass spectrometry (LC-MS/MS) using multiple reaction monitoring acquisition, algorithm reported as likelihood of adenomatous polyps
Overa (OVA1 Next Generation), Asprira Labs, Inc, Vermillion, Inc	0003U	Oncology (ovarian) biochemical assays of five proteins (apolipoprotein A-1, CA 125 II, follicle stimulating hormone, human epididymis protein 4, transferrin), utilizing serum, algorithm reported as a likelihood score
	▶(0004U has been deleted)◀	
ExosomeDx® Prostate (IntelliScore), Exosome Diagnostics, Inc	0005U	Oncology (prostate) gene expression profile by real-time RT-PCR of 3 genes *(ERG, PCA3,* and *SPDEF)*, urine, algorithm reported as risk score
▶Drug-drug, Drug-substance Identification and Interaction, Aegis Sciences Corporation◀	▲0006U	▶Detection of interacting medications, substances, supplements and foods, 120 or more analytes, definitive chromatography with mass spectrometry, urine, description and severity of each interaction identified, per date of service◀
ToxProtect, Genotox Laboratories Ltd	#0007U	Drug test(s), presumptive, with definitive confirmation of positive results, any number of drug classes, urine, includes specimen verification including DNA authentication in comparison to buccal DNA, per date of service ▶(For additional PLA code with identical clinical descriptor, see 0020U. See Appendix O to determine appropriate code assignment)◀
AmHPR Helicobacter pylori Antibiotic Resistance Next Generation Sequencing Panel, American Molecular Laboratories, Inc	0008U	Helicobacter pylori detection and antibiotic resistance, DNA, 16S and 23S rRNA, gyrA, pbp1,rdxA and rpoB, next generation sequencing, formalin-fixed paraffin-embedded or fresh tissue, predictive, reported as positive or negative for resistance to clarithromycin, fluoroquinolones, metronidazole, amoxicillin, tetracycline and rifabutin

★ = Telemedicine   ✛ = Add-on code   ⚡ = FDA approval pending   # = Resequenced code   ⊘ = Modifier 51 exempt

Appendix O

Proprietary Name and Clinical Laboratory or Manufacturer	Alpha-Numeric Code	Code Descriptor
DEPArray™ HER2, PacificDx	0009U	Oncology (breast cancer), *ERBB2* (HER2) copy number by FISH, tumor cells from formalin-fixed paraffin-embedded tissue isolated using image-based dielectrophoresis (DEP) sorting, reported as *ERBB2* gene amplified or non-amplified
Bacterial Typing by Whole Genome Sequencing, Mayo Clinic	0010U	Infectious disease (bacterial), strain typing by whole genome sequencing, phylogenetic-based report of strain relatedness, per submitted isolate
Cordant CORE™, Cordant Health Solutions	0011U	Prescription drug monitoring, evaluation of drugs present by LC-MS/MS, using oral fluid, reported as a comparison to an estimated steady-state range, per date of service including all drug compounds and metabolites
MatePair Targeted Rearrangements, Congenital, Mayo Clinic	0012U	Germline disorders, gene rearrangement detection by whole genome next-generation sequencing, DNA, whole blood, report of specific gene rearrangement(s)
MatePair Targeted Rearrangements, Oncology, Mayo Clinic	0013U	Oncology (solid organ neoplasia), gene rearrangement detection by whole genome next-generation sequencing, DNA, fresh or frozen tissue or cells, report of specific gene rearrangement(s)
MatePair Targeted Rearrangements, Hematologic, Mayo Clinic	0014U	Hematology (hematolymphoid neoplasia), gene rearrangement detection by whole genome next-generation sequencing, DNA, whole blood or bone marrow, report of specific gene rearrangement(s)
	▶(0015U has been deleted)◄	
BCR-ABL1 major and minor breakpoint fusion transcripts, University of Iowa, Department of Pathology, Asuragen	0016U	Oncology (hematolymphoid neoplasia), RNA, *BCR/ABL1* major and minor breakpoint fusion transcripts, quantitative PCR amplification, blood or bone marrow, report of fusion not detected or detected with quantitation
JAK2 Mutation, University of Iowa, Department of Pathology	0017U	Oncology (hematolymphoid neoplasia), *JAK2* mutation, DNA, PCR amplification of exons 12-14 and sequence analysis, blood or bone marrow, report of *JAK2* mutation not detected or detected
▶ThyraMIR™, Interpace Diagnostics, Interpace Diagnostics◄	●0018U	▶Oncology (thyroid), microRNA profiling by RT-PCR of 10 microRNA sequences, utilizing fine needle aspirate, algorithm reported as a positive or negative result for moderate to high risk of malignancy◄
▶OncoTarget/OncoTreat, Columbia University Department of Pathology and Cell Biology, Darwin Health◄	●0019U	▶Oncology, RNA, gene expression by whole transcriptome sequencing, formalin-fixed paraffin-embedded tissue or fresh frozen tissue, predictive algorithm reported as potential targets for therapeutic agents◄

(Continued on page 238)

▲ = Revised code   ● = New code   ▶ ◄ = Contains new or revised text   ✕ = Duplicate PLA test

Proprietary Name and Clinical Laboratory or Manufacturer	Alpha-Numeric Code	Code Descriptor
▶ToxLok, InSource Diagnostics, InSource Diagnostics◀	✂●0020U	▶Drug test(s), presumptive, with definitive confirmation of positive results, any number of drug classes, urine, with specimen verification including DNA authentication in comparison to buccal DNA, per date of service (For additional PLA code with identical clinical descriptor, see 0007U. See Appendix O to determine appropriate code assignment)◀
▶Apifiny®, Armune BioScience, Inc◀	●0021U	▶Oncology (prostate), detection of 8 autoantibodies (ARF 6, NKX3-1, 5'-UTR-BMI1, CEP 164, 3'-UTR-Ropporin, Desmocollin, AURKAIP-1, CSNK2A2), multiplexed immunoassay and flow cytometry serum, algorithm reported as risk score◀
▶Oncomine™ Dx Target Test, Thermo Fisher Scientific◀	●0022U	▶Targeted genomic sequence analysis panel, non-small cell lung neoplasia, DNA and RNA analysis, 23 genes, interrogation for sequence variants and rearrangements, reported as presence/absence of variants and associated therapy(ies) to consider◀
▶LeukoStrat® CDx FLT3 Mutation Assay, LabPMM LLC, an Invivoscribe Technologies, Inc Company, Invivoscribe Technologies, Inc◀	●0023U	▶Oncology (acute myelogenous leukemia), DNA, genotyping of internal tandem duplication, p. D835, p.I836, using mononuclear cells, reported as detection or non-detection of FLT3 mutation and indication for or against the use of midostaurin◀
▶GlycA, Laboratory Corporation of America, Laboratory Corporation of America◀	●0024U	▶Glycosylated acute phase proteins (GlycA), nuclear magnetic resonance spectroscopy, quantitative◀
▶UrSure Tenofovir Quantification Test, Synergy Medical Laboratories, UrSure Inc◀	●0025U	▶Tenofovir, by liquid chromatography with tandem mass spectrometry (LC-MS/MS), urine, quantitative◀
▶Thyroseq Genomic Classifier, CBLPath, Inc, University of Pittsburgh Medical Center◀	●0026U	▶Oncology (thyroid), DNA and mRNA of 112 genes, next-generation sequencing, fine needle aspirate of thyroid nodule, algorithmic analysis reported as a categorical result ("Positive, high probability of malignancy" or "Negative, low probability of malignancy")◀
▶JAK2 Exons 12 to 15 Sequencing, Mayo Clinic, Mayo Clinic◀	●0027U	▶JAK2 (Janus kinase 2) (eg, myeloproliferative disorder) gene analysis, targeted sequence analysis exons 12-15◀
▶CYP2D6 Genotype Cascade, Mayo Clinic, Mayo Clinic◀	●0028U	▶CYP2D6 (cytochrome P450, family 2, subfamily D, polypeptide 6) (eg, drug metabolism) gene analysis, copy number variants, common variants with reflex to targeted sequence analysis◀
▶Focused Pharmacogenomics Panel, Mayo Clinic, Mayo Clinic◀	●0029U	▶Drug metabolism (adverse drug reactions and drug response), targeted sequence analysis (ie, CYP1A2, CYP2C19, CYP2C9, CYP2D6, CYP3A4, CYP3A5, CYP4F2, SLCO1B1, VKORC1 and rs12777823)◀
▶Warfarin Response Genotype, Mayo Clinic, Mayo Clinic◀	●0030U	▶Drug metabolism (warfarin drug response), targeted sequence analysis (ie, CYP2C9, CYP4F2, VKORC1, rs12777823)◀

★=Telemedicine ✚=Add-on code ✖=FDA approval pending #=Resequenced code ⊘=Modifier 51 exempt

Proprietary Name and Clinical Laboratory or Manufacturer	Alpha-Numeric Code	Code Descriptor
▶Cytochrome P450 1A2 Genotype, Mayo Clinic, Mayo Clinic◀	●0031U	▶*CYP1A2 (cytochrome P450 family 1, subfamily A, member 2) (eg, drug metabolism) gene analysis, common variants (ie, *1F, *1K, *6, *7)*◀
▶Catechol-O-Methyltransferase (COMT) Genotype, Mayo Clinic, Mayo Clinic◀	●0032U	▶*COMT (catechol-O-methyltransferase) (eg, drug metabolism) gene analysis, c.472G>A (rs4680) variant*◀
▶Serotonin Receptor Genotype (HTR2A and HTR2C), Mayo Clinic, Mayo Clinic◀	●0033U	▶*HTR2A (5-hydroxytryptamine receptor 2A), HTR2C (5-hydroxytryptamine receptor 2C) (eg, citalopram metabolism) gene analysis, common variants (ie, HTR2A rs7997012 [c.614-2211T>C], HTR2C rs3813929 [c.-759C>T] and rs1414334 [c.551-3008C>G])*◀
▶Thiopurine Methyltransferase (TPMT) and Nudix Hydrolase (NUDT15) Genotyping, Mayo Clinic, Mayo Clinic◀	●0034U	▶ *TPMT (thiopurine S-methyltransferase), NUDT15 (nudix hydroxylase 15) (eg, thiopurine metabolism) gene analysis, common variants (ie, TPMT *2, *3A, *3B, *3C, *4, *5, *6, *8, *12; NUDT15 *3, *4, *5)*◀
▶Real-time quaking-induced conversion for prion detection (RT-QuIC), National Prion Disease Pathology Surveillance Center◀	●0035U	▶Neurology (prion disease), cerebrospinal fluid, detection of prion protein by quaking-induced conformational conversion, qualitative◀
▶EXaCT-1 Whole Exome Testing, Lab of Oncology-Molecular Detection, Weill Cornell Medicine-Clinical Genomics Laboratory◀	●0036U	▶Exome (ie, somatic mutations), paired formalin-fixed paraffin-embedded tumor tissue and normal specimen, sequence analyses◀
▶FoundationOne CDx™ (F1CDx), Foundation Medicine, Inc, Foundation Medicine, Inc◀	●0037U	▶Targeted genomic sequence analysis, solid organ neoplasm, DNA analysis of 324 genes, interrogation for sequence variants, gene copy number amplifications, gene rearrangements, microsatellite instability and tumor mutational burden◀
▶Sensieva™ Droplet 25OH Vitamin D2/D3 Microvolume LC/MS Assay, InSource Diagnostics, InSource Diagnostics◀	●0038U	▶Vitamin D, 25 hydroxy D2 and D3, by LC-MS/MS, serum microsample, quantitative◀
▶Anti-dsDNA, High Salt/Avidity, University of Washington, Department of Laboratory Medicine, Bio-Rad◀	●0039U	▶Deoxyribonucleic acid (DNA) antibody, double stranded, high avidity◀
▶MRDx BCR-ABL Test, MolecularMD, MolecularMD◀	●0040U	▶*BCR/ABL1 (t(9;22))* (eg, chronic myelogenous leukemia) translocation analysis, major breakpoint, quantitative◀
▶Lyme ImmunoBlot IgM, IGeneX Inc, ID-FISH Technology Inc (ASR) (Lyme ImmunoBlot IgM Strips Only)◀	●0041U	▶Borrelia burgdorferi, antibody detection of 5 recombinant protein groups, by immunoblot, IgM◀
▶Lyme ImmunoBlot IgG, IGeneX Inc, ID-FISH Technology Inc (ASR) (Lyme ImmunoBlot IgG Strips Only)◀	●0042U	▶Borrelia burgdorferi, antibody detection of 12 recombinant protein groups, by immunoblot, IgG◀

(*Continued on page 240*)

Proprietary Name and Clinical Laboratory or Manufacturer	Alpha-Numeric Code	Code Descriptor
▶Tick-Borne Relapsing Fever (TBRF) Borrelia ImmunoBlots IgM Test, IGeneX Inc ID-FISH Technology◀	●0043U	▶Tick-borne relapsing fever Borrelia group, antibody detection to 4 recombinant protein groups, by immunoblot, IgM◀
▶Tick-Borne Relapsing Fever (TBRF) Borrelia ImmunoBlots IgG Test, IGeneX Inc, ID-FISH Technology Inc (Provides TBRF ImmunoBlot IgG Strips)◀	●0044U	▶Tick-borne relapsing fever Borrelia group, antibody detection to 4 recombinant protein groups, by immunoblot, IgG◀
▶The Oncotype DX® Breast DCIS Score™ Test, Genomic Health, Inc, Genomic Health, Inc◀	●0045U	▶Oncology (breast ductal carcinoma in situ), mRNA, gene expression profiling by real-time RT-PCR of 12 genes (7 content and 5 housekeeping), utilizing formalin-fixed paraffin-embedded tissue, algorithm reported as recurrence score◀
▶*FLT3* ITD MRD by NGS, LabPMM LLC, an Invivoscribe Technologies, Inc Company◀	●0046U	▶*FLT3 (fms-related tyrosine kinase 3)* (eg, acute myeloid leukemia) internal tandem duplication (ITD) variants, quantitative◀
▶Oncotype DX Genomic Prostate Score, Genomic Health, Inc, Genomic Health, Inc◀	●0047U	▶Oncology (prostate), mRNA, gene expression profiling by real-time RT-PCR of 17 genes (12 content and 5 housekeeping), utilizing formalin-fixed paraffin-embedded tissue, algorithm reported as a risk score◀
▶MSK-IMPACT (Integrated Mutation Profiling of Actionable Cancer Targets), Memorial Sloan Kettering Cancer Center◀	●0048U	▶Oncology (solid organ neoplasia), DNA, targeted sequencing of protein-coding exons of 468 cancer-associated genes, including interrogation for somatic mutations and microsatellite instability, matched with normal specimens, utilizing formalin-fixed paraffin-embedded tumor tissue, report of clinically significant mutation(s)◀
▶NPM1 MRD by NGS, LabPMM LLC, an Invivoscribe Technologies, Inc Company◀	●0049U	▶*NPM1 (nucleophosmin)* (eg, acute myeloid leukemia) gene analysis, quantitative◀
▶MyAML NGS Panel, LabPMM LLC, an Invivoscribe Technologies, Inc Company◀	●0050U	▶Targeted genomic sequence analysis panel, acute myelogenous leukemia, DNA analysis, 194 genes, interrogation for sequence variants, copy number variants or rearrangements◀
▶UCompliDx, Elite Medical Laboratory Solutions, LLC, Elite Medical Laboratory Solutions, LLC (LDT)◀	●0051U	▶Prescription drug monitoring, evaluation of drugs present by LC-MS/MS, urine, 31 drug panel, reported as quantitative results, detected or not detected, per date of service◀
▶VAP Cholesterol Test, VAP Diagnostics Laboratory, Inc, VAP Diagnostics Laboratory, Inc◀	●0052U	▶Lipoprotein, blood, high resolution fractionation and quantitation of lipoproteins including all five major lipoprotein classes and the subclasses of HDL, LDL, and VLDL by vertical auto profile ultracentrifugation◀
▶Prostate Cancer Risk Panel, Mayo Clinic, Laboratory Developed Test◀	●0053U	▶Oncology (prostate cancer), FISH analysis of 4 genes (*ASAP1, HDAC9, CHD1* and *PTEN*), needle biopsy specimen, algorithm reported as probability of higher tumor grade◀

★ =Telemedicine   ✚ =Add-on code   ⁄ =FDA approval pending   # =Resequenced code   ⦸ =Modifier 51 exempt

Proprietary Name and Clinical Laboratory or Manufacturer	Alpha-Numeric Code	Code Descriptor
▶AssuranceRx Micro Serum, Firstox Laboratories, LLC, Firstox Laboratories, LLC◀	●0054U	▶Prescription drug monitoring, 14 or more classes of drugs and substances, definitive tandem mass spectrometry with chromatography, capillary blood, quantitative report with therapeutic and toxic ranges, including steady-state range for the prescribed dose when detected, per date of service◀
▶myTAIHEART, TAI Diagnostics, Inc, TAI Diagnostics, Inc◀	●0055U	▶Cardiology (heart transplant), cell-free DNA, PCR assay of 96 DNA target sequences (94 single nucleotide polymorphism targets and two control targets), plasma◀
▶MatePair Acute Myeloid Leukemia Panel, Mayo Clinic, Laboratory Developed Test◀	●0056U	▶Hematology (acute myelogenous leukemia), DNA, whole genome next-generation sequencing to detect gene rearrangement(s), blood or bone marrow, report of specific gene rearrangement(s)◀
▶RNA-Sequencing by NGS, OmniSeq, Inc, Life Technologies Corporation◀	●0057U	▶Oncology (solid organ neoplasia), mRNA, gene expression profiling by massively parallel sequencing for analysis of 51 genes, utilizing formalin-fixed paraffin-embedded tissue, algorithm reported as a normalized percentile rank◀
▶Merkel SmT Oncoprotein Antibody Titer, University of Washington, Department of Laboratory Medicine◀	●0058U	▶Oncology (Merkel cell carcinoma), detection of antibodies to the Merkel cell polyoma virus oncoprotein (small T antigen), serum, quantitative◀
▶Merkel Virus VP1 Capsid Antibody, University of Washington, Department of Laboratory Medicine◀	●0059U	▶Oncology (Merkel cell carcinoma), detection of antibodies to the Merkel cell polyoma virus capsid protein (VP1), serum, reported as positive or negative◀
▶Twins Zygosity PLA, Natera, Inc, Natera, Inc◀	●0060U	▶Twin zygosity, genomic-targeted sequence analysis of chromosome 2, using circulating cell-free fetal DNA in maternal blood◀
▶Transcutaneous multispectral measurement of tissue oxygenation and hemoglobin using spatial frequency domain imaging (SFDI), Modulated Imaging, Inc, Modulated Imaging, Inc◀	●0061U	▶Transcutaneous measurement of five biomarkers (tissue oxygenation [StO_2], oxyhemoglobin [$ctHbO_2$], deoxyhemoglobin [ctHbR], papillary and reticular dermal hemoglobin concentrations [ctHb1 and ctHb2]), using spatial frequency domain imaging (SFDI) and multi-spectral analysis◀

Rationale

In accordance with the changes (addition of new codes, including the PLA codes) in the Pathology and Laboratory section, Appendix O has been revised to reflect these changes. Three new administrative MAAA codes (0011M, 0012M, 0013M) have been added and one administrative MAAA code (0001M) deleted. Two new Category I MAAA codes (81596, 81518) have been added. All PLA codes (0001U-0061U) with their procedure's proprietary name have been included in Appendix O too.

Refer to the codebook and the Rationale for codes 81596, 81518, and 0001U-0061U for a full discussion of these changes.

Indexes

Instructions for the Use of the Changes Indexes

The Changes Indexes are **not** a substitute for the main text of *CPT Changes 2019* or the main text of the CPT codebook. The changes indexes consist of two types of content—coding changes and modifiers—all of which are intended to assist users in searching and locating information quickly within *CPT Changes 2019*.

Index of Coding Changes

The Index of Coding Changes does not list existing codes unless they are new, revised, or deleted, or if the code may be affected by revised and/or new guidelines and parenthetical notes. Also included are codes described in the Rationales. This index enables users to quickly search and locate the codes within a page(s), in addition to discerning the status of a code (new, revised, deleted, or textually changed) because the status of each new, revised, or deleted code is noted in parentheses next to the code number:

Index of Modifiers

A limited Index of Modifiers, ie, limited to only the modifiers that are in new and/or revised parenthetical notes and guidelines in this book, as well as limited to only those modifiers that appear in the Rationales, is provided to help users quickly locate these modifiers and to know where in the book these modifiers are listed or mentioned.

Indexes

Index of Coding Changes

★ = Telemedicine   + = Add-on code   ✗ = FDA approval pending   # = Resequenced code   ⊘ = Modifier 51 exempt

Indexes

★ = Telemedicine   ✚ = Add-on code   ✗ = FDA approval pending   # = Resequenced code   ⊘ = Modifier 51 exempt

Indexes

Indexes

★ = Telemedicine   ✛ = Add-on code   ✎ = FDA approval pending   # = Resequenced code   ⊘ = Modifier 51 exempt

Index of Modifiers

Modifier, Descriptor

Page Numbers

NOTES

NOTES

NOTES

NOTES

NOTES

NOTES

NOTES

NOTES

NOTES